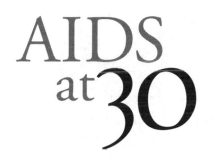

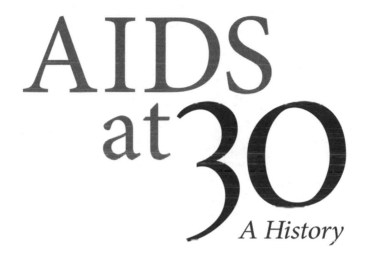

AIDS at 30

A History

Victoria A. Harden

Potomac Books
Washington, D.C.

Library of Congress Cataloging-in-Publication Data
Harden, Victoria Angela.
AIDS at 30: a history / Victoria A. Harden.—1st ed.
    p. cm.
 Includes bibliographical references and index.
 ISBN 978-1-59797-294-9 (hardcover: alk. paper)
 ISBN 978-1-61234-516-1 (electronic edition)
1. AIDS (disease)—History. I. Title. II. Title: AIDS at thirty.
 RA643.8.H37 2012
 616.97'92—dc23

                                                    2011028331

Printed in the United States of America on acid-free paper that meets the American National Standards Institute Z39-48 Standard.

Potomac Books
22841 Quicksilver Drive
Dulles, Virginia 20166

First Edition

10 9 8 7 6 5 4 3 2 1

for Sibyl Victoria McDonell-Leslie

Contents

List of Illustrations		ix
List of Abbreviations		xi
Preface		xiii
Prologue	Emergence in Silence	1
1	What Is This New Disease?	11
2	Searching for the Cause of AIDS	39
3	Clinical Research, Epidemic of Fear, and AIDS in the Worldwide Blood Supply	71
4	AIDS as a Cultural Phenomenon	95
5	AIDS Therapy	125
6	Communicating AIDS	159
7	The Global Epidemic	185
8	The Third Decade	213
Epilogue	AIDS at 30	245
Glossary		253
Notes		261
Index		307
About the Author		323

Illustrations

1.1	Humoral immune system	18
1.2	Cellular immune system	19
1.3	City of New York Department of Health AIDS team	27
1.4	James Curran	28
2.1	Components of the U.S. Department of Health and Human Services, 1981	43
2.2	Replication of an RNA virus (hepatitis C virus)	46
2.3	HIV replication cycle	47
2.4	Robert C. Gallo	48
2.5	Laboratory of Tumor Cell Biology, U.S. National Cancer Institute, 1985	49
2.6	Jean-Claude Chermann, Françoise Barré-Sinoussi, and Luc Montagnier	52
2.7	Koch's postulates	56
3.1	H. Clifford Lane and Anthony S. Fauci	74
3.2	1983 voluntary blood-donor disqualification form	88
3.3	1985 Abbott Laboratories diagnostic AIDS test kit	91
4.1	Surgeon General C. Everett Koop	100
4.2	*Surgeon General's Report on AIDS* (1986) and *Understanding AIDS* (1988)	103
4.3	Final report of the National Commission on AIDS, 1993	113
4.4	ACT UP "Storm the NIH" protest, May 21, 1990	116

4.5   "Storm the NIH" protester, May 21, 1990   116
4.6   Needle exchange, Seattle, Washington, 2007   118
4.7   AIDS quilt   121
5.1   HIV virion   128
5.2   HIV life cycle, 1987   129
5.3   Hiroaki "Mitch" Mitsuya, Samuel Broder, and Robert Yarchoan   131
5.4   Process of bringing a drug to market   134
5.5   HIV life cycle, 2009   153
5.6   "No Obits," *Bay Area Reporter*, San Francisco, California,
      August 13, 1998   156
6.1   "*Pneumocystis* Pneumonia—Los Angeles," *MMWR*,
      June 5, 1981   162
6.2   Larry Kramer   169
6.3   AIDS awareness trading cards   179
6.4   Australian AIDS poster, 1980s   180
7.1   Projet SIDA team, 1986   189
7.2   Trans-African highways based on 2000–2003 data   195
7.3   Global prevalence of AIDS, 2010   201
8.1   Peter Piot, 2000   218
8.2   United Nations Building with AIDS red ribbon   220
9.1   Annual AIDS-related deaths by region, 1990–2009   246
9.2   Human immunodeficiency virus in three dimensions   248

Abbreviations

ACT UP	AIDS Coalition to Unleash Power
amfAR	American Foundation for AIDS Research
ANC	African National Congress
APHA	American Public Health Association
ASH	assistant secretary for health, DHHS
BBC	British Broadcasting Corporation
CDC	U.S. Centers for Disease Control and Prevention
CIA	U.S. Central Intelligence Agency
DHHS	U.S. Department of Health and Human Services
DOH	Department of Health (New York City)
EIS	Epidemic Intelligence Service (CDC)
FDA	U.S. Food and Drug Administration
FOIA	U.S. Freedom of Information Act
FWG	French Working Group
GHESKIO	Haitian Group for the Study of Kaposi's Sarcoma and Opportunistic Infections
GLAAD	Gay and Lesbian Alliance against Defamation
GMHC	Gay Men's Health Crisis
GPA	Global Programme on AIDS (WHO)
IAVI	International AIDS Vaccine Initiative
ICD	International Classification of Diseases (WHO document)

ICMR	Indian Council of Medical Research
INRB	National Institute of Biomedical Research (Zaire)
INSERM	National Institute for Health and Medical Research (France)
ITM	Institute of Tropical Medicine (Belgium)
MAP	Multicountry AIDS Program (World Bank)
MCC	Medicines Control Council (South Africa)
NAT	National AIDS Trust (United Kingdom)
NCI	U.S. National Cancer Institute
NEI	U.S. National Eye Institute
NIAID	U.S. National Institute of Allergy and Infectious Diseases
NIDR	U.S. National Institute of Dental Research
NIH	U.S. National Institutes of Health
NINCDS	U.S. National Institute of Neurological and Communicative Disorders and Stroke
OAR	Office of AIDS Research, NIH
PAHO	Pan American Health Organization (Western Hemisphere branch of WHO)
PEPFAR	U.S. President's Emergency Plan for AIDS Relief
PHS	U.S. Public Health Service
SABC	South African Broadcasting Corporation
SVCP	Special Virus Cancer Program
TAC	Treatment Action Campaign (South Africa)
TAG	Treatment Action Group (United States)
TASO	The AIDS Support Organization (Uganda)
UCLA	University of California–Los Angeles
UCSF	University of California–San Francisco
UN	United Nations
UNAIDS	Joint United Nations Programme on HIV/AIDS
UNDP	United Nations Development Programme
UNGASS	United Nations General Assembly Special Session
UNICEF	United Nations International Children's Emergency Relief Fund
USAID	U.S. Agency for International Development
VRC	Vaccine Research Center, NIH
WHO	World Health Organization

Preface

This book had its origin in September 1984, when I arrived at the U.S. National Institutes of Health (NIH) to write about another infectious disease for the National Institute of Allergy and Infectious Diseases (NIAID) and found myself housed in an office with Ruth Guyer, an immunologist turned science writer who was producing a newsletter called the *AIDS Memorandum*. Talk around the NIH campus was intense with regard to the new disease AIDS, and a number of NIAID scientists working on AIDS were next door or downstairs from our office. Confessing that I had never heard of T cells and B cells, which seemed to be involved somehow with AIDS, I asked Guyer to enlighten me, and so began my education into molecular immunology and virology. As a historian, I wondered who was collecting materials such as the *AIDS Memorandum* and conducting interviews with scientists working on AIDS, and I found out that no formal historical process existed at NIH. Here was a new disease, key investigators working around me, important discoveries going on, and no one was capturing this? It seemed a dereliction of duty for a historian not to make some sort of attempt to document what was occurring.

In 1986 I had the good fortune to become the founding director of the Office of NIH History and Stetten Museum, a position from which I was able to include what by then was beginning to be called HIV/AIDS documentation efforts alongside other initiatives to document biomedical research history at the United States' foremost medical research institution. Because my research on HIV/AIDS was conducted over more than a quarter century, however, I have incurred more debts to more people than I can possibly acknowledge. The number of NIH staff who went out of their way to assist me at various times is far too large for me to name every person, but to them all I am most grateful. My colleagues in the Office of Communications at NIH, mostly trained as journalists, were welcoming to a historian and taught me much about excellence in writing and thinking about a public audience. Don Ralbovsky collected ephemera for the Stetten Museum during the 1990 "Storm the NIH" ACT UP protest. Dennis Rodrigues worked with me for some years on the AIDS oral history project, bringing his expertise as a former staff member of the NIH AIDS Executive Committee. The communications staff in the NIAID and the National Cancer Institute (NCI) worked intensely with me in 2001 to prepare the website "In Their Own Words: NIH Scientists Recall the Early Years of AIDS," which was launched to mark the twentieth anniversary of the AIDS epidemic.

My own staff in the Office of NIH History and Stetten Museum also helped in many different ways. Archivist Brooke Fox worked heroically to organize the mountain of AIDS materials generated at NIH, including photos, oral histories, and documents. Her successor, Barbara Harkins, responded to every request for access to these materials as the writing was in progress. Michele Lyons curated the artifacts collected by the Stetten Museum. Caroline Hannaway expertly edited many of the AIDS oral histories. The historical offices at the Public Health Service (PHS) and the Food and Drug Administration (FDA), working to preserve different aspects of the history of HIV/AIDS, were always available for consultation and advice. FDA historian Suzanne Junod took the initiative to send the Stetten Museum one of the earliest HIV test kits approved by the FDA for our collection.

History colleagues around the world also pointed me to materials and worked to preserve historical documents for future histories of AIDS. Initially, I had hoped to include an appendix listing repositories of interest to other scholars in this book, but in short order I realized that such a list would merit a book of its own. In addition, many new documentary materials are just now beginning to be organized. After my research on U.S. federal policy on HIV/AIDS in the 1980s was complete, for example, the U.S. National Library of Medicine (NLM) acquired a chronological file of correspondence about AIDS that covers all agencies in the Department of Health and Human Services that will be of great use for future scholars.

In 1988, a group of scholars in the American Association for the History of Medicine formed the AIDS History Group and elected Guenter Risse and me cochairs. In 1995 Caroline Hannaway took over as cochair with me. Until 1999 we published the *AIDS History Group Newsletter*, which aimed to keep people around the world—including community activists, journalists, archivists, health care personnel, and others in addition to historians—in touch with each other. In 1989 the group held a conference, "AIDS and the Historian," at the NIH, and Guenter Risse and I edited a conference proceedings volume. Courtesy of organizational efforts by William Helfand and his late wife, Audrey, the group was also able to hold a second conference in 1993, "AIDS and the Public Debate: Historical and Contemporary Perspectives," which brought together historians, public health officials, physicians, and pharmaceutical company officials to assess where the epidemic stood. Caroline Hannaway and John Parascandola coedited the conference proceedings volume with me. All the participants in these efforts deserve thanks for broadening and deepening my understanding of aspects of HIV/AIDS.

The scientists, physicians, public health officials, administrators, nurses, technicians, and social workers who participated in the NIH oral history project provided in-depth information over the years about how the epidemic was viewed from different professional perspectives and patiently tutored me in the science, medicine, and politics of AIDS. At the National Institute of Allergy and Infectious Diseases, I owe special thanks to Greg Folkers for assistance on many issues over two decades.

Two colleagues who also pursued AIDS oral history programs in the United States generously shared their interviews. Gerald Oppenheimer gave me access to the oral histories he and Ronald Bayer conducted with AIDS physicians in New York, and Mary Marshall Clark, director of the Columbia University Oral History Research Office, arranged for me to have digital access to them. Sally Smith Hughes, the historian who conducted and edited oral histories to document the response to the AIDS epidemic in the San Francisco Bay area, not only worked with the Regional Oral History Program at the University of California–Berkeley to make the interviews available on the Internet but also provided comments on a portion of my manuscript.

My thanks also go to the following people for reading and commenting on chapter drafts, especially for helping me clarify the science involved in AIDS research: James Curran, David Sencer, Roberto Trujillio, Anthony Fauci, H. Clifford Lane, Robert Yarchoan, Thomas Quinn, Peter Piot, and David Morens. James Mason, Harold Jaffe, and Donald Resio also guided me in understanding the details of particular issues. Their comments have made the text more accurate. Any errors that remain are mine alone.

My editor at Potomac Books, Elizabeth Demers, worked very hard to make this book happen, even in the face of the economic downturn in 2008–2009. Thanks are due to my family, especially my daughter, Emily McDonell, who transcribed some of the oral histories, and my daughter-in-law, Thyra Leslie, who helped me locate key sources. My son, Durward McDonell, and stepson, David Berger, bailed me out—twice—after computer crashes. Most of all I owe thanks to my husband, Robert Berger, who has always been my first reader and rock of stability, and who may now get to see more than the back of my head toiling at the computer on the manuscript.

Anyone who engages with the HIV/AIDS epidemic is overwhelmed by the suffering and death wreaked by HIV. Most writers hope to have a positive impact on the state of the world, and if this book can help to spur decisions that will save lives, I will be more than repaid for the effort. The book is dedicated to my granddaughter Sibyl, in the hope that she will live to see a world in which HIV/AIDS is no longer a threat to human health.

Prologue:
Emergence in Silence

"We will never escape the ecosystem and the limits of the ecosystem. Whether we like it or not, we are caught in the food chain, eating and being eaten. It is one of the conditions of life."

—WILLIAM H. MCNEILL.[1]

On June 5, 2011, the world observed the thirtieth anniversary of the disease known as acquired immune deficiency syndrome, or AIDS. The term "AIDS" was coined to summarize a medical phenomenon whose cause was initially not known but that is now understood to embody the end-stage signs and symptoms that emerge after long infection with the human immunodeficiency virus (HIV). The actual number of people who have died of AIDS is not known. As of December 2010, some 33.3 million people were living with HIV infection. In three decades, this virus and the manifestation of opportunistic infections and cancers known as AIDS have left children without parents and countries without a sizable portion of young adults who could have served as leaders in the future. The very specific date of June 5, 1981, records the moment when medically trained individuals had become sufficiently aware that a new disease existed that they published what they knew to alert other physicians and public health officers.[2] Six physicians—five in the Department of Medicine at the University of California–Los Angeles and one at Cedars-Sinai Hospital in Los Angeles—reported on the cases of five young men who suffered from a disease normally seen only in patients whose immune systems had been severely damaged.[3]

This publication marked the beginning of a new era in medicine. For a generation, humans had enjoyed the illusion that infectious diseases had been conquered with antibiotics and vaccines. Between the 1950s and 1981, physicians whose practice focused on infectious diseases almost always saw their patients get well. Penicillin and broad spectrum antibiotics, coupled with vaccines against polio and other childhood diseases, freed most patients and physicians in the industrialized world from the fear of death by diseases caused by bacteria, viruses, and other types of microbes. Defeating infections in undeveloped nations appeared to be largely a challenge of moral and economic will, not of medical knowledge. By the late 1970s, the main problem faced by those who were less optimistic about human triumph over microbes was convincing their colleagues, research funding organizations, and the public that their concerns had any value. Within a decade after June 5, 1981, however, it became clear that the "triumph" of humans over microbes was merely a victory in one skirmish marking the timeless competition of life-forms on earth.[4]

What Is AIDS?

Diseases get their names in a variety of ways. Malaria, a very old malady, took its name from the Italian for "bad air." People living near Rome believed that illness was contracted from the bad smells, or *miasmas,* arising from nearby swamps long before they had any notion about microbes and mosquito transmission. Hepatitis comes from the Greek word for "liver" and means an inflammation of the liver. Today it is designated as "hepatitis A," "hepatitis B," etc., depending on which of several hepatitis viruses has caused the liver inflammation. Hemophilia was named from the Latin word for "blood" and the Greek word for "affection," or "tending toward," and describes the hemophiliac's characteristic of bleeding easily. As a new disease, AIDS was named by the physicians, scientists, and public health leaders who were attempting to respond to it. As we will see in chapter 1, the earliest cases of what came to be known as AIDS were linked to an immune deficiency—the "ID" part of the abbreviation. These early cases were clustered into groups suffering from opportunistic infections such as a pneumonia caused by *Pneumocystis carinii*, a widely spread organism usually held in check by the normal immune system, and by Kaposi's sarcoma (KS), a rare cancer seen in kidney transplant patients whose immune system had been suppressed to prevent rejection of the donor organ.[5] When it became clear that the immune deficiency was not caused by an inherited genetic mutation like the one that caused hemophilia, the "A" for "acquired" immune deficiency was added. Finally, people suffering from AIDS came to their doctors with many other problems as well as pneumonia and Kaposi's sarcoma. Some had candidiasis, sometimes called thrush, in their mouths. Some had widespread herpes cold sores or genital sores or other viral infections usually controlled by the immune system. What physicians saw, then, was a "syndrome," a predictable group of several symptoms, the "S" in AIDS.

When AIDS was first recognized, physicians defined the syndrome according to those infections and cancers that they saw initially. As it became clear that AIDS was afflicting many more people than originally thought and that women often had different symptoms from men, and children had different symptoms from adults, the particular problems that fell into the syndrome "S" of AIDS were expanded. Today two systems exist side by side for classifying what is exactly encompassed by the name of any particular disease, one system published by the U.S. Centers for Disease Control and Prevention (known by its historic moniker, CDC) and another by the World Health Organization (WHO). The first definition of AIDS, utilized by the CDC in 1981, was based only on clinical signs limited to the groups of people already encountered with AIDS. Over the next few years, the clinical definition was expanded as more was learned about the disease. (This will be discussed in detail in chapter 1.) In 1986 the CDC and WHO moved cautiously to define AIDS as the end-stage manifestation of infection with a particular virus. Because diagnostic tests that were appropriate and cost-effective for many different geographical locations were still being developed, the CDC was willing to define AIDS by clinical symptoms in the absence of laboratory tests for the causative virus.[6] In 1993 infection with HIV was defined as essential for classifying the disease as AIDS. In 1994 WHO's International Classification of Diseases (ICD) likewise defined AIDS as the result of HIV infection. The two systems differed with respect to the method for determining when full-blown AIDS appeared: the CDC linked it to a specific level of affected immune-system cells that could be tested for. When the level fell below two hundred cells per microliter of blood, a person was said to have AIDS. The WHO's standard was oriented toward populations in which laboratory testing might not be readily available. It continued to utilize well-known clinical manifestations of AIDS such as recurrent pneumonias, invasive cervical cancer, neurological deterioration, and Kaposi's sarcoma to mark the onset of AIDS.[7]

More recently, the definition of AIDS has changed as physicians and researchers have learned new details about the types of opportunistic infections and cancers that long-term infection with HIV permits. Ill-defined conditions such as "cardiac arrest, unspecified hypotension, unspecified disorders of the circulatory system, acute or unspecified respiratory failure, and respiratory failure in a newborn" also complicate the AIDS picture. Deaths from such conditions are now defined as caused by HIV infection if it existed as an underlying condition.[8] In 1995, with the meeting of the first White House Conference on HIV/AIDS, the name of the disease shifted from "AIDS" to "HIV/AIDS," the form in which it is now known, thirty years after it was first detected. HIV/AIDS is an infection with the human immunodeficiency virus. After a long incubation period without treatment, that infection leads to the various opportunistic infections, cancers, and other organ failures that are called the syndrome of acquired immunodeficiency.

HIV/AIDS Is a Zoonosis

HIV/AIDS is a *zoonosis*, a disease caused by a microscopic pathogen transmitted from other animals to humans.[9] These tiny pathogens, which usually exist harmlessly in their animal hosts, may experience a mutation or a recombination of genetic materials and thereby become able to infect human beings. More than half the human diseases caused by infectious pathogens are shared between animals and humans.[10] Rocky Mountain spotted fever microbes, for example, coexist happily with particular ticks. *Rickettsia rickettsii*, the spotted fever germ, is passed from infected female tick to her offspring via her eggs with no apparent ill effects on the ticks. If an infected tick bites a human, however, *R. rickettsii* organisms pass into the human's body, where they cause a high fever and attack the cells of the circulatory system, causing leakage in capillaries that appear as spots on the skin of the victim and may, in the most severe cases, lead to circulatory collapse and death.[11]

Many types of pathogens cause human disease. Bacteria, viruses, protozoa, and prions are known as "infectious" because they must infect, or enter the human body, to cause illness. They are transmitted from one human host to another in several different ways. Influenza and measles viruses can be transmitted in the air between an infected person and someone else. A healthy person is bitten by an infected mosquito to become infected with yellow fever or malaria. The bacteria that cause typhoid fever must be ingested in contaminated water, milk, or food. Some pathogens, such as the hepatitis B virus, are transmitted primarily by sexual contact or via blood—through injection with a contaminated needle, through accidental blood-to-blood contact as in a multiperson auto accident, or by transfusion with infected blood or blood products.

HIV, like the hepatitis B virus, is overwhelmingly transmitted through sexual contact or via blood. HIV is called a *retrovirus* because as it replicates, one step in the replication process includes a reversal of the action by which other viruses reproduce themselves (see chapter 2 for more details). Initially, the retroviruses that became HIV strains inhabited nonhuman primates such as chimpanzees and sooty mangaby monkeys. In retrospect, scientists named these retroviruses simian immunodeficiency viruses (SIV). HIV appeared after a genetic change in SIV made it possible for the altered virus to "jump species" to infect and kill human hosts.[12] Viruses are constantly mutating and changing, and those that resulted in the creation of HIV strains are believed to have emerged on many different occasions. Molecular research in 2006 traced the first strain of HIV identified (HIV-1) to a recombined version of a SIV of a specific type of chimpanzee, *Pan troglodytes troglodytes,* that evolved on three separate occasions. A second strain, HIV-2, was traced to a different SIV of sooty mangabys (*Cercocebus atys*).[13] Between 2007 and 2010, additional research defined the origin of HIV strains even more specifically and suggested that particular SIV strains caused immunodeficiency in chimpanzees, thus making the disease AIDS not solely a human affliction.[14]

HIV is made up of a single strand of ribonucleic acid (RNA), which carries the genes that govern the way the virus infects a host cell and replicates itself. Around that RNA is a protein coat and an envelope of lipids, or fat, punctuated with protuberances that fit into receptor molecules in human immune-system cells and serve as keys in locks to let the virus infect the cell (see figure 5.1 for a diagram of HIV). Transmission of HIV from one host to another is not at all easy, unlike the transmission of the measles virus in aerosol droplets from an infected person's cough or sneeze. The most common ways HIV is transmitted are via sexual relations that permit the virus to enter tiny tears in the body's mucosal surfaces and by the kind of blood-to-blood contact that can occur when a drug user injects himself with a needle already used by someone with HIV or when a health care provider reuses a contaminated, nonsterile instrument. Transfusion with HIV-contaminated blood is another way the virus may travel from host to host, but once HIV was identified, donor screening and testing for the virus and discarding contaminated blood products became one of the highest priorities of medicine, and today blood products—at least in the industrialized world—are safe.[15]

The Silent Emergence of HIV/AIDS

The virus that causes the devastating symptoms of AIDS had killed the rare human host for nearly a century before physicians recognized its existence. In 2008 laboratory analysis of genetic material from HIV-infected patients indicated that HIV began infecting humans as early as 1910 around the African city Léopoldville, capital of what was then called the Belgian Congo. Today the city is called Kinshasa, and it is capital of the Democratic Republic of Congo. In the early twentieth century, Léopoldville was growing as the major navigable port on the Congo River above rapids between it and the sea. In 1898 a portage railway had been completed to transport goods around the rapids, enabling the city's rapid expansion. Increased traffic along the Congo River may have contributed to the initial spread of HIV, but it is impossible to track down the case-by-case progress of HIV infection. Scientists now estimate that by the 1960s only about one thousand Africans had been infected with HIV.[16]

The most common strain of HIV outside of sub-Saharan Africa is one known as HIV-1, group M, subtype B. The group and subtype are only important in that scientists have been able to trace the movement of this particular strain backward from the United States, where it arrived in the 1970s, to Haiti, where it arrived in the 1960s, and then back to Africa, where the virus originated. Haiti was found to have the oldest AIDS epidemic outside sub-Saharan Africa, and although individual infections cannot be traced, it is known that many French-speaking Haitians with sufficient resources to flee the repressive political regime of François Duvalier ("Papa Doc"), who took power in 1957, moved to French-speaking African countries. In 1960 the Belgian Congo was granted independence and became the Democratic Republic of Congo. The Belgians left without having trained Congolese to run the machinery of government (the first Congolese graduated from college only in 1956). To help the new republic, its leaders recruited French-speaking Haitian managers from among the exiles who had fled Haiti, and for five years, Haitians essentially made the country function. By 1970 native citizens were in place to manage the bureaucracy, and with the death of Duvalier in 1971, some of the worst practices of his regime were lifted. Haitians living in Africa began to return home about the same time as the African country was renamed Zaire.[17]

Based on historical association, it appears that Haitians were infected with HIV while in Africa in the 1960s and unknowingly passed it along to their sexual contacts when they visited Haiti. The rate of transmission increased in the 1970s as expatriate Haitians returned from Africa to take up residence again in Haiti. In the 1970s and into the 1980s, the Haitian capital, Port-au-Prince, became a popular vacation site for some homosexual men from the United States who took advantage of the willingness of some Haitian men to engage in sex with other men to earn a living. Two groups of scientists believe that HIV was transmitted to the United States and other countries in the Western Hemisphere via Haiti, but this argument has been challenged by others who believe the Haitian AIDS epidemic was seeded by tourists coming into Haiti from other places and seeking paid sexual encounters. What is certain, however, is that Haiti has a higher prevalence of HIV than the Dominican Republic, which shares the same island of Hispaniola.[18]

Recognition of AIDS as a New Disease in Humans

The recognition of AIDS as a new disease in humans is much clearer in hindsight than it was as it unfolded. Knowing now that the origin of the causative virus was in sub-Saharan West Africa raises the question of why AIDS was not first identified there but instead in the gay communities of major cities in the United States. The answer undoubtedly lies in the difference between how medicine is practiced by physicians and experienced by patients in Africa and in the United States. Africans who succumbed to AIDS in the decades before 1981 were likely poor, rural people who rarely consulted physicians who practiced Western medicine. The Haitians and Europeans who contracted AIDS in Africa may have consulted Western-trained doctors, but they represented too few cases at any one time to alert physicians that a new pattern had emerged.

Conversely, physicians and nurses, seeing an African with a fever and wasting, would likely attribute the symptoms to any of a host of fevers present in tropical countries.

Peter Piot, who headed the Joint United Nations Programme on HIV/AIDS (UNAIDS) from 1994 through 2008, recalled the first case of AIDS he saw in Antwerp, Belgium. He had been participating in a postmortem exam in the late 1970s of "a Greek sailor, who came from what was then called Zaire [now Democratic Republic of Congo] and who had been a fisherman in Lake Tanganyika—he had died with something very unusual, with disseminated cryptococcal meningitis; in other words, an infection with a fungus that is very rare, and certainly if it's disseminated. And that was the first time [I saw a case of AIDS]. We knew afterwards because we had kept all the specimens, including blood, and he was HIV positive."[19]

Judith Williams, a medical social worker at the National Institutes of Health, described her experience in 1964 with an African she believed had AIDS. While working in children's health in Nigeria, where her husband had been posted with the U.S. State Department, Williams recalled,

> I was in the village, doing the well-baby clinic, and they [the people] said, "Would you come with us to see this man who is very ill?" So we walked to a little hut that they had built outside of the town, and I said, "What is the problem with this man? What is wrong with him?" They said, "He has slimming disease." I said, "Oh, slimming disease. But what does he do for a living?" They said, "Well, he was a monkey hunter. That is who gets slimming disease, monkey hunters." . . . So we went to this little shack that they had made for him, and the man was completely emaciated, just bones, and probably suffering from diarrhea and all sorts of problems. There was not really much that could be done for him. The villagers said, "No, no, they always die. What happens is, when they start to get sick, we bring them out here and then we take care of them until they die."[20]

In contrast, most of the earliest AIDS patients in the United States were largely Caucasian, upper-middle-class homosexual men with health insurance who regularly consulted physicians when they fell ill. The physicians who treated these individuals saw an increasing number of unusual opportunistic infections and cancers among their patients, who had not experienced such problems in the past. These physicians thus recognized a disruption in the medical history of their patient populations that led them to question idiosyncratic diagnoses and wonder about the possibility of a novel disease process.

AIDS History Tells Us about Ourselves

The history of AIDS, like the histories of all epidemics, tells us much about the medical ideas, political organization, and cultural beliefs that define human social organizations as they face the challenge of epidemic disease. These ideas and beliefs also shaped the actions of physicians seeing patients in daily practice and of public health physicians attempting to reduce disease incidence on a societal scale. Religious and other cultural beliefs contributed significantly to how communities helped or shunned those infected and how those not infected might be taught to avoid the disease. Books, movies, newspaper articles, and even ephemera such as AIDS-prevention posters and messages on matchbook covers have been shaped by the cultural beliefs of their authors. Commercial interests, primarily pharmaceutical companies, developed therapies under the dual demands of profit making and ethical responsibility. The marketers of quack remedies also appeared shortly after the new disease was identified and have continued to prey on desperate people for three decades. Alternative ideas about the cause of AIDS took hold at high political levels in some cases and created roadblocks to effective treatment of people with AIDS in entire countries. Those who spread urban legends and conspiracy theories about AIDS exploited the developing Internet and World Wide Web to gain support for their ideas. Demands for cures and prevention by social groups affected by AIDS changed the way that health lobbying was accomplished and altered some aspects of medical research protocols for new drugs.

Sources of Information

The AIDS epidemic unfolded just as the computer was revolutionizing communications throughout the world. This means that documentation of the earliest years of the epidemic exists largely in paper records—books, newspapers, magazines, official reports, government hearings, memos, letters, and the like. Some of these have been digitized; others have not. Other sources include still photographs, video recordings from television, artifacts collected in museums, and oral histories. As the transition from letters written on paper to e-mail messages occurred, many important communications were deleted and are thus unavailable for review. Once electronic record archival policies were implemented, the digital documentary record improved. With the advent of the World Wide Web, a great deal of information, both old and new, gravitated to the Internet. Major AIDS organizations—whether for-profit, nonprofit, governmental, or international—developed websites to convey current information, and over time, they also made archival materials available. The Internet also permitted real-time discussion of ideas concerning AIDS. The free online encyclopedia Wikipedia, for example, contains in its editorial section on AIDS discussions that still rage about various aspects of the disease.

For the historian, the sheer volume of materials available is overwhelming. It would be impossible to provide details on every event and every important person in AIDS history, or even every archival repository with materials about the pandemic, and the result would be unreadable. This great mass of facts is best understood via a historical narrative that attempts to sort out and highlight particular issues relevant to AIDS today. Thus my account is "a" history of AIDS as opposed to "the" history of AIDS. I witnessed the unfolding epidemic as the agency historian at the U.S. National Institutes of Health (NIH) during a period when NIH medical researchers worked to understand how HIV affected the human body and to devise some intervention to prevent or treat the disease process. My personal interest is thus strongest in conveying how mainstream science and medicine came to understand this disease and responded to it within the social and political contexts of the last decades of the twentieth century and the first decade of the twenty-first. Much more about the economic, political, and social dimensions of the AIDS epidemic has been written by others, and I have followed the work of many other scholars in preparing the chapters dealing with those matters. It is my hope that this book will help illuminate how those in the health care professions responded to this new disease in our time, especially those who sought to comprehend and describe AIDS, to identify its cause, and to develop preventive and therapeutic interventions to slow or stop the devastation wreaked by HIV on the human species.

1

What Is This New Disease?

"The work in AIDS was very difficult because we didn't know where we were going. We were blind people in a dark room, and if we had seen the light, we didn't know if we would recognize it."

—Selma Dritz[1]

How does a physician know that a medical condition in one of his or her patients constitutes a new disease? Why would a physician even think that a new disease has emerged rather than that he or she is simply not recognizing the signs and symptoms of an existing disease? AIDS has been identified in retrospect as a disease caused by a retrovirus that gained the ability to infect humans after the recombination of genetic material in a virus that infected nonhuman primates, but when the first article describing a potentially new disease was published in 1981, AIDS was no more than five documented cases of an unusual opportunistic infection normally seen only in people whose immune systems had been suppressed for organ transplantation or cancer therapy.

In the thirty years between June 1981 and June 2011, the disease AIDS has been defined in different terms by the medical community, by the groups of people who suffered from AIDS, by cultures and religions around the world, and by people charged with making political decisions within those cultures. In this chapter, I explore how a new disease is recognized and defined, because that changing consensus holds powerful consequences for those who contract the disease as well as their families, friends, employers, and fellow citizens.

What Is a Disease?

In the *Oxford English Dictionary,* the word *disease* is defined first as "an absence of ease . . . a cause of discomfort or distress" and second as "a condition of the body, or some part or organ of the body, in which its functions are disturbed or deranged; a morbid physical condition; a departure from the state of health."[2] Both definitions describe a sense of illness, but neither provides details for how diseases are identified or named. Since the time of the ancient Greeks, one way physicians have named diseases is by describing their physical manifestations: what we call epilepsy, for example, was known to them as the *falling sickness* because of the seizures that caused a person to fall down. Fevers, themselves a reflection of the physical state of being hotter than normal, were described with adjectives such as "relapsing" and "spotted," according to observable symptoms.

It is important to understand that thinking about any disease always develops within larger intellectual concepts about how the human body works. Until the last decades of the nineteenth century, there was no place in medical thinking for the idea that microscopic pathogens could cause specific diseases or even that the fever one person had was necessarily caused by the same thing that caused similar fever symptoms in someone else. The balance of body fluids, or "humors"; the individual constitution inherited from parents; the good or bad influences of environment and diet; foul-smelling *miasmas* thought to carry disease—these were the principal features of a physician's intellectual framework for explaining fevers, digestive problems, balance difficulties, vision, hearing, wasting, reproductive, and all other disease issues.

Toward the end of the nineteenth century, new medical ideas and laboratory technology fostered a radical change in the understanding of infectious diseases. Individual researchers, such as Louis Pasteur in France and Robert Koch in Germany, conducted studies that convinced other scientists and physicians that particular bacteria and protozoa (germs) caused anthrax, cholera, and tuberculosis. In the 1880s Koch published several versions of a laboratory method, which he called postulates that had to be satisfied, by which scientists might demonstrate that a particular germ caused a particular disease (see figure 2.7 for the classic version of Koch's postulates).[3] By the turn of the new century, most mainstream physicians, public health officers, and scientists who studied microorganisms accepted the germ theory of infectious disease.

The general public was slower to accept this new concept of disease causation.[4] Some groundwork had been laid at the end of the eighteenth century by the introduction of vaccination against smallpox, although widespread vaccination was not common in many locales and no one could explain exactly how or why vaccination worked. Pasteur's demonstration that his vaccine against rabies would protect against that deadly disease further promoted his argument that microscopic pathogens caused disease, as did Joseph Lister's success in preventing death from "putrefaction," which we would call infection, by using carbolic acid to kill germs in the operating theater.

The single event that finally convinced the public of the germ theory's merit was the 1891 demonstration by Emil von Behring that serum, the liquid part of blood, taken from someone who had recovered from diphtheria, could be injected into a person suffering from the disease, and afterward, the patient would be restored to health. Behring's work was based on the similar results of Japanese scientist Shibasaburo Kitasato, who had previously developed a successful serum therapy against tetanus. In 1894 Behring began producing "serum therapy" commercially with the Hoechst pharmaceutical company. Soon, parents who had perhaps watched one child die from diphtheria while a physician held its hand witnessed the miracle of seeing another dangerously ill child sit up and function again within a day or so after receiving an injection of diphtheria antiserum. Such a powerful demonstration won strong public converts to the new thinking.[5] Power to cure disease, not the publications and logic of laboratory science, convinced the public that the germ theory was correct. Both laboratory evidence and the ability to restore sick people to a healthier state, if not to cure them, became important in the history of AIDS at different moments and with different consequences, as we shall see in chapters 2 and 5. In 1901 Behring was awarded the first Nobel Prize in Physiology or Medicine for his work on serum therapy in diphtheria.[6] It is generally believed that the Nobel committee should also have honored Kitasato but that European nationalism and perhaps racism led to Kitasato's being excluded.[7] The awarding of the Nobel prize for the work demonstrating the cause of AIDS was similarly limited to researchers of one European country and produced a scientific controversy, as we shall see in chapter 2.

First Encounters: Defining AIDS as a New Disease

The fable of the elephant and the blind men, each of whom felt a different part of the large beast and insisted that what he felt represented the entirety of the animal, accurately reflects the first human encounters with the new disease AIDS. Those suffering from its symptoms and their caregivers perceived AIDS in the most direct and painful way, but as a group, they had no way of understanding that what was happening within their bodies represented a new disease entity. The practicing physicians who treated these patients served as the front line in recognizing a new disease and attempting to ameliorate its symptoms. Close behind them came public health officials who sought to understand the disease on a population-based scale and to protect society at large from a new disease about which very little was known. Physicians and scientists who worked in medical research collaborated with their colleagues in an effort to understand the *pathophysiology*—the disease process in the human body— and to devise interventions to ease the suffering. Both public health and medical research personnel needed funding for their work, however, so city, state, and national governments were faced with decisions about how much money and effort to expend on research, monitoring, and treatment. This political calculus occurred many times in societies around the world, some of which held different views about illness, about who got sick and why, and about the role of governments in responding to disease outbreaks.

Fear of infection, a very old response to disease, fueled the reactions of many in these societies. When AIDS was shown to be sexually transmitted, religions and cultures around the world responded according to their own views of appropriate sexual behavior. Businesses, ethical and unethical, realized that a new disease offered an opportunity to develop treatments that would generate income. Newspapers, magazines, television, and eventually the Internet provided information about AIDS, sometimes helpful, sometimes exploitative. An ever-active culture of paranoia saw sinister plots in the advent of a new disease and disseminated urban legends and allegations that provided a constant counterpoint to the efforts of mainstream medicine to address AIDS. In this chapter, I will look at the initial response to the advent of AIDS.

Patient and Caregiver Experiences

Between the time HIV emerged through a change in a virus that infected other primates and the late 1970s, those people who suffered from AIDS certainly knew they were ill but had no understanding that their afflictions were the symptoms of a new disease. In the late 1970s enough people who previously had been healthy consulted Western physicians about AIDS symptoms to raise the possibility in the minds of those doctors that a new disease had appeared. Looking backward, many physicians remembered seeing patients or receiving puzzling telephone calls asking for consultations about unusual cases. These cases were noted in Africa, Haiti, the United States, and Europe, especially in countries such as Belgium, with former colonial ties to French-speaking African countries.[8]

AIDS was first recognized among homosexual men in large cities in the United States. About three weeks before the first medical publication about AIDS appeared, the *New York Native* reported on rumors of a "gay cancer" circulating in New York's gay community but, relying on knowledge purportedly relayed from the CDC, stated that the rumors had no substance.[9] Randy Shilts, in his book *And the Band Played On: Politics, People, and the AIDS Epidemic*, wrote movingly in 1987 about the initial appearance of AIDS from the perspective of someone who lived in the gay community in San Francisco and, as he later revealed, was infected with the AIDS virus himself.[10] His book articulated an agonizing cry of Why? Why the gay community? Why now, just as gay life had become open after such a long period of oppression? Who was to blame? In detail, Shilts chronicled the efforts of individuals to care for their friends and lovers who suffered from AIDS. He described the tragedies of some patients whose families rejected them and a caring, end-of-life reconciliation of other patients with families who reconnected with their sons after the onset of AIDS.

Shilts and others have written about the impact of AIDS on the gay communities in the United States, and it is important to understand the status of homosexuals in U.S. society at the time that AIDS appeared. In the heady period of the 1970s, ignited by riots that occurred in June 1969 in response to a police raid at Greenwich Village's Stonewall Inn bar in New York (a meeting place for homosexual men), the gay community resolved to demand civil rights rather than be treated as second-class citizens.[11] For many in the gay community, freedom from the fear of discrimination also meant freedom to enjoy their sexuality with few or no concerns about disease. Physicians, both gay and straight, who saw an increase in sexually transmitted diseases among their gay male patients worried about the increasing toll repeated infectious diseases took on the bodies of men who had a large number of sexual partners.[12] Shortly after the AIDS epidemic began, some leaders of the gay community likewise began counseling caution in sexual activities. Larry Kramer, a founder of the Gay Men's Health Crisis (GMHC) group in New York City, wrote in 1981 in the *New York Native*:

> It's easy to become frightened that one of the many things we've done or taken over the past years may be all that it takes for a cancer to grow from a tiny something-or-other that got in there who knows when from doing who knows what. But *something* we are doing *is* ticking off the time bomb that is causing the breakdown of immunity in certain bodies, and while it is true that we don't know what it is specifically, isn't it better to be cautious until various suspected causes have been discarded, rather than be reckless?[13]

Kramer's warning that gay men should reassess their sexual behavior was received with hostility and derision by some in the gay community, even as friends and colleagues fell ill.

Practicing Physicians Who First Recognized AIDS

A striking characteristic of the recognition of AIDS as a new disease—far different from the recognition of most new diseases before it—is that although it presented as unusual infections and cancer, its essence as an immunological disorder was perceived rapidly by most physicians who encountered a patient. Beginning in the 1970s, a century of immunological study, coupled with the emergence of laboratory techniques for studying living things at the molecular level, produced new knowledge about the two arms of the immune system and how they were related. As figure 1.1 shows, humoral immunity is made up of immune system cells called B cells (because they originated in the bone marrow). When a B cell encounters an antigen, a molecule or substance that is foreign to the body (such as an invading virus), it engulfs the invader and "presents" a protein from the invader to another immune-system cell, the helper T cell. The helper T cell secretes chemicals called lymphokines that enable the B cell to multiply into plasma cells that secrete specific antibodies, proteins used by the immune system to identify and neutralize foreign molecules, that lock onto the invader. The helper T cell also triggers the development of memory B cells, which "remember" that particular invader's immunological signature. If it again attempts to invade the body, those memory cells signal other B cells to ramp up production of antibodies that neutralize the invaders before they can cause disease.

This immunological process is the basis for making vaccines such as those against polio and measles. Disease-causing viruses are grown in a laboratory and then killed or rendered harmless. The material thus produced and containing the viruses is injected into people who have not suffered from the disease, and the B cells perform their memory process so that if a person encounters live, virulent viruses, antibodies will be produced to stop the virus from causing disease. Although the theory of vaccine production is simply stated, actually producing effective vaccines is a long and arduous process. For most viral diseases, however, from West Nile fever to the common cold, no preventive vaccine has ever been successfully produced.

Cellular immunity is the second arm of the immune system. Figure 1.2 shows how helper T cells (named because they are processed through the thymus gland as they mature) are also activated when macrophages "present" an antigen to them. In cellular immunity, the helper T cells secrete lymphokines that direct other macrophages, granulocytes, and even some other T cells to identify and destroy infected cells. Still other T cells, called suppressor T cells, recognize when the microbial threat has been defeated and shut down the immunological response.

The key, or master, cell in both humoral and cellular immunity is the helper T cell. This cell is relentlessly destroyed by HIV, which explains why the immune system cannot respond to opportunistic infections and cancers when most of the helper T cells have been destroyed. In the late 1970s the ability to characterize the cells of the immune system and describe their actions was in its infancy and was one of the most exciting new intellectual fields in medicine. Damage caused to the immune system in the process of organ transplant or chemotherapy for cancer had made physicians aware that certain infections and cancers normally kept in check by the immune system became life threatening to patients undergoing these procedures.[14]

In early 1981, therefore, when physicians in Los Angeles encountered patients with fevers, weight loss, and infections such as *Pneumocystis carinii*

Antibodies are triggered when a B cell
encounters its matching antigen.

The B cell takes in the antigen
and digests it,

then displays antigen fragments
bound to its own distinctive
marker molecules.

The combination of antigen
fragment and marker molecule
attracts the help
of a mature,
matching T cell.

Lymphokines secreted by the T cell
allow the B cell to multiply and mature
into antibody-producing plasma cells.

Released into the bloodstream, antibodies lock onto matching
antigens. These antigen-antibody complexes are soon eliminated,
either by the complement cascade or by the liver and the spleen.

Figure 1.1. Humoral immune system. In addition to triggering the production of antibodies, the helper T cell instructs some B cells to remember the invader so that antibodies may be produced quickly if the body encounters it again. This diagram also shows that the helper T cell is the master cell governing humoral immunity. HIV destroys these T cells, leaving the body unable to mount a humoral response against invading microorganisms. *Figure from* Understanding the Immune System, *National Institutes of Health, NIH Publication No. 88-529, 1988.*

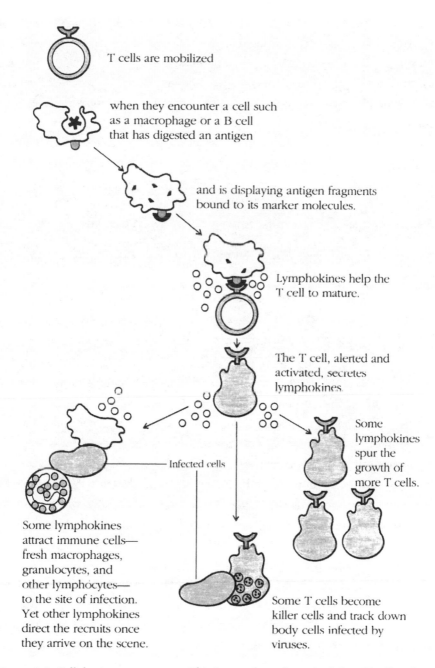

T cells are mobilized

when they encounter a cell such as a macrophage or a B cell that has digested an antigen

and is displaying antigen fragments bound to its marker molecules.

Lymphokines help the T cell to mature.

The T cell, alerted and activated, secretes lymphokines.

Infected cells

Some lymphokines spur the growth of more T cells.

Some lymphokines attract immune cells—fresh macrophages, granulocytes, and other lymphocytes—to the site of infection. Yet other lymphokines direct the recruits once they arrive on the scene.

Some T cells become killer cells and track down body cells infected by viruses.

Figure 1.2. Cellular immune system. This image shows how the helper T cell orchestrates the cellular immune response. HIV destroys these T cells, leaving the body unable to mount a cellular response against invading microorganisms. *Figure from* Understanding the Immune System, *National Institutes of Health, NIH Publication No. 88-529, 1988.*

pneumonia (PCP) and thrush (oral candidiasis), they realized that the immune systems of their patients must be damaged. What had caused the damage was puzzling because these patients previously had been generally healthy and had no history of organ transplant or cancer chemotherapy. By June 1981 several California physicians were ready to suggest that the symptoms represented a syndrome not previously seen. Michael Gottlieb, a thirty-three-year-old assistant professor of allergy and immunology at the medical school of the University of California–Los Angeles (UCLA), was one of these physicians. He had personal knowledge of five cases, one of which he learned about from a former student, Wayne Shandera, who in 1981 was the epidemic control officer in Los Angeles for the CDC.[15] Gottlieb initially hoped to write about these cases as a possible new disease and publish the article in the distinguished *New England Journal of Medicine*, but he discovered that its publication schedule precluded quick reporting. He stated,

> In April 1981, I telephoned Dr. Arnold S. Relman, who was then the editor of the *Journal,* to request information about the speed of the review process and to ask his advice about how to inform doctors rapidly about a development that might have important public health implications. I also thought that the report of a new immune deficiency with a possible infectious cause might merit publication in the *Journal.* I recall describing the outbreak—in what now seems a colossal understatement—as "possibly a bigger story than Legionnaires' disease." Relman said that the peer review process took a minimum of three months and suggested publication of a brief report in *MMWR* [*Morbidity and Mortality Weekly Reports*, published by the CDC], noting that this would not preclude the publication of a full article later.[16]

Gottlieb and Shandera sketched out an article that appeared in the *MMWR* on June 5. Authored with his colleagues Howard M. Schanker, Peng Thim Fan, Andrew Saxon, Joel D. Weisman, and Irving Pozalski, Gottlieb's article noted that all five of the patients were homosexual men, but the title of the paper addressed only the unusual infection and its location: "*Pneumocystis* Pneumonia—Los Angeles."[17] In 1981 the *MMWR* was not widely read by physicians, but when the Gottlieb paper was followed in July and August by two more *MMWR* papers linking the rare cancer called Kaposi's sarcoma to patients in San Francisco, California, and in New York, some of whom also suffered from PCP, the word about a possible new disease began to spread rapidly.[18] By December, detailed studies of defects in the immune systems of patients suffering from these ailments were published in mainstream journals such as the *New England Journal of Medicine*.[19]

The July *MMWR* paper emerged from a different medical specialty, dermatology. Practicing dermatologists in New York and San Francisco saw unusual purple skin lesions that were surprisingly diagnosed as Kaposi's sarcoma, a rare cancer but one known to be relatively benign and which usually affected aging males of Eastern European or Mediterranean heritage. There was some speculation, not proven, that cytomegalovirus (CMV) might be involved in its causation. Alvin Friedman-Kien, a dermatologist practicing in New York, was one of the people who first recognized that the unusual cases of KS in young men signaled something new. "There were three cases in the medical center during the year before I saw my first three cases," he stated in an interview, noting that none of his colleagues who saw those cases "thought [they were] unusual enough to write up" for a medical publication.[20] By early March 1981 Friedman-Kien had personally seen two cases, and after consulting with colleagues, especially oncologist Linda Laubenstein, he learned that at least twenty cases in gay men could be identified in New York. He then contacted colleagues in San Francisco, particularly his longtime colleague Marcus Conant. Conant discussed the situation with other San Francisco dermatologists and rapidly identified six more KS cases in gay men, including the editor of San Francisco's gay newspaper, the *Advocate*. Some of these patients also suffered from *Pneumocystis* pneumonia. With twenty-six cases documented, Friedman-Kien and more than forty of his colleagues submitted a report to the CDC that was published on July 3 as "Kaposi's Sarcoma and *Pneumocystis* Pneumonia among Homosexual Men—New York City and California."[21]

On August 28, a third *MMWR* paper referencing reviews of the literature on *Pneumocystis* pneumonia and Kaposi's sarcoma reported that since the July 3 paper came out, seventy additional cases of KS or PCP or both had been reported in individuals with no known underlying condition. The summary table in this article noted that one woman, suffering only from PCP, was included in the seventy cases. The race of the woman was not noted, nor was her sexual preference. Of the men, the racial composition included Caucasian, African-American, Hispanic, and "unknown." A large majority of these patients were homosexual, but some declared themselves to be heterosexual and, for others, the information was not collected.

AIDS was thus identified first by U.S. physicians trained in immunology, infectious diseases, dermatology, and oncology. The rapid circulation of information by telephone and by word of mouth at professional meetings, in addition to the articles in the *MMWR* during the summer of 1981, ensured that news of this new disease came to be known quickly within U.S. medicine. Word also spread around the world via the same mechanisms and because of the authority inherent in peer-reviewed medical literature. Physicians also accepted that the malady being described was an immune deficiency problem. In September, physicians at Hvidovre Hospital, University of Copenhagen, Denmark, reported two cases of Kaposi's sarcoma in homosexual men, one of whom had had contact with the gay community in New York City.[22] In December, British physicians reported a case of PCP in a forty-nine-year-old homosexual male admitted to the Royal National Hospital, Bournemouth, who had contact within the previous year with gay friends in Miami, Florida. In France, a group of young clinicians led by an infectious disease specialist, Willy Rozenbaum, and immunologist Jacques Leibovitch, formed a Working Group to collect and disseminate information about the incidence of AIDS in France.[23]

The exception that perhaps proves the rule of how quickly and widely the new disease characterized by immunological deficiency was becoming accepted came in a paper about a patient who reported having profuse diarrhea for nearly nine months. He was found to have intestinal cryptosporidiosis, a waterborne disease caused by a one-celled protozoan organism. During treatment, he developed an infection with cytomegalovirus, a virus that also soon became associated with AIDS symptoms. The paper's authors, a group of investigators at Harvard Medical School, had seen five patients with intestinal cryptosporiosis. Four others were confirmed to be immune deficient; this had not been confirmed in the fifth patient before death.[24] Retrospectively, this paper was classified by the U.S. National Library of Medicine as an "AIDS paper," and the symptoms reported certainly reflect what was later learned about various manifestations of AIDS. Because the patients did not present with PCP or KS, however, the authors did not suggest that they were suffering from the new disease.

AIDS was first identified within the gay communities of Los Angeles, San Francisco, and New York, hence its first appellations linked the disease to homosexual men. Michael Gottlieb noted that he and his colleagues "called it GRID, Gay Related Immune Deficiency, out of no disrespect, out of no wish to stigmatize. But in our little microcosm that's all we saw. We have five gay men, so why not be out there and say 'Yes, this is gay-related in our experience.'"[25] In December 1981 two physicians at Duke University reported a case of the new disease in *The Lancet* and proposed the name "gay compromise syndrome." Thus, even though in retrospect physicians recall seeing women and heterosexual men with the symptoms of AIDS, the first reported cases all described gay males and indelibly linked AIDS in the minds of many as a disease of homosexual men.

The initial responses of physicians in Los Angeles, San Francisco, and New York to the new disease were twofold. First, physicians attempted to ameliorate their patients' symptoms with existing therapies. Pentamidine isethionate was one of the drugs available to suppress the ravages of *Pneumocystis* pneumonia when first-line drugs were ineffective, and traditional cancer chemotherapy was available to treat Kaposi's sarcoma. What physicians quickly realized, however, was that their patients improved from KS or PCP only to fall ill to some other opportunistic infection. Because of this, these physicians knew that a great deal more information was needed in order to help their patients. They thus sought secondly to educate their peers and people judged to be at risk in how to recognize the new disease. They also joined with public health agencies to conduct pilot studies that would provide more data about the disease.

In San Francisco, Marcus Conant and his colleagues organized a Kaposi's sarcoma study group that held its first clinic on September 21, 1981, to treat patients and discuss cases. San Francisco General Hospital, a part of the School of Medicine at the University of California–San Francisco (UCSF), expanded this work into an AIDS clinic that became a widely known and respected center for treatment and research.[26] In April 1982 attorney Frank Jacobson pressed Conant to raise money for AIDS education in the gay community. The result was the formation of the Kaposi's Sarcoma Research and Education Foundation.[27]

In Los Angeles, Michael Gottlieb collaborated with the dean of the School of Public Health at UCLA to sponsor an educational workshop about the new disease for physicians from Los Angeles and surrounding counties. An "ongoing dialog with leaders of the gay community, physicians associated with gay organizations," and student groups at UCLA was also supported by the UCLA Center for Interdisciplinary Research in Immunological Diseases, headed by Gottlieb's colleague John Fahey.[28] The administration of UCLA, however, in contrast to that at UCSF, was not anxious to have the UCLA hospital known as a center for AIDS patients. The clinic for AIDS patients at UCLA was "officially and deliberately named the Adult Immunodeficiencies Clinic," a reflection of UCLA's concern that patients and medical students might not come to a hospital where they thought they might contract AIDS.[29] Eventually, Michael Gottlieb left UCLA to continue his AIDS practice in the private sector.

Public Health Officials

The practicing physicians who first recognized that something new was occurring turned to two government institutions for help: first, their own city or county public health department and, second, to the U.S. Centers for Disease Control. The individuals who led these agencies were trained in epidemiology, the study of epidemics on a large scale, and they had learned on the job how to work with legislators to promote public health policies for their jurisdictions. Public health physicians differed from private practitioners in that they wanted to pursue a career that would have an impact on large populations instead of focusing on individual patients one at a time.

In the decades after the polio vaccine was introduced in the 1950s—following soon on the heels of the development of penicillin and broad spectrum antibiotics in the 1940s—complacency about epidemic infectious diseases resulted in their study being neglected and in loss of funding and prestige for public health agencies. One lecturer at the 1971 annual meeting of the American Public Health Association commented on the sad state of public health departments in the United States: "Fragmentation of programs is rampant," he said. In many locales "the hospitals with their outpatient departments and other public services are becoming the centers of health activities. In New York City, for example, the once famous Health Department has become a pale shadow of its former self."[30] Dedicated public health officers were still needed in the United States, but they were rarely viewed as being at the forefront of medicine. Serious epidemics and new diseases were thought to occur primarily in undeveloped areas of the world, such as sub-Saharan Africa. The appearance of Lassa fever in 1969 in Nigeria and Ebola fever in Zaire in 1976 reinforced this view. Even the surprise outbreak of an exotic and deadly fever in Marburg, Germany, was traced to infections from laboratory African Grivet monkeys, whose habitat was the savannahs of Sudan, Eritrea, and Ethiopia.[31]

One of the singular exceptions in the United States to this decline was the teaching program of King K. Holmes at the University of Washington. In the 1960s Holmes had followed his interest in microbiology and medicine into the field of sexually transmitted disease epidemiology. In an interview with historian Gerald Oppenheimer, Holmes described the excitement of working in a field where there were no "wise old people at the top to say, 'That's a stupid idea. Don't do it.'"[32] Holmes also held a commission in the U.S. Public Health Service and was connected to the CDC while doing research at the University of Washington funded by grants from the NIH, so he had an insider's knowledge of the federal government's public health and medical research activities. During the 1970s fellows in his program spread out to academic and governmental positions in sexually transmitted disease epidemiology that positioned many of them to move into AIDS public health and medical research leadership positions.[33]

In the late 1970s, moreover, two new diseases appeared in the United States that slightly shook the American public's complacency about the dangers of infectious diseases. In 1976 at an American Legion convention in Philadelphia, Pennsylvania, a mysterious respiratory malady struck 182 Legionnaires or members of their families; 29 of them died. This disease outbreak led to "an investigation of unprecedented magnitude" by the CDC, conducted under the critical eyes of the mass media, which raised questions about the ability of biomedicine to respond to unknown pathogens. Six months later, however, CDC microbiologists identified a bacterium, *Legionella pneumophila*, as the etiological agent. Its affinity for growing in modern air-handling systems led to its distribution through the air to unwary victims.[34] In 1980 a toxin-producing organism, *Staphylococcus aureus*, was identified by a CDC task force as the culprit in sickening nearly a thousand menstruating women and causing the deaths of forty. Toxic-shock syndrome was linked to infection via highly absorbent tampons.[35] As types of microorganisms already known to medicine, the germs that caused Legionnaires' disease and toxic-shock syndrome were identified by existing laboratory investigative methods and were treatable with antibiotics.

The agency that handled the outbreaks of Legionnaires' disease and toxic-shock syndrome was the U.S. Center for Disease Control. Created in 1946 in Atlanta, Georgia, as the Communicable Disease Center, the CDC trained epidemiologists for rapid response to infectious, primarily communicable, epidemic outbreaks such as typhoid fever and measles. As the belief that infectious diseases had been conquered became widespread in the 1960s and 1970s, CDC leadership responded by broadening the agency's mission and changing its name to Center for Disease Control. In October 1980 the CDC underwent a reorganization that made the name of the umbrella organization plural (*Centers for Disease Control*), and its mission statement was broadened to "developing and applying disease prevention and control, environmental health, and health promotion and health education activities designed to improve the health of the people of the United States."[36] The Center for Infectious Diseases and laboratories specializing in tuberculosis and sexually transmitted diseases remained devoted to the agency's historic mandate to respond to communicable disease outbreaks. Other components focused on health promotion and education, environmental health, prevention services, professional development and training, and occupational health and safety. The CDC, like the rest of the U.S. medical establishment, was not expecting to face a new and deadly infectious disease like AIDS.

Many close personal ties existed between CDC personnel and staff at state and local health departments. The CDC trained physicians, nurses, and other allied health personnel in its highly regarded Epidemic Intelligence Service (EIS). When they completed their training, EIS officers were posted to state health departments around the country, and many leaders on the local and state levels had taken the EIS training in Atlanta. As noted previously, Wayne Shandera was the CDC's epidemic control officer in Los Angeles when Michael Gottlieb, his former teacher, asked about the possibility of getting the word out quickly about the *Pneumocystis* pneumonia cases via the CDC's *Morbidity and Mortality Weekly Report*. Similarly, in New York City, the new health commissioner appointed in 1981 to improve the city's health department was David J. Sencer, a former director of the CDC (see figure 1.3).

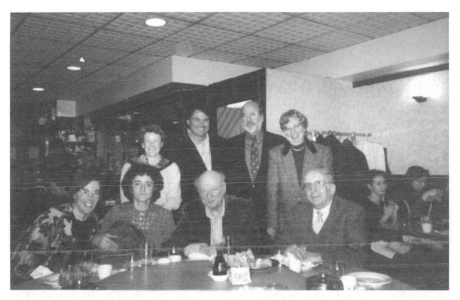

Figure 1.3. City of New York Department of Health team that responded to AIDS, with Mayor Edward Koch in 1998. Seated, left to right: Polly Thomas, Anastasia Lekatsas, Mayor Koch, Commissioner David Sencer. Standing, left to right: Mary Chamberland, Rand Stoneburner, Irwin Davison, Katherine Lord. *Courtesy of Polly Thomas, MD, photograph by Fredric Bell.*

Legionnaires' disease and toxic-shock syndrome were fresh in the minds of public health epidemiologists called in to address the apparently new disease characterized by opportunistic infections and Kaposi's sarcoma. The CDC's initial response to AIDS was described by James Curran, who headed the agency's AIDS effort for fourteen years: it started with a meeting "convened in the CDC director's conference room. People from all parts of the CDC got together. . . . We had scientists from Cancer, Parasitic Diseases, STDs, Viral Diseases, and other people. We talked about what this meant and what we thought it was."[37] They organized a task force on Kaposi's sarcoma and opportunistic infections and elected Curran chair (figure 1.4). The project was initially funded for three months.[38]

The first goal of the task force was to determine that this apparently new syndrome was real, that it was occurring in the populations and geographical areas reported, and that the CDC could verify these things. In this effort, members contacted major hospitals, "all State and local health departments, as well as academicians throughout the world, predominantly in Europe and Latin

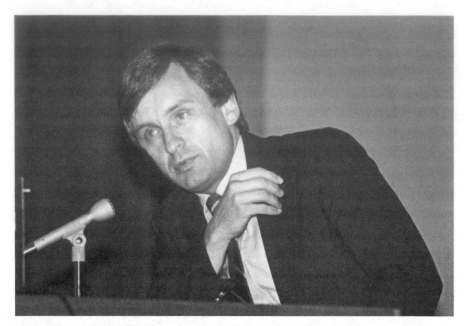

Figure 1.4. James Curran, leader of the CDC AIDS Task Force, 1986. *Courtesy of Centers for Disease Control and Prevention.*

America, and universities to inquire about whether they were also seeing these cases." The task force also contacted cancer registries—databases holding information about cancer types seen in particular geographical areas—in New York and California, as well as the registry maintained by the U.S. National Cancer Institute (NCI), to verify that Kaposi's sarcoma "was not occurring in young men in the United States prior to 1980."[39] As the sole supplier of the second-tier antibiotic used to treat *Pneumocystis carinii* pneumonia, the CDC held in its own records evidence that between 1967 and 1980, in spite of thousands of requests for the drug pentamidine isethionate, "there were no requests for this drug in persons, adults without underlying illness." By April 1982, however, 50 percent of the demand came from patients with the new disease.[40]

The next step for the CDC was to assign the EIS officers currently serving in the eighteen largest metropolitan areas in the country to investigate and characterize individual cases that had been identified. To this end, a case definition for this new syndrome was established; this became the first of many "definitions" of AIDS. It was defined as "life-threatening opportunistic infections or Kaposi's sarcoma in people with no case of underlying immunosuppression."

The most important characteristic of the case definition, Curran noted, "was that it was *specific*. It was not so important that it be sensitive initially. But it was important that it be specific because when you are determining whether a problem is new and looking for the etiology, you have to make sure that you do not over diagnose it."[41]

The task force initially excluded other manifestations of AIDS that were not recognized as such in the beginning. An unintended consequence of the first definition of AIDS was that, although it was designed for epidemiologic surveillance purposes, some federal agencies utilized it to determine which AIDS patients qualified for Social Security disability payments. Those with different manifestations were excluded because their symptoms did not fit the narrow definition being used to study the disease epidemiologically.[42] Within a year, in September 1982, the CDC expanded the case definition to "a disease, at least moderately predictive of a defect in cell-mediated immunity, occurring in a person with no known cause for diminished resistance to that disease" and noted the difficulty of differentiating manifestations of AIDS from other immune deficiencies. This editorial comment also pointed out that in ignorance of the cause of AIDS, there was no "reliable, inexpensive, widely available test" to diagnose it, reflecting the reliance of late-twentieth-century medicine on laboratory tests that produced some observable change to confirm existence of a disease entity.[43]

In New York City, the CDC worked with Alvin Friedman-Kien and other physicians who had seen the first KS and PCP cases and with the New York City Department of Health (DOH). Polly Thomas, a pediatrician and CDC-trained EIS officer assigned to the DOH, described the initial activities of the department:

> We proceeded to go talk to as many people with this syndrome as we could, and they were all gay men. The men were identified by physicians who were calling illness reports in to Dr. Friedman-Kien. And then at some point in the autumn of '81, we formalized the way New York City doctors could notify us of this unusual syndrome. We sent letters to all the infectious disease doctors, infection control officers, cancer doctors, telling them that the health department needed to hear about these cases in order to get them recorded. We used some simple forms and the doctors were eager to report their cases.[44]

In San Francisco, Selma Dritz, assistant director of disease control for the San Francisco Health Department and the person on the front line of the city's public health response to AIDS, noted that the San Francisco Health Department enjoyed an advantage at the beginning of the AIDS epidemic that other large urban health departments did not. The geography of the city of San Francisco made it a "compact city . . . just fifty square miles; it's a square seven miles on each side. . . . The compactness of the city made it possible for us in the health department, police department, fire department, to know practically everybody active there," she told historian Sally Smith Hughes in an interview.[45] The Health Department also had a coordinating office for gay and lesbian health services, which met every week with members of that group. "Each week I would report to them how many more new cases there were, how many more new deaths," Dritz said.[46]

In addition to surveillance work in Los Angeles, New York City, San Francisco, and Atlanta, the CDC conducted a case control study comparing 50 patients with 120 homosexual men who were not ill. The results from Los Angeles were published the following June; the results of the national study were delayed until 1983 because budget constraints at the CDC slowed the analysis.[47] The epidemiological study showed that the single variable most closely associated with illness was a large number of male sex partners per year. Those sick with the new disease "were also more likely to have been exposed to feces during sex, have had syphilis and non-B hepatitis, have been treated for enteric parasites, and have used various illicit substances."[48]

The first peer-reviewed results from the CDC's surveillance work were published in January 1982 in the *New England Journal of Medicine*. Focusing on 159 cases of Kaposi's sarcoma or opportunistic infections between June and November 1981, the task force noted that the one woman and several men who stated that they were not homosexual did admit to being injecting drug users. For the first time, it was clear that the new disease might be transmitted in blood as well as by sex.[49] In January 1982 the CDC's hemophilia expert, Bruce Evatt, learned that an elderly hemophilia patient in southern Florida had died of *Pneumocystis* pneumonia. The doctor suspected that the Factor VIII the patient received—that is, the clotting factor derived from pooled blood that permitted him to live a normal life—might have been contaminated with something, perhaps a virus, and was the source of the infection. By the early summer, two more hemophiliacs, in Ohio and Colorado, also developed *Pneumocystis* pneumonia.[50] By July 9, the CDC had reports of thirty-four cases of AIDS in five states.[51] To the epidemiologists at the CDC, these data indicated very strongly that a blood-borne pathogen, probably a virus, was causing the disease. In December 1982, when a case of AIDS was identified in a baby who had received a transfusion at UCSF from a donor who was subsequently diagnosed with AIDS, it represented "the nail in the coffin" as proof that AIDS was transmissible by blood, according to Selma Dritz.[52]

On July 13 a meeting about the new disease, sponsored by the National Institute of Environmental Health Sciences, one of the NIH institutes, took place. All interested parties were scheduled to present updates and propose hypotheses about the disease's cause. William Foege, CDC director, presented information about the disease in three hemophiliacs. Foege's data were so compelling in support of a transmissible, blood-borne, and sexually transmitted agent, probably a virus, that all other presenters, who had planned to discuss the possibilities that the disease was caused by environmental toxins, drugs, immune overload, and other agents, changed their presentations to indicate that these environmental factors might be cofactors to a causative virus.[53]

Two weeks later, at similar meeting sponsored by the New York City Department of Health, cases of AIDS were reported in all of what the media termed "4-H" groups: heroin addicts (injecting drug users), heterosexual hemophiliacs, Haitians, and homosexual men.[54] Knowing that diseases did not single out countries or ethnic groups, the attendees were concerned as to why Haitians should appear as a risk group, but the data collected identified enough Haitians who fit the case definition to make "Haitian" appear as a category. The correlation between Haitians and AIDS, as opposed to any other national group and AIDS, would not be explained for more than two decades, and before more was known about AIDS, Haitians suffered from discrimination because of this initial finding.[55] The late July meeting, which was attended by a number of NIH researchers, prompted one attendee to recommend that NIH mount "a most urgent response," including the commitment of monies "in excess of our one million dollars."[56] Within two weeks, an NIH-wide working group on the "epidemic of acquired immunosuppression, opportunistic infections, and Kaposi's sarcoma" had been established to disseminate information among interested investigators at NIH and to maintain liaison with the CDC.[57]

At the higher administrative level of the Department of Health and Human Services (DHHS), findings about AIDS were circulated through regular meetings of U.S. Public Health Service (PHS) agency heads with the assistant secretary for health.[58] Discussions at these meetings were aimed at responding to the emerging disease as health professionals within the context of the political realities of the newly inaugurated administration of President Ronald Reagan. Worldwide, new reports continued to be published in the medical literature about the occurrence of Kaposi's sarcoma and opportunistic infections. Cases were reported in Japan, Spain, Denmark, and the Netherlands.[59]

Medical Researchers

During the first two years of the AIDS epidemic, 1981 and 1982, the new syndrome was described epidemiologically. Until there was some understanding about what exactly constituted the illness, it was impossible to determine a cause and devise an effective intervention. Nonetheless, some medical scientists who devoted their careers to laboratory and clinical research were drawn to explore the mysterious immune deficiency. Those scientists who were physicians had chosen a third pathway within medicine. Rather than treating individual patients with known remedies as practicing physicians did or studying, planning, and executing population-wide interventions, such as mass vaccinations, as public health physicians did, medical researchers worked in laboratories and clinics trying to understand how the human body works in health and disease. These physicians and their scientist colleagues valued the intellectual rewards of solving highly complex biological problems. In contrast, practicing physicians valued most highly the satisfaction of healing individual patients or at least ameliorating their pain, whereas public health physicians chose the rewards of identifying health threats to entire populations and devising interventions to prevent or treat them.[60] From the earliest days of the epidemic, medical researchers consulted with their counterparts among practicing physicians and public health officials, a result of longstanding relationships formed during medical training and frequent attendance at professional association meetings. Alvin Friedman-Kien, for example, had spent two years at NCI in Bethesda, Maryland, as a clinical associate while discharging his military obligation, so he was familiar with NIH scientists and policies.[61]

When William Foege asked Vincent T. DeVita, director of NCI, to assign a liaison to the CDC's task force on AIDS, DeVita chose William D. DeWys, chief of the Clinical Investigations Branch, Cancer Therapy Evaluation Program, Division of Cancer Treatment.[62] A young investigator interested in the possible connections between viruses and cancer, DeWys also chaired the first national conference on the new disease cosponsored by NCI and CDC.[63] This meeting was held in September 1981, with the goal of developing "a coordinated strategy regarding the etiology and treatment" of the disease.[64] Participants realized that at that time, they faced a chicken-and-egg problem. Which came first, the wasting syndrome or the cancer and/or opportunistic infections?[65] What did emerge from this conference was the conviction that studies of this new disease should be conducted systematically, under a common protocol, with all patients enrolled in the CDC case-control study.[66]

Many who have written about the AIDS epidemic have strongly criticized governments or the medical establishment for not devising a way to halt the epidemic immediately and for having some members who expressed homophobic personal feelings or who did not resign their positions in public health and medical research to protest the lack of interest in AIDS by the conservative political administration of Ronald Reagan. These criticisms embody the frustration at mainstream medicine's inability to live up to a public image that, however overstated in fact, had come to be expected of it because of antibiotics, the polio vaccine, organ transplants, and other high profile achievements. It also indicates that physicians, public health officials, and medical researchers were expected not to embody human frailties such as desire for prestige or wealth. They were also assumed to enjoy political clout to change local, state, and national health policies that they largely did not have. Many physicians, public health officers, and medical researchers absolutely deserved to be called "heroes" for their efforts on behalf of early AIDS patients. Others harbored personal antipathy against homosexual men, just as they and others had not valued women or minorities in the years before AIDS. In short, the medical community was made up of fallible human beings. What is striking in retrospect, however, is how steadfast the majority of public health and medical research physicians and scientists who addressed AIDS were in the face of criticism from all sides. AIDS patients and their caregivers demanded cures that could not be produced. Conservative politicians, religious groups, and voters demanded that money be spent on diseases they did not connect with sex and sin. These ongoing battles will be discussed in more detail in chapter 4.

In retrospect, the most disturbing aspect of the medical response during 1981 and 1982 came from those physicians who oversaw the blood supplies in the United States and in other countries. Their reaction to the suggestion by infectious disease and public health physicians that the new disease might be blood-borne reflects the starkly different concerns of medical subcultures. On July 17, 1982, the CDC's assistant director, Jeffrey Koplan, presided over a meeting of twenty-eight people representing government, blood banks, pharmaceutical manufacturers, the Hemophilia Foundation, and the National Gay Task Force. Despite the compelling evidence of the hemophiliac cases that AIDS had a blood-borne cause, virtually all of the participants outside the government wanted more definitive proof that a blood-borne infectious agent was present before altering any procedures that might threaten a steady supply of blood for the nation.[67] They viewed blood banks as a national resource, repository of "a gift given by one citizen for the welfare of another, unknown."[68] To blood bankers, excluding groups such as homosexual men or Haitians smacked of the old racial discrimination that denied African Americans the right to donate blood for a Caucasian recipient. Harvey Klein, chief of the Department of Transfusion Medicine at the National Institutes of Health, noted that blood bankers feared any decision that would remove large numbers of donors to blood banks. "Without pretty good proof that you were helping the blood supply, you might, in fact, end up with people dying because there was not enough blood available."[69] The struggle over the safety of the blood supplies in countries around the world will be discussed in detail in chapter 3. A small positive footnote to the contentious July 1982 meeting was that participants agreed to name the disease Acquired Immune Deficiency Syndrome, or AIDS.[70]

Social and Political Context

"Medicine is a social science," wrote nineteenth-century physician Rudolf Virchow, "and politics is nothing more than medicine on a grand scale."[71] The AIDS epidemic, like all other medical and scientific phenomena, occurred not as an abstract biological phenomenon but as a disease in human societies that had diverse political and cultural views. In retrospect, many of the views of people with AIDS, assumptions about how to prevent and treat diseases, how

to allocate economic resources within health systems, and what roles governments should play, are easily sorted into decisions that contributed to easing
the epidemic or to making it worse. One of the hallmarks of literature and other
media relating to AIDS is a strident tone reflecting a desire to allocate blame
and hold someone or some institution accountable for the suffering.

In the United States, the year 1981 marked not only the recognition that a
new disease had emerged but also a new political and social era of conservatism. The previous decade had witnessed a transition from the economic secu
rity of the 1960s to inflation triggered by the guns-and-butter policies of the
administrations of Lyndon Johnson and Richard Nixon during the Vietnam
War; from the political liberalism that produced the civil rights laws of the
1960s to a conservative backlash at particular elements of change, such as school
busing and affirmative action to promote racial integration. The country had
been deeply shocked by the Watergate scandal in the early 1970s. During President Jimmy Carter's administration, an economic condition called stagflation—
inflation in a stagnant economy—and a new sense of international vulnerability, resulting from the abduction of U.S. hostages by Iranian militants in Tehran,
further eroded public confidence in the federal government.

In January 1981 Ronald Reagan was inaugurated as the fortieth U.S. president. In his inaugural speech, he asserted, "Government is not a solution to
our problem. Government *is* the problem." The Reagan administration moved
quickly to downsize executive branch agencies, including the health agencies.
The hospitals run by the U.S. Public Health Service since 1798 were closed in
1981. The CDC's budget was slashed. Efforts were launched to reduce FDA
regulatory oversight and rein in medical research spending by the NIH. One
policy analyst at the time observed that the most striking gap in Reagan administration health policy was "the absence of any positive agenda to address
pressing problems in the health care sector."[72]

A political philosophy that aimed to reduce the role of government in
American life—with the exception of spending for national defense—was not
conducive to a rapid response by the White House to news of a new disease
outbreak, and indeed, none was forthcoming during 1981. In January 1982 C.
Everett Koop was confirmed as U.S. surgeon general after a contentious public
relations battle focusing on Koop's published opposition to abortion. Within
the Reagan administration, however, Koop had little power. With very few

resources and instruction from the White House that AIDS was not a topic the administration wished to engage, Koop was not permitted to provide national leadership as a spokesperson on AIDS until 1986, during Reagan's second term.[73]

In 1982 Congressman Henry Waxman, representative of California's thirtieth district, which included much of Los Angeles, where the first AIDS cases were reported, held a hearing about the new disease. Waxman listened to statements from officials involved with AIDS at the CDC and the NCI, from physicians involved with the care of the earliest AIDS patients, from an AIDS patient who spoke about his and others' suffering from the disease, and from the president of the American Public Health Association (APHA). A Democrat, the congressman repeatedly asked about funding for epidemiological studies and research grants related to the new disease, and repeatedly, he heard that these had been cut by the Reagan administration. The APHA president was blunt: "In the last two years, the Centers for Disease Control has lost twenty-seven percent of its coping capacity, ultimately its ability to respond to problems of disease and contagions in this country. The NIH, which is supposed to be producing the scientific research that guides this Nation's curative interventions, has lost thirty percent of its real funding, and this next year can grant only twenty-seven percent of the approved new and competing research awards."[74] Waxman was pleased to get this information on record and endorsed the need for Congress to do more to respond to AIDS. It would be five years, however, before substantial AIDS funding emerged from the U.S. Congress (see chapter 4 for detailed discussion of this).

Another outcome of this first political hearing on AIDS was an image that came to dominate medical understanding of AIDS. James Curran told Waxman, "Recent studies in New York and California would suggest that this is merely the tip of the iceberg, that there may be tens of thousands of men who have milder breakdowns or milder compromises in their immune systems."[75] The iceberg image was used by speakers three more times before the hearing ended to indicate that identified cases of AIDS represented only one-eighth of the number of people infected with the presumed causative pathogen. There was little question that less than one year after the existence of the disease had been recognized, epidemiologists feared that AIDS could become a worldwide scourge.

The End of the Beginning

Between 1981 and 1983 AIDS was recognized as a disease occurring predominately in the gay communities of urban centers in the United States but also among injecting drug users, recipients of blood and blood products, and, unaccountably at the time, people from Haiti. Those who suffered the debilitating infections and cancers and those who cared for them, both health care personnel and caregivers at home, were stunned by the inability of modern medicine to restore them to health. The advent of AIDS stands as a watershed in medical history, a humbling reminder that after less than four decades of apparent triumph over microbial pathogens, humans will never be able to divorce themselves from the exigencies of being a part of the natural world.

During these two years, the medically trained personnel who made the greatest contributions were the practicing physicians who recognized that something new needed to be addressed and the federal, state, and local public health officials who worked together to describe as exactly as possible what was happening. The discipline of epidemiology provided the tools they used and guided their conclusions that AIDS was most likely caused by some pathogen, probably a virus that was transmissible by sex, by injections with contaminated needles, and in blood products. The skepticism of other physicians and scientists not schooled in epidemiology led them to demand more persuasive evidence—some sort of laboratory demonstration of causality—before they were willing to endorse complex and expensive measures such as changes in the way blood and blood products were handled. By March 1983, however, public health officials felt sufficiently confident that a transmissible agent was responsible for AIDS that the CDC issued guidelines for prevention even in the absence of knowledge of the cause. These guidelines basically advised prudence: people should not have sex with those who are ill with AIDS, gay men should know that multiple sexual partners increases their likelihood of acquiring AIDS, populations at high risk of AIDS should abstain from donating blood, physicians should recommend that people about to undergo surgery donate their own blood in advance in case it should be needed, and safer blood products should be developed for hemophiliacs.[76]

James Curran pointed to June 1981 through March 1983 as the period in which he believes the CDC made its "most difficult, but also most productive and important contributions." It was not just the agency's ability to gather epidemiologic data of a high quality quickly and to develop consensus in the scientific community that AIDS was caused by some infectious agent. It was "also in convincing and communicating to people and getting people together, especially scientists, blood bankers, and the gay community. These were a lot of unnatural partners," he stated.[77]

During this same two-year period, members of the gay communities in large U.S. cities established organizations to support AIDS patients and their caregivers and to stay in contact with public health officials to learn new information that might help halt or diminish new cases of the disease. Larry Kramer and a number of other leaders in New York's gay community met in the fall of 1981 to discuss strategies to help. In 1982 they founded the Gay Men's Health Crisis.[78] In San Francisco, a similar self-help plan played out. One of the earliest people in San Francisco to be diagnosed with AIDS was a registered nurse named Bobbi Campbell. In April 1982 Campbell described how he and a fellow patient at the Kaposi's Sarcoma Clinic at the University of California–San Francisco had started a support group for others in San Francisco struggling with KS.[79] Also in this period, the beginnings of political advocacy on behalf of more funding for surveillance, research, and care of AIDS patients emerged. Their flowering in the years that followed would change the way other groups conducted health lobbying as well. This phenomenon will be discussed in greater detail in chapter 4.

In the spring of 1983 Campbell and others rallied in Denver, Colorado, on behalf of self-empowerment for people suffering from AIDS. Taking the civil rights movement of the 1950s and '60s and the feminist movement of the 1970s as their precedents, they issued the Denver Principles, demanding that they not be treated as patients but as "people with AIDS (PWAs)." In addition, they strongly urged that PWAs be included on any government or medical committee addressing the AIDS epidemic at any level and that PWAs practice and support safer sexual practices and inform any partners of their health status.[80] Never before had those with a disease self-identified as a distinct interest group, but people with AIDS used the label PWA to empower themselves and demand dignity in a largely unaccepting social climate.[81]

2

Searching for the Cause of AIDS

"The history of science, like the history of all human ideas, is a history of irresponsible dreams, of obstinacy, of error. But science is one of the very few human activities—perhaps the only one—in which errors are systematically criticized and fairly often, in time, corrected . . . in other fields there is change but rarely progress."

—KARL R. POPPER[1]

Between the summers of 1981 and 1983, AIDS was established as a new transmissible disease that interfered with the immune system's ability to fight off opportunistic infections and cancers. The next critical step, begun even as AIDS was still being defined, was finding out what was causing this devastating illness. Was a single microscopic pathogen responsible—a virus, a bacterium, a fungus, or another type of microorganism? Was the cause an environmental toxin like a pesticide or drug? Was it a nutritional deficiency? As medical researchers began to search for the cause of AIDS, they first tested for and excluded known agents such as the bacterium that caused Legionnaires' disease. Next, they explored possibilities raised by the epidemiological evidence. AIDS was transmissible by blood and sex, but could it be transmitted in other ways? In the United States, AIDS was predominately showing up in the gay communities of large urban centers. Was there some aspect of gay life, especially gay sex, that might be causing the disease? Then there were those outlier cases— women, babies, heterosexual hemophiliacs, drug addicts, and, most curiously,

Haitians. This suggested that something not specifically connected with the gay community was at work.

This chapter focuses on the search to find the cause of AIDS. It will examine the institutional and intellectual frameworks in which researchers searched and the technology available in the early 1980s. Within two short years after epidemiologists determined that AIDS was most likely caused by a transmissible agent—between mid-1982 and the early fall of 1984—most of the worldwide medical community was persuaded that the cause of AIDS had been found. Compared with the history of most diseases, this is a breathtakingly short time. The information gained during this period, moreover, had immediate application for developing a tool to diagnose AIDS, for safeguarding the worldwide blood supply, and for supplying a rational basis from which therapies and a preventive vaccine for AIDS might be sought.

The research to identify the cause of AIDS became a race among individual laboratories and nations for the prestige of being first. Personal animosities and Murphy's law—if things can go wrong, they will—exacerbated the tensions. Fallible human beings, despite their expertise and keen intelligence, were searching for the cause of AIDS. Although these research scientists often nursed hurt feelings, anger, or frustration when their efforts weren't recognized, they were able to collaborate sufficiently to identify the causative retrovirus, characterize it, and develop clinical tests from their laboratory assays to enable diagnosis and blood screening.

Early Research Routes: The Value of Dead Ends

Immediately after AIDS was identified, researchers started to "rule out" possible causes. For example, cytomegalovirus, a virus that infects almost everyone by the time they become adults, is normally held in check by the immune system. In AIDS patients, however, it caused severe symptoms, including blindness, gastrointestinal ulcers and bleeding, and inflammation of the brain. In addition some evidence implicated CMV in Kaposi's sarcoma, and one early theory was that AIDS was also caused by this virus.[2] It turned out that the unusually harsh symptoms caused by cytomegalovirus infection in AIDS patients were simply the result of their severely suppressed immune status—cytomegalovirus was opportunistic, like *Pneumocystis carinii* pneumonia. Similar conclusions were drawn about other unusually severe infections seen in AIDS patients that rarely appeared in healthy people, such as toxoplasmosis, cryptosporidiosis, and candidiasis.

A second line of research was pursued by immunologists who explored the possibility that some type of microorganism other than a virus might be the cause or a necessary cofactor to the cause of AIDS. A group at the National Institute of Allergy and Infectious Diseases (NIAID) led by Kenneth Sell argued for a fungus that released a potent cyclosporin-like immunosuppressive agent. Three different strains of this fungal toxin were isolated from AIDS patients, all containing a compound similar to the powerful agent used to prevent patients from rejecting transplanted organs.[3] Although the fungal toxin theory was strongly suggestive as a possible source of immune suppression, the researchers dropped it after persuasive evidence for a retroviral cause was presented.

Another line of etiological research came out of a group investigating what appeared to be "outbreaks" of cancer in particular environmental settings. James Goedert and William Blattner, both in the Epidemiology and Biostatistics Program at the National Cancer Institute, set up a pilot study of fifteen gay men in Manhattan. Their study showed an apparent connection between the immune deficiency and the use of amyl nitrites, drugs colloquially known as "poppers" that enhanced sexual orgasm, by the study population. "We went wrong in our analysis in that paper," Blattner stated. In retrospect, the use of these drugs "was a mark of a high risk behavior for HIV infection"; there was no direct link between the drugs and the disease.[4]

As these and other early theories were ruled out, many scientists endured ridicule about their wrongheadedness in discerning the cause of AIDS. These dead ends, however, should not be viewed in the perfect clarity of hindsight but rather in the complex and frightening situation in which AIDS patients and physicians found themselves. Blattner commented, "You have to understand that when you are going through this kind of process and living it, as opposed to looking back on it, things were not that clear. There were very few of us who were living it, because there were not very many people working in the area. It is very clear to people in retrospect how 'stupid' we were, but ultimately the problem got solved through the process of scientific research."[5]

Each of these lines of research provided information that helped to rule them out as the exclusive cause of AIDS. Another concern was that a single cause might not be found or that one or more cofactors to a causative agent might be necessary to produce AIDS; potential cofactors were identified well into the 1990s.[6] The value of investigations such as these is in illuminating the self-correcting mechanism of scientific research. A scientific argument and the evidence for it must stand up to the most rigorous criticism before it is accepted as correct, and this sets science apart from political maneuvering, arguments based on emotion, and faith-based causal claims. This point is sometimes missed by people who write about AIDS, but it is key to understanding why medical researchers worldwide so quickly agreed in 1984 that the cause of AIDS had been found.

Institutional Settings for Early AIDS Research

NATIONAL INSTITUTES OF HEALTH

A great deal of the earliest research on AIDS in the United States was conducted in the intramural, or in-house, laboratories and clinics at the National Institutes of Health in Bethesda, Maryland. This happened for two reasons. First, the NIH intramural program had historically been tasked with responding to medical and public health crises, although it had done less of this since the creation of the Centers for Disease Control after World War II. Nonetheless, many NIH investigators were members of the U.S. Public Health Service and felt a sense of duty about addressing medical problems affecting the United States. (See figure 2.1 for a schematic describing the health agencies of the U.S. Department of Health and Human Services in 1981.)

Second, the intramural NIH program was sufficiently flexible to permit scientists and physicians to shift their research focus quickly to address the new problem. When AIDS appeared, most medical research in the United States was conducted at universities and funded by NIH grants in aid of research through the extramural, or grants program. To ensure scientific quality, these grants were awarded only after winning approval via a two-step process that required nearly two years to complete. After submitting a grant proposal, a scientist would wait to see what score the proposal received from a committee of scientists in the same field—a process known as peer review. If the proposal scored well enough, it moved forward to a different vetting process in the NIH institute related to its subject matter (e.g., research on eye diseases went to the National Eye Institute [NEI] and infectious diseases research went to NIAID). This second committee, known as the advisory council to an institute, comprised both

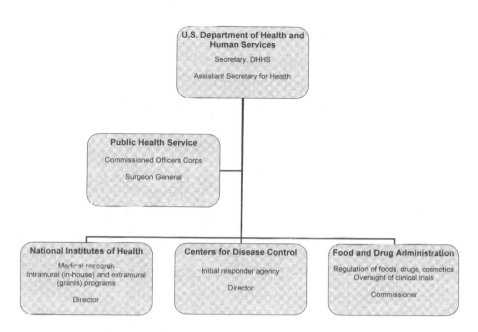

Figure 2.1. Organizational chart of the public health components of the U.S. Department of Health and Human Services, 1981. *Courtesy of the author.*

nonfederal scientists and laypeople and was charged with determining broad areas of research for each institute to support if there were too many excellent grant proposals and too little money to fund them all. Once a proposal had gained approval from an institute advisory council, the money would be made available to the institution in which the scientist worked. To attract large numbers of scientists to work on a particular problem such as AIDS, Congress could also designate research dollars specifically for the problem, but until 1986 large amounts of money were not appropriated for AIDS. The reason for this will be discussed more in chapter 4.

The NIH intramural program permitted the chiefs of laboratories and clinical branches to determine the direction of their research projects and to change that direction overnight, if necessary. These laboratories and clinics were subject to review every three years by an external committee of scientists, but once approval of that group had been obtained, the laboratory or branch chief controlled the research agenda for the next three years.

Since 1946, when the NIH grants program was launched, many committees had evaluated the intramural program to see if it should be allowed to exist in such a different configuration from the extramural structure.[7] With the advent of AIDS, the flexibility inherent in the intramural program was proved, as it enabled investigators to reorient their research to the problem of AIDS rapidly.[8]

Another aspect of the NIH organizational structure that is important to understand when thinking about the research response to AIDS is the structure of many separate components under the NIH umbrella. In 1981 there were eleven institutes, two centers, three divisions, and the Office of the NIH Director, for a total of seventeen components of the NIH. By 2010 the NIH had grown to twenty-seven components. Once AIDS was known to be an infectious disease, it seemed obvious that the National Institute for Allergy and Infectious Diseases would be the logical location for AIDS research, and indeed, it eventually became the lead institute for AIDS research.

NIAID had a distinguished tradition in virological research, but in the late 1960s, Robert Huebner, one of its leading virologists, became interested in viruses as possible causes of cancer and moved to the NCI. Thus both NIAID and NCI had active programs in virological research. When AIDS appeared in 1981, NIAID emphasized research on whether AIDS might be caused by a non-tumor-causing virus or a fungus and on the study of how AIDS destroyed the immune system, which will be discussed in detail in chapter 3. In 1983 NIAID also launched the publication of the *AIDS Memorandum,* "to provide a centralized forum for the rapid but informal dissemination of new clinical and experimental findings on AIDS." It was modeled on previous memoranda for hepatitis, leprosy, and interferon and presented preliminary data, negative findings, single-case reports, and other information that might be useful to the community of researchers but not suitable for publication in mainstream journals. "Ground rules" printed in each issue by NIAID specified that the articles had not been peer reviewed, were subject to change before publication, and could not be cited without permission of the authors.[9]

As it happened, however, NCI played the leading role in the United States in research on the cause of AIDS. The reason for this lies in characteristics of AIDS and in the field of research for which Huebner had left NIAID for NCI. Kaposi's sarcoma, a cancer seen in otherwise healthy young males, was one of the first diseases that came to be identified with AIDS.[10] When it became clear that a virus, possibly a retrovirus, was the likely cause of AIDS, NCI was the location of the laboratory that had first identified the existence of a human retrovirus, the Laboratory of Tumor Cell Biology, headed by Robert C. Gallo. Gallo's work on human retroviruses had grown out of a program in the 1960s and 1970s that sought to determine whether viruses might cause some cancers (see figures 2.2 and 2.3 on what makes retroviruses unique among viruses).

The Special Virus Cancer Program (SVCP) was created in 1958 at the urging of scientists, and funding was sustained throughout the 1960s for research on all types of viruses that might cause cancer. With the passage in 1971 of the National Cancer Act, Congress and President Richard Nixon created a National Cancer Program and launched a "war on cancer."[11] The act vastly expanded resources for cancer research, including those for the SVCP. Scientists from around the world were attracted to the question of whether viruses caused cancer, and the availability of funding for fellowships drew many of them to the National Cancer Institute to work in laboratories searching for such viruses. All the major AIDS retrovirologists—including Robert Gallo, Françoise Barré-Sinoussi, Jean-Claude Chermann, and Jay Levy—had been trained in the ideas and methods fostered by this program as postdoctoral or visiting international fellows in Bethesda.[12]

The search for human retroviruses that would cause tumors like those caused by retroviruses in animals was a key element of SVCP, but none were found by 1974. Because no viruses at all had been linked to specific cancers under the program, it was shut down.[13] Subsequently, a number of viruses were indeed identified as the cause of malignancies, such as hepatitis B virus as a cause of liver cancer and the human papilloma virus as the cause of cervical cancer. The SVCP, in addition to training the retrovirologists who led world AIDS research, resulted in the development of commercially available biological reagents, substances that are used in the study of immunological and other processes in laboratories of molecular and cell biology. Previously, scientists had been forced to spend a great deal of time preparing reagents individually for each experiment. These reagents would prove vitally important in AIDS research.

LABORATORY OF TUMOR CELL BIOLOGY, NATIONAL CANCER INSTITUTE, NATIONAL INSTITUTES OF HEALTH

Robert C. Gallo had been drawn into cancer research initially because of the death of his sister and only sibling from leukemia (figure 2.4). After completing

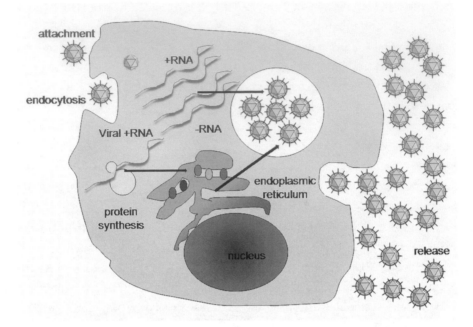

Figure 2.2. Replication of an RNA virus (hepatitis C virus). (1) Attachment. The virus attaches to the host cell receptors. (2) Endocytosis, the virus is taken into the cell. (3) Virus takes over particular components of cell machinery to produce new viral genomes and proteins. (4) New viral particles are formed and released from the cell. *Courtesy of Graham Colm at Wikimedia Commons.*

medical school at Jefferson Medical College and a residency at the University of Chicago, Gallo came to NCI in 1965 as a postdoctoral fellow, a "clinical associate" in NIH terminology. There he became interested in the Special Virus Cancer Program's research on possible retroviral causation of cancers. In 1972 he was promoted to laboratory chief, after which he devoted his laboratory, named the Laboratory of Tumor Cell Biology, to searching for a human retrovirus even as the scientific community began to abandon its belief that viruses might be involved in cancer causation. In 1975 Gallo presented evidence that a human retrovirus existed, but his work was shown to be the result of a laboratory contamination, a humiliating scientific experience that made him insist on experiments that produced multiple types of data to demonstrate a putative retrovirus definitely as the cause of AIDS.[14]

In 1976, with his colleagues Doris Morgan and Frank Ruschetti, Gallo reported the discovery that a protein called interleukin-2 was a T-cell growth

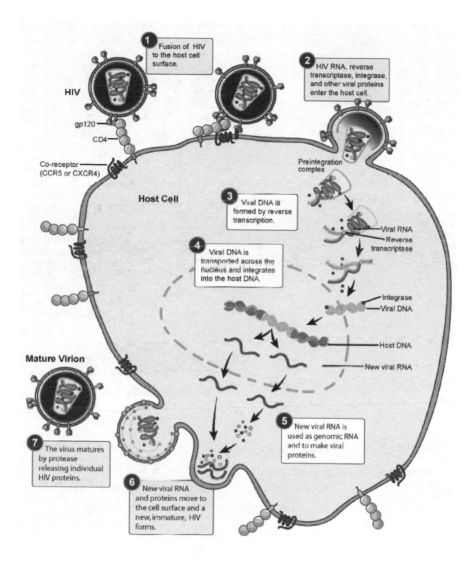

Figure 2.3. What makes a retrovirus different? HIV replication cycle. Unlike the hepatitis C virus, the HIV virus includes an enzyme called reverse transcriptase, which causes it to transcribe its RNA into DNA after attaching to and entering a host cell. This action is the reverse of usual genetic transcription, which moves from DNA to RNA, hence the name retrovirus. *Courtesy of the U.S. National Institute of Allergy and Infectious Diseases.*

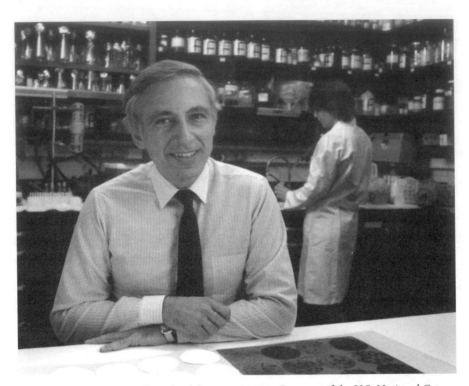

Figure 2.4. Robert C. Gallo in his laboratory, 1985. *Courtesy of the U.S. National Cancer Institute.*

factor that made it possible to maintain a culture of T cells for various experiments, something that had not previously been possible and that became essential to cultivating the AIDS virus in the laboratory.[15] In 1980, utilizing the ability to maintain T-cell lines in conjunction with highly sensitive assays, or tests, to determine the presence of an enzyme that was exclusive to retroviruses, Gallo and members of his laboratory published persuasive evidence for the existence of a human retrovirus, which they called HTLV, for human T-cell Lymphoma virus.[16] The following year HTLV-II was identified.[17] This work positioned Gallo and his laboratory as the most well-known group of scientists working in the field of retrovirology. In sum, the laboratory was located at the NIH, the premier biomedical research institution in the United States whose mission was to address the problems of human health and disease, in NCI, the best-funded institute at NIH. It was an intramural laboratory, and thus it could quickly redirect its focus to AIDS research. These factors made the Laboratory of Tumor

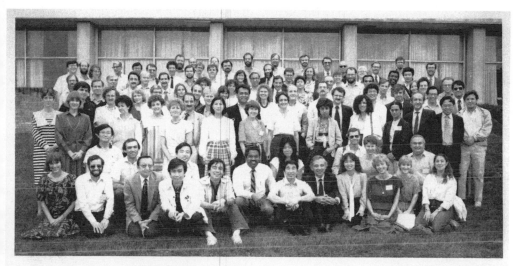

Laboratory of Tumor Cell Biology

Annual Meeting 1985

Figure 2.5. Annual Gallo laboratory meeting, 1985. This meeting to discuss research interests included members of the Laboratory of Tumor Cell Biology, U.S. National Cancer Institute, and collaborators from around the world. Key colleagues in research on AIDS: Robert C. Gallo, chief of the laboratory, in a suit, is fifth from the right in the front row. M. G. Sarngadharan, in white shirt and tie, is seventh from the right in the front row. Flossie Wong-Staal is standing in the second row, behind and slightly to the left of Sarngadharan, wearing a white blouse and plaid skirt. Mikulas Popovic is standing in the back row, sixth from the left. Jörg Schüpbach is in the center of the back row, seventh from the right. Marvin Reitz, in a white shirt, is second from left in the second row of people standing. Samuel Broder, wearing a suit, is in the second row of people standing, behind and slightly to the right of Gallo. Myron Essex, visiting from the Harvard School of Public Health, is also in the second row of people standing, third from right, wearing a suit. Jacques Leibovitch, visiting from the Raymond Poincare Hospital in France, is the person in a white shirt standing farthest on the right. *Courtesy of the U.S. National Institutes of Health.*

Cell Biology the most logical place for extensive U.S. research on a retrovirus as the cause of AIDS.(See figure 2.5 for a photo of the 1985 group attending the annual meeting of Gallo's laboratory and collaborators.)

UNIVERSITY OF CALIFORNIA–SAN FRANCISCO

A second site in the United States where the search for the AIDS virus was conducted was the laboratory of the Department of Medicine at the University of California at San Francisco (UCSF), headed by Jay Levy. Levy had also done postdoctoral work as a clinical associate at NIH, with Robert J. Huebner and with Huebner's NIAID colleagues Wallace Rowe and Janet Hartley. During his NIH tenure, Levy discovered the xenotropic viruses. Xenotropic (literally, "foreign-attracted") viruses live normally in one species, but if cultured in the laboratory, they will not reinfect the host species but instead will infect another species.

When he moved to San Francisco, Levy maintained his interest in research on potentially carcinogenic viruses. At UCSF, however, he was embedded in an educational institution that depended primarily on U.S. federal government funding to support research projects. He thus worked with only a few postdoctoral students in a small, basic-virology research laboratory. By 1981, according to an interview with historian Sally Smith Hughes, he was on the verge of being terminated by UCSF if he couldn't win a new grant to support his research.[18] In August 1981 he was contacted by Paul Volberding, who had studied as a postdoctoral fellow under Levy and was then working as an oncologist at San Francisco General Hospital, where he saw cases of Kaposi's sarcoma in young homosexual men. He invited Levy to conduct grand rounds and discuss possible viral causation of KS, and although Levy was intrigued and wanted to pursue the question in his laboratory, he had no funding to do so.[19]

PASTEUR INSTITUTE

The second major institution involved in the search for the cause of AIDS was the Pasteur Institute in Paris, France. Historically, the Pasteur Institute had produced vaccines—it was built with funds from a nation grateful for Louis Pasteur's pioneering work against anthrax and rabies. From revenues produced, it supported new research, and one of the principal areas it focused on was virology. In 1972 virologist Luc Montagnier was invited to create a viral oncology research unit in the Pasteur Institute's Virology Department. Trained at the Universities of Poitiers and Paris, Montagnier qualified for a doctorate in medicine in 1960, then spent the next three years studying with virologist Kingsley Sanders in the Medical Research Council laboratories at Carshalton, England. When Sanders left for a position at the Sloan-Kettering Institute in New York City, Montagnier moved to the Institute of Virology at Glasgow, Scotland, where the team of Michael Stoker and Ian MacPherson were studying tumor viruses in animals, viruses now called retroviruses. Montagnier also benefited from association with Renato Dulbecco, who spent a sabbatical year in Glasgow and whose work on the mechanism of retroviruses was recognized with a Nobel prize in 1975. Montagnier himself developed a method using agar culture to demonstrate the carcinogenic power of a virus.[20] In 1964 Montagnier moved to the Pasteur Pavilion of the Curie Institute in Paris. There he joined in the study of the Rous sarcoma virus, examining how retroviruses were able to become a part of the host cells' DNA (a double helix–shaped strand of deoxyribonucleic acid), their genetic material. In his memoir, *Virus,* he noted the mid-1960s entry of many new researchers in the field, including Robert Gallo at the National Cancer Institute, and the 1970 discovery by Howard Temin and David Baltimore of the enzyme reverse transcriptase as the solution to the problem Montagnier had been studying from a different approach: how a retrovirus with RNA (a single helix–shaped strand of ribonucleic acid) as its genetic material transforms itself into a DNA form that can integrate into its host's nuclear DNA.[21]

In 1972, when Montagnier was asked to create a viral oncology unit at the Pasteur Institute, he personally was interested in the study of host defenses, the production of interferon (a protein produced by cells), and cell membranes. To head a section on retrovirology, therefore, he recruited Jean-Claude Chermann, who had trained with scientists at the National Cancer Institute in Bethesda. Chermann had led a group studying the relationship between retroviruses and mice at the Pasteur Institute's laboratory at Marne-la-Coquette.[22] There, he was joined by Françoise Sinoussi (after her marriage, Françoise Barré-Sinoussi), who had arrived in the early 1970s as a graduate student. After completing her PhD at the University of Paris, Barré-Sinoussi spent one year at the National Cancer Institute in Bethesda as a visiting postdoctoral fellow with Robert Bassin in the Viral Leukemia and Lymphoma Branch. She was then offered a position funded by the National Institute for Health and Medical Research in France (INSERM), which made it possible for her to return to Paris and rejoin Chermann at the Pasteur Institute (figure 2.6 shows the Pasteur Institute investigators).[23]

The structure of the Pasteur Institute's governance did not make it easy for Montagnier's group to shift quickly to work on AIDS. As are grant monies in the United States, funds for research at the Pasteur Institute are awarded for specific projects, and investigators are not free to follow promising leads that deviate from approved protocols. With few exceptions, they must simply pro-

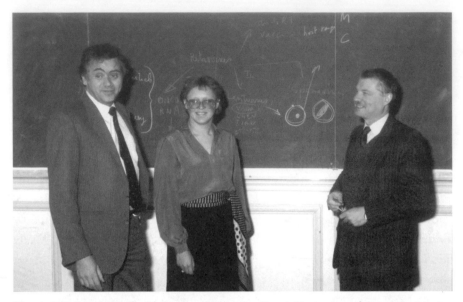

Figure 2.6. Jean-Claude Chermann, Françoise Barré-Sinoussi, and Luc Montagnier, Pasteur Institute, 1985. *Courtesy of Institut Pasteur.*

pose a new line of research at the time new proposals are considered and wait for funding before the idea can be pursued. There also was no national mandate for the Pasteur Institute to address public health threats in France similar to the mission that enabled the NIH to shift quickly to address AIDS.[24]

Intellectual Framework: Molecular Biology

Between the 1968–1969 "Hong Kong flu," the previous pandemic (worldwide epidemic), of an infectious disease and the advent of AIDS, a major intellectual shift occurred within biomedical research.[25] In the 1970s decades of biochemical research came to fruition, enabling scientists to begin to tease out how living things functioned at the molecular level. As researchers around the world assessed the disease process in AIDS and searched for the causative agent, their mental images were of cells with specific molecular receptors on the surface and viruses with particular surface proteins that fit into the receptors on cells like keys into locks. With this mindset to guide them and with the laboratory tools they had at hand, they searched for the cause of AIDS.

What laboratory tools were available in 1981 to help researchers test their molecular concepts and, in the case of AIDS, to demonstrate that some proposed cause might be real while others were just coincidental? Electron micro-scopes could provide images of viruses budding from cells. A catalog of such images was beginning to change the way viruses were categorized.[26] Various diagnostic tests utilizing radioactive or fluorescent "tags" permitted scientists to detect a physical change, such as a change in color, when these substances at-tached to proteins from a particular virus. An instrument to sort cells into their subsets automatically using fluorescent tags, called a fluorescence-activated cell sorter (a FACS machine, pronounced like the ubiquitous office fax machine), had just become available in the early 1980s. It was so expensive, however, that only a few laboratories had access to one. At the NIH, scientists in the well-funded National Cancer Institute had a FACS machine. Those in the more poorly funded National Institute of Allergy and Infectious Diseases did not. They had to utilize older, more tedious methods to identify and count different cell types. Computer analysis of cell-sorting data, however obtained, was done with the limited computer technology available in 1981. In one of the first texts to discuss the use of computers to analyze data, the author suggested that an en-tire computer, which could be expected to have "64 K core memory" and a disk that would store at least "10 megawords," be dedicated to the task.[27] One of the technologies that was not available in the early 1980s was the polymerase chain reaction (PCR), which permitted the amplification of a tiny piece of DNA into an amount easily studied. PCR was not cited in AIDS publications until 1988.[28]

The Search Begins

From the moment it became clear that AIDS was infectious and transmitted through blood and sex, epidemiologists began pressing more virologists to be-come involved. In the fall of 1982, Robert C. Gallo, as chief of the NCI Labo-ratory of Tumor Cell Biology, turned his laboratory's work toward AIDS. As Gallo and James Curran, head of the Centers for Disease Control's task force on AIDS, tell the story, Gallo's decision came after the two of them chatted in an anteroom in Bethesda, awaiting their turns to appear before the National Cancer Advisory Board. Curran was to give an update on the epidemiology of AIDS. Gallo was to be recognized for having been awarded the Albert Lasker Prize for basic research for his discovery of the first human retrovirus. Curran pressed Gallo to start working on the etiology, or cause, of AIDS. "Where the heck are the virologists in this?" Curran asked him. In his memoir about AIDS,

Virus Hunting, Gallo stated that after listening to Curran, he decided to run some tests to see if the AIDS agent might be a retrovirus. The method to do this is to test for an enzyme called reverse transcriptase, which is utilized by a retrovirus to covert its RNA into DNA. A positive test for this enzyme means that a retrovirus is present in the sample. The results suggested further research, and soon Gallo's laboratory was deeply involved in the search for the etiological agent of AIDS.

The entry of Luc Montagnier's laboratory at the Pasteur Institute also happened because of pressure from other physicians working with AIDS patients. In the winter of 1982 the vaccine-production component of the Pasteur Institute had asked Montagnier to test blood plasma used in making the hepatitis B vaccine for possible contamination with the newly identified human retrovirus HTLV-1. To accomplish this study, Montagnier needed and obtained T-cell growth factor, interleukin-2. He knew nothing about AIDS, however, when he agreed to undertake the vaccine analysis.

He was drawn into the search for the cause of AIDS by members of the French Working Group (FWG) whose leader, Jacques Leibovitch, in August 1982 had read a review article about AIDS in which Robert Gallo had suggested that one of the two human T-cell leukemia viruses (HTLV-I and HTLV-II)—the only two known human retroviruses—were good candidates for the cause of AIDS. Gallo pointed out that the AIDS agent attacked T cells, as did the HTLVs; was prevalent in the Caribbean, as were the HTLVs; and was transmissible by blood and sex, as were the HTLVs.[29] Leibovitch and his colleagues lacked laboratory experience with retroviruses, so they began looking for a retrovirologist who would test French AIDS samples for the presence of reverse transcriptase. Initially, several French retrovirologists rebuffed the FWG's request because they were not interested in investigating the cause of the new disease. Finally, one member of the FWG approached Jean-Claude Chermann in Montagnier's Viral Oncology Unit, and Chermann agreed to test the AIDS sample.[30] In December, Montagnier himself was approached by a former student, Françoise Brun-Vézinet, who had become director of the virology laboratory at Claude Bernard Hospital in Paris. She asked Montagnier to test a lymph node sample from an AIDS patient for the possible presence of a retrovirus.[31] Having learned that the previous sample tested positive for reverse transcriptase, Montagnier and his colleagues at the Pasteur Institute entered what became a race to identify the AIDS virus.

Who Discovered the Cause of AIDS and How Did They Do It?

Often in scientific research on health problems of the highest public importance, several researchers arrive at solutions about the same time. Because of the prestige involved in being first, disputes erupt as nationalism and personality clashes lead to ad hominem attacks in an effort to gain credit for oneself or to discredit competitors. Examples abound in the history of medicine and science. In the 1840s three men and their partisans claimed priority for discovering anesthesia, one of two discoveries that made modern surgery possible.[32] Similar controversy emerged from the laboratories of Louis Pasteur and Robert Koch over priority in discoveries about the germ theory and prompted bitter nationalistic rivalries between the French and Germans and their allies following the Franco-Prussian War of 1870–71. The contentiousness was so bad that it limited research in immunology for some fifty years because of nationalistic differences over approaches to cellular and humoral immunity.[33] Author Hal Hellman has published a series of books on *Great Feuds in . . .* , detailing many of these controversies.[34]

Research aimed at finding the cause of AIDS produced another great feud. Sadly, the expertise brought to bear by the laboratories that worked on the etiology of AIDS was overshadowed by personal, nationalistic, and popular culture antagonisms. In sociological terms, finding the AIDS virus was an example of multiple discovery, because all three leading laboratories had the knowledge and skills necessary to detect the virus and demonstrate its connection to AIDS, although they varied greatly in the resources available to them to accomplish this. In reality, however, scientific problems are not solved by science in the abstract but by individual people or groups within laboratories. For this reason, we must examine what "discovery" means with respect to assigning credit for discovering the cause of AIDS.

One first thinks of "discovery" as something new that a scientist finds in a eureka moment. With respect to microscopic pathogens, it is hardly that simple; the human body is host to billions of microscopic life forms even when completely healthy. The human gut, for example, houses large colonies of bacteria that help digest food. Even when the body is suffering from disease symptoms, there are likely multiple microscopic life forms present, some known and others never before seen. They might be the cause of the disease, or they may have nothing to do with it. In the late nineteenth century, as bacteriologists began thinking about germs as the cause of infectious diseases, many studied microscopic slides of tissue or fluids taken from sick people and claimed that whatever bacteria they saw were the cause of the disease, when, in fact, they were not. Robert Koch, one of the foremost bacteriologists of the time, was concerned about wild claims and sought to bring rigorous thinking to the new science. Koch developed standards of proof to establish a causal relationship between one germ and one disease that became known as Koch's postulates. Koch actually put forth several versions of his rules, but the best known version was the one associated with his demonstration that a particular bacterium was the cause of tuberculosis (figure 2.7 contains this 1884 version of Koch's postulates).[35] Philosopher of science K. Codell Carter described the first three postulates as state-

Koch's Postulates, 1884

1. An alien structure must be exhibited in all cases of the disease.

2. The structure must be shown to be a living organism and must be distinguishable from all other microorganisms.

3. The distribution of microorganisms must correlate with and explain the disease phenomena.

4. The microorganism must be cultivated outside the diseased animal and isolated from all disease products which could be causally significant.

5. The pure isolated microorganism must be inoculated into test animals and these animals must then display the same symptoms as the original diseased animal.

Figure 2.7. Koch's postulates as stated in his 1884 paper identifying the tubercle bacillus as the cause of tuberculosis. *Figure from "Koch's Postulates in Relation to the Work of Jacob Henle and Edwin Klebs," by K. Codell Carter,* Medical History *29 (1985): 353–74.*

ments affirming that if you do not have a particular microorganism present, you will not have disease. In logical terms, that is a "necessity argument": it is necessary for this particular organism to be present in order for someone to have the disease. The last two of the five postulates are weaker philosophically, but they are the best known and first invoked by most people.

"Cultivation outside the diseased animal" was rigidly defined in Koch's time as cultivation of bacteria on media in laboratory glassware, and during the early study of viruses, many scientists maintained that they could not possibly exist because they could not be cultured in a laboratory petri dish. The definition what constitutes "culture" of a pathogen, therefore, has changed many times. Further, a person does not get sick every time he or she encounters a disease organism because of differences in individual immunity. This means that disease will not be produced 100 percent of the time when an organism is inoculated into an experimental animal or human. Many diseases are also species specific, so animal models are sometimes impossible to identify. Smallpox is one example of a disease limited to human hosts for which there is no animal model. In the case of such diseases, it is impossible to prove causation by inoculating any other animal with the putative disease germs to produce a new case of the disease, and for diseases like smallpox and AIDS, it is ethically unacceptable to use humans as the experimental animals to prove causation. This means that, for AIDS, a great deal of different types of evidence needed to be presented to demonstrate persuasively that what is now called the human immunodeficiency virus was the single cause of AIDS. With this in mind, let us examine the steps taken by each laboratory engaged in the search for the cause of AIDS.

LABORATORY OF TUMOR CELL BIOLOGY, NATIONAL CANCER INSTITUTE

In March 1983 Gallo's group reported evidence of reverse transcriptase in two of thirty-three samples from AIDS patients, and they suggested that if, as expected, the cause of AIDS was a retrovirus that targeted T cells, their sensitive molecular probes should be of help in identifying it.[36] In the same issue of *Science,* two other papers addressing AIDS appeared. One was from Myron (Max) Essex, discoverer of the feline leukemia virus (also a retrovirus) and his colleagues at Harvard University School of Public Health as well as two physicians, Cirilo (Cy) Cabradilla and Donald Francis, from the Centers for Disease Control. Their paper also suggested that a retrovirus might be the cause of

AIDS.[37] The third paper was from the Pasteur Institute and will be discussed in more detail below.

PASTEUR INSTITUTE

In Paris, Luc Montagnier's group took a different approach. After detecting reverse transcriptase in the sample obtained from the FWG, Françoise Barré-Sinoussi and Jean-Claude Chermann began looking for a new virus and planned to characterize it once it had been identified. When a lymph node from a French homosexual man who had pre-AIDS symptoms was given to them, they isolated a virus from the lymph node. Their thinking was that an AIDS retrovirus would behave like other viruses; that is, it would be easier to find in a person recently infected than one suffering from full-blown AIDS. As it turned out, this was not true, and their misconception contributed to the great difficulty the French experienced in obtaining large quantities of virus. They called the virus they identified LAV for "lymphadenopathy-associated virus," since it came from a person with swollen lymph nodes, which is often, but not necessarily, a symptom of recent infection with HIV. Their research on the virus showed some similarity to the only other two known human retroviruses, HTLV-I and HTLV-II, which the Gallo group had identified the previous year, but the major core protein found in the new virus, p25, did not cross-react with the core protein, p24, of HTLV-1. The virus was cultured for only a short time in T lymphocytes of normal donors before the cell line could no longer be maintained. These findings were also published in the May 20, 1983, issue of *Science* and listed Françoise Barré-Sinoussi as first author and Luc Montagnier as last, or senior, author and included ten other members of their laboratory as coauthors, including Jean-Claude Chermann, the chief of the retrovirology section; Willy Rozenbaum of the French Working Group; and Françoise Vézinet-Brun, who supplied the lymph node from the patient at the Claude Bernard Hospital in Paris.[38]

This paper describing LAV provided the basis for the French claim of discovery of the AIDS virus, as the virus they described turned out to be what became known as HIV. The paper, however, made no claim of causation, and it did not provide evidence that the virus was the cause of AIDS. Without evidence of causation, LAV might well have turned out to be another dead end. Subsequently, the Montagnier group was first to observe correctly that the

AIDS virus killed its host cells instead of transforming them into malignant cells as HTLV-1 and HTLV-2 had done. In addition, they were first to present data showing correlation, although not conclusive causative evidence, of a viral protein with antibodies in patients with AIDS.[39]

LABORATORY OF TUMOR CELL BIOLOGY, NATIONAL CANCER INSTITUTE

In May 1984 members of the Gallo laboratory published four papers in *Science* presenting evidence that a virus they identified as HTLV-III—the third retrovirus known to attack T cells—was the cause of AIDS. What evidence was contained in these papers? The first paper, whose lead author was Mikulas (Mika) Popovic, a physician and scientist trained in the former Czechoslovakia, showed that the laboratory had been able to develop a cell culture in which the putative AIDS virus, which previously had killed the cells it infected, would grow and that it could be kept going by transferring samples to new cultures of these type cells.[40] This meant that sufficient quantities of the virus could be produced for studies to be done.

Gallo himself was lead author on the second paper, which reported multiple detections and isolations of the virus. This paper illustrated that the same virus could be found in many, but not all, people with AIDS, mothers whose babies had AIDS, and some of those in high-risk groups. It found no virus in the group at low risk. Among multiple methods used to detect the virus, the laboratory reported imaging with an electron microscope and an indirect immune fluorescence test and reported that the virus had a cylindrical-shaped core instead of the spherical cores of the earlier HTLVs.[41]

The third paper, for which Jörg Schüpbach, a physician trained in Switzerland, was the lead author, provided detailed analysis of the antigens—molecules that provoke a response by the immune system, usually proteins or strings of carbohydrate molecules—found in the HTLV-III virus. Using a technique called the "Western blot" in which the multiple proteins separate out as they travel through a base substance and are then identified by specific antibodies, the authors provided photos of the bands produced and compared them with those produced by already-known human retroviruses.[42]

The final paper, whose lead author was M. G. (Sarang) Sarngadharan—a biochemist and virologist educated at Delhi University, India—reported that a very high percentage of AIDS patients (88 percent) and high-risk patients with symptoms of what was called "pre-AIDS" (79 percent) had antibodies in their blood that reacted with the antigens identified in HTLV-III, but that less than 1 percent of heterosexual control group patients demonstrated such antibodies.[43] Shortly thereafter, another paper, published in the *Lancet* jointly with investigators in New York and Boston, took the phrase "very high percentage" in the correlation between viral antigens and serum antibodies in AIDS patients to 100 percent correlation. The authors reported thirty-four out of thirty-four AIDS patients as positive for HTLV-III antibodies, sixteen out of nineteen lymphadenopathy syndrome (pre-AIDS) patients as positive to HTLV-III antibodies, and zero out of fourteen controls positive.[44]

The four *Science* articles were accompanied by an editorial stating that Gallo's evidence "appeared to settle the matter." The editorial also quoted Jerome Groopman of New England Deaconess Hospital and Harvard University as saying, "I think that Dr. Gallo has identified the cause of AIDS, and I am a very cautious, skeptical person who has been involved with AIDS from the start." Groopman had provided Gallo with the serum tested in the double-blind study published in the *Lancet*. "There were no false positives and no false negatives. I can tell you it was remarkable," Groopman said.[45] In fact, after the publication of these papers, most of the medical science community was persuaded that the cause of AIDS had indeed been identified. It is important to note, however, that some scientists remained skeptical. We will examine the case of the AIDS doubters in chapters 6 and 8.

UNIVERSITY OF CALIFORNIA–SAN FRANCISCO AND OTHER LABORATORIES
Later in August 1984 Jay Levy published a *Science* paper that also identified what he termed an "AIDS-associated retrovirus" (ARV) in San Francisco AIDS patients.[46] Later that year, in collaboration with colleagues at Chiron Corporation and with Spanish colleagues, Levy published additional papers. They reported the cloning of the virus and detection of antibodies to ARV in hemophiliacs and people in other risk groups in southern Spain.[47] Similarly, Robin Weiss's group in England and Giovanni Battista Rossi and his colleagues in Italy isolated retroviruses from AIDS patients in September 1984, and the CDC reported positive antibody tests from major cities throughout the United

States.[48] Levy's publications, supported by a grant from NCI that he had finally obtained in 1983, came too late for him to compete seriously for priority in the discovery contest. They stand, however, as evidence that highly trained retrovirologists at this time had the knowledge and skills to do such research if given the resources.

PERSUASIVENESS OF EVIDENCE

In terms of scientific logic, what did the papers from the Gallo laboratory say that was so convincing? They did not attempt to show that animals or humans could be actively infected with AIDS.[49] They did report the ability to culture the virus in the laboratory, and this achievement was key to being able to do other studies. They described the composition of the viral antigens, and they used sensitive and specific tests to look for antibodies in the sera of individuals to antigens exclusive to this virus. What they found was that if the viral antigens were not detected, the person did not have AIDS or pre-AIDS. The evidence linking one particular virus to patients with AIDS or pre-AIDS convinced the scientific community that the cause of AIDS had been found.

A Controversy Begins

With the demonstration that a particular virus caused AIDS came the controversy that enveloped and overshadowed the medical research issues. The controversy had two taproots that intertwined to render it even more intractable than it might have been. The first root was personal animosities and resentments within the scientific community over credit for the discovery of the cause of AIDS. The second was the money to be made under patent rights to the adaptation of a viral assay into a test for the presence of the AIDS virus in people and in donated blood and blood products.

The scientists who headed the two laboratories involved in the race for priority in finding the cause of AIDS were by their own estimation ambitious. Luc Montagnier, in his account of research on AIDS, described the triumphs and disappointments of the work in these words: "One must have the mentality of a gambler or a fisherman. As for me, I am only interested in big fish. But they are rather rare."[50] Virtually everything written about Robert Gallo refers to his competitive nature and his volatile, emotional personality. Among scientists, even those who have suffered under his sometimes sharp tongue, Gallo is extolled for his intensity and brilliance in addressing research problems. Gallo might best be described as a "Mozart of science among the many Salieris in biomedicine," to use the terminology of Bernadine Healy, director of NIH from 1991 to 1993. "Salieri," Healy recalled, "was talented in a workmanlike sort of way. He could compose and get the job done with competence. Mozart was a mercurial, brilliant, difficult genius. The music he composed was not merely competent; it was sublime."[51] Because his strong personality alienated many people who were in positions to foster controversy, however, Gallo himself became the primary focus of criticism. The attacks on his laboratory procedure and ethics will be analyzed in chapter 6. Interestingly, although they frequently had their differences, Montagnier and Gallo collaborated on research throughout the controversies and still advise each other after thirty years.

The Heckler Press Conference, April 23, 1984

Weeks before the four papers in *Science* were to be published, Gallo gave an interview to a British freelance writer that included confidential information about the upcoming publications that would identify a virus as the cause of AIDS. The writer, Martin Redfearn, passed along the information to colleagues at the *New Scientist*, who decided to breach the confidentiality request and announce the findings ahead of the peer-reviewed articles scheduled for May publication. When word about this impending story reached NCI and the Department of Health and Human Services, Margaret Heckler, secretary of DHHS, decided to call a press conference immediately so that the U.S. government might be the first to announce that the cause of AIDS had been found. The presidential administration of Ronald Reagan, for which she worked, had been severely criticized for not speaking out about AIDS. Announcing that Gallo, a federal employee, had found the cause of the disease would go a long way toward silencing critics. Gallo was summarily called back to the United States from a conference in Italy, and he briefed the secretary on his work and that of the Pasteur Institute, making sure that acknowledgment of both laboratories was included in the prepared text of her announcement. The text of her speech included the following: "I especially want to cite the efforts of the Pasteur Institute in France, which has in part been working in collaboration with the National Cancer Institute. They have previously identified a virus which they have linked to AIDS patients, and within the next few weeks we will know with certainty whether that virus is the same one identified through the NCI's work. We believe it will prove to be the same."[52]

Shortly before this, one of the people who especially disliked Robert Gallo's style, Donald Francis—an epidemiologist on the staff of the Centers for Disease Control in Atlanta, Georgia—had briefed James O. Mason, director of the CDC, about the Pasteur Institute's isolation of a putative AIDS virus. Francis had trained with Max Essex at Harvard and had hired a former contract retrovirologist from Gallo's laboratory, V. S. (Kaly) Kalyanaraman, to provide expertise at the CDC in setting up a retrovirological laboratory. Gallo was not pleased about losing Kalyanaraman but was unable to match the CDC's offer, and Francis felt the sting of Gallo's displeasure over the telephone. Similarly, during a meeting at the Pasteur Institute at which Francis was present along with Gallo and Montagnier, Gallo pointedly excluded Francis from discussions with Montagnier and his group about plans for the two laboratories to move forward jointly in analyzing the viruses each had found related to AIDS.[53] In April, Lawrence K. Altman, a former CDC epidemiologist who had become the chief medical writer at the *New York Times* and who was a friend of Francis's, stopped by the CDC to inquire from Mason how work on AIDS was progressing. Mason told him about the work done at the Pasteur Institute but asked him to delay publishing until after the DHHS press announcement had been made, an announcement about which Mason had just learned. According to Francis, after Altman read the news release issued describing the press conference, he called Mason to say that he would have to break his agreement to delay publication. Thus, on Sunday, April 22, 1984, the day before the DHHS press conference, the *New York Times* ran a page one story stating that the Pasteur Institute had discovered the AIDS virus; it made no mention of research at the NCI.[54]

On Monday morning, April 23, Gallo; Vincent DeVita; and James Wyngaarden, director of NIH, were greeted by one of Secretary Heckler's assistants who was livid about the Altman story and what he saw as its preemption of the DHHS announcement. Gallo was mystified at why the article was written since the Montagnier laboratory had no new publications coming out, but Donald Francis, who had briefed Mason on the Pasteur Institute's work, apparently wanted to see the Montagnier group rather than the Gallo group get credit for discovery. Francis also believed that peer-reviewed publication should not be

required before medical research breakthroughs were announced, a topic frequently debated hotly by scientists and the press.[55]

Secretary Heckler proudly announced that DHHS funds and resources had
produced results: the probable cause of AIDS had been found. Further, she emphasized that the technique to grow the virus developed in Gallo's laboratory
would make possible a blood test to diagnose people infected with the AIDS
virus, to render the blood supply safe, and to provide the basis for making a vaccine against AIDS. "We hope to have such a vaccine ready for testing in about
two years," she stated.[56] Unfortunately, because of a cold, she lost her voice and
was unable to read the paragraph crediting the work of the Pasteur Institute
on camera. Gallo's adversaries blamed him for the omission. The Montagnier
group in Paris felt insulted. The lack of a spoken acknowledgment about the
work of the French "left a bitter taste in my mouth," wrote Montagnier.[57]

Patent Rights to AIDS Blood Test

The second root of controversy was directly related to money. The first clinical
application that resulted from the demonstration of a single virus as the cause of
AIDS was a laboratory test that could identify the virus in the blood of infected
people. This test would not only inform individuals whether or not they were
infected and alert them to the need to protect their sexual partners if they tested
positive but also could be used to test donated blood so that infected batches
could be discarded. This test was critical for hemophiliacs receiving Factor VIII
replacement therapy and important also for anyone who might need a blood
transfusion after an accident or during surgery.

Such a test was developed from a laboratory assay for antibodies to one of
the viral proteins in the AIDS virus. In early 1984 both the Gallo laboratory and
the Montagnier laboratory developed such assays but used different viral proteins. The Gallo laboratory prepared an enzyme-linked immunosorbant assay
(ELISA) against gp41 (glycoprotein 41, a protein of molecular weight 41,000
daltons with sugar chains attached), which, as it was later found, was detectable
in all HIV-infected patients, from early infection through full-blown AIDS.[58]
The Montagnier laboratory's test utilized p24 and p25, proteins that were found
to appear only in the early stages of HIV infection and that decreased over time.
The French test was granted a U.S. patent in 1987, but Gallo's was the more useful test.[59]

After developing these tests, the individual laboratories were not involved directly in the granting of patents or the negotiating of profits from the licensing of the patents. Legal offices at the NIH and the Pasteur Institute handled these matters. In 1984 most NIH scientists thought of their discoveries as being in the public domain, since they were funded by the American taxpayer. Any company could pick up the knowledge and use it to patent a product. In the 1970s, however, with the rise of biotechnology and its promise of large profits from patents on knowledge produced in federal laboratories, the U.S. government became more interested in having federal scientists patent scientific discoveries so that royalties would come back to the Treasury—i.e., the people of the United States—instead of going to the private firms that produced commercial versions of the technique, instrument, or drug. In 1980 the Bayh-Dole Act required scientists at universities conducting research with taxpayer funds to grant the U.S. government a nonexclusive license to the invention. In 1986 the Technology Transfer Act required federal scientists to submit discoveries for possible patenting. During the period of 1984–1986, before this law was enacted, both the AIDS blood test and the first AIDS antiretroviral drug, azidothymidine (AZT), were developed, and both ended up in patent disputes.[60] The AZT story will be discussed in chapter 5.

In France, the Pasteur Institute was accustomed to patenting discoveries because it depended on patent royalties and the sale of biologicals to fund its research work. When the U.S. Patent Office granted the U.S. AIDS blood test patent to its developers, Robert Gallo and two NCI colleagues, and his institution, the National Institutes of Health, before the earlier-filed French patent application, the Pasteur Institute cried foul. Gallo recounted a meeting with François Jacob, the president of the Pasteur Institute, in which Gallo was asked to intervene and ensure that monies from the patent were shared. Even though Gallo agreed to try to help, the administration of the patent was in the hands of officials in the U.S. Department of Health and Human Services, who were not inclined to share the monies or the credit with the French. The Board of Directors for the Pasteur Institute, therefore, hired attorneys and a public relations firm that moved aggressively to argue the French case, which included suggesting that Gallo had based his work on the virus discovered by the French in 1983.[61] In its most severe form, the story said that Gallo "stole the French virus."

This allegation led to two legal inquiries regarding ethical and legal misconduct by the Gallo laboratory, which will be discussed in chapter 6.

After several wrenching years of accusations and international legal maneuvering, the issue was resolved at the highest levels—the first time a scientific dispute had been settled by heads of state. On March 31, 1987, U.S. president Ronald Reagan and French prime minister Jacques Chirac signed an agreement at the White House in Washington, D.C., stating that equal parts of the royalties from Gallo's blood test, which had become the standard test used, would be awarded to the NIH and the Pasteur Institute for research purposes. The actual amounts were to be based on sales of test kits prepared by each country, which had the effect of providing greater income to the NIH than to Pasteur Institute because the kits produced by the French company were bought primarily in France and those by American-licensed companies were bought throughout the rest of the world. One-third of the royalties were to be given to the newly created World AIDS Foundation. In 1994 the agreement was modified to ensure that the French would receive an equal share of the royalties by the time the patent expired in 2002. Under this arrangement, each country kept 20 percent of the royalties generated by test kits developed by its own laboratories. Eighty percent of the royalties were pooled. A quarter of the pool would go to the World AIDS Foundation. Of the remaining monies, the French received two-thirds and the Americans one-third.[62]

How much money was generated in royalties for individuals by this blood test? The information is available for the NIH scientists. The three who developed the test—Gallo, Popovic, and Sarngadharen—each received nothing before 1986, when the Technology Transfer Act was signed and permitted scientist inventors to receive up to US$10,000 per year. In October 1989 the limit was increased to US$100,000 per year, and in 1998 it was increased again to US$150,000 annually. In 2002 the patent expired, and thus the royalties ended for both institutions.[63]

After the question of money was settled, in 1987 Gallo and Montagnier published an article in the April 2 issue of *Nature* titled "The Chronology of AIDS Research," in which they set out their views of who did what in the search for the AIDS agent. Basically, they stated that in 1983 Montagnier's laboratory was the first to isolate the virus that turned out to be the AIDS agent and to recognize that, unlike the other two known human retroviruses, it did not cause cancer but instead killed its host T cells. The Montagnier laboratory, however, had no way of sustaining a culture of their virus or demonstrating its relationship to AIDS. In 1984 the Gallo laboratory provided evidence that persuaded the scientific community that a single virus was the cause of AIDS.[64] The answer to the question of who discovered the AIDS virus leads back to the definition of "discovery." Montagnier's group at the Pasteur Institute first isolated a virus that turned out to be HIV, but Gallo's group marshaled the evidence that a single retrovirus was the cause of AIDS. In my opinion as a historian of science evaluating both contributions, they made the correct decision when they agreed to be considered codiscoverers of AIDS.

LAV, HTLV-III, and ARV All Become HIV

Between 1984 and 1986, another tempest flared in the scientific literature over the name of the AIDS virus. Each laboratory that had isolated the virus by 1984 had given it a name. Montagnier's laboratory called it LAV, for lymphadenopathy-associated virus, because it had been isolated from a patient with swollen lymph nodes, not one with full-blown AIDS. Montagnier argued that the person who first discovered a virus got to name it. Gallo's laboratory called it HTLV-III, for human T-cell lymphotropic virus number three, viewing it as the third human retrovirus that attacked T cells. Jay Levy's laboratory called it ARV, for AIDS-associated retrovirus, which perhaps seemed to be the most logical name, since it identified the virus with the disease.

No standard actually existed, however, for naming viruses. Some, such as measles, were named after the disease they caused. Some, such as tobacco mosaic virus, were named after their host animal or plant. Some, such as Rous sarcoma virus, were named after their discoverer. Between 1984 and 1986, as the U.S.-French dispute over patent rights raged, nationalistic biases surfaced in the scientific literature whenever the AIDS virus was referenced. French authors or those who sympathized with Montagnier's claim to naming the virus always referred to LAV/HTLV-III. Authors in the United States or those who sympathized with Gallo's claim to naming the virus always referred to HTLV-III/LAV. Jay Levy's ARV was not widely used during this international nomenclature tug-of-war.[65]

By the mid-1980s molecular techniques had made it possible to classify viruses according to how they were related genetically, and although it had not previously been standard procedure, this method offered a rational basis for deciding on a name for the AIDS virus. In 1985 a multinational subcommittee on retroviruses of the International Committee on the Taxonomy of Viruses was asked to resolve the dispute. Both Luc Montagnier and Jay Levy were added as members of the special committee. Robert Gallo was already a standing member, as were Nobel laureates Howard Temin and Harold Varmus. Varmus chaired the committee. Since the patent dispute had not yet been resolved, members were wary of choosing among the names proposed by Gallo, Montagnier, and Levy for fear of appearing to back one person. The committee decided to choose a neutral name, human immunodeficiency virus, and published the announcement simultaneously in *Science* and *Nature* in May 1986. Gallo did not sign the original published letter but accepted the nomenclature within six weeks, after examining new genetic sequence data for the virus that convinced him it was a lentivirus (a slowly incubating virus), not an oncovirus (a cancer-causing virus) as he originally believed.[66]

It was not until the early 1990s, however, that a final twist to the story of the discovery of the AIDS virus was revealed. During those frenetic days of research in 1983 and 1984, laboratories working on the AIDS virus routinely swapped viral samples. In late 1990 newly developed PCR technology made it possible to analyze the original viral samples more closely. The Gallo laboratory had called its AIDS virus HTLV-III, specifically one isolate known as HTLV-IIIB. The Montagnier laboratory's virus was LAV and was obtained from a patient whose name began with BRU; hence it was known as LAV-BRU. In 1985 both laboratories had published papers giving the nucleotide sequences of their virus samples and confirming that they were identical.[67] Surprisingly, the 1990 PCR studies showed that HTLV-IIIB and LAV-BRU were *not* identical. LAV-BRU was not only different from HTLV-IIIB but also different from the description of LAV-BRU published by the Montagnier laboratory in 1985. In fact, the viral samples in both laboratories had been contaminated with a virus taken from a patient whose name began with LAI. Both the Gallo and Montagnier laboratories had actually identified a virus revealed to be LAV-LAI. They acknowledged this contamination in 1991 publications. As it turned out, LAI grew much more luxuriantly than other cultures, thus enabling quicker progress than would have been possible otherwise.[68]

The 2008 Nobel Prize

In 2008 the Nobel committee awarded half its prize in Physiology or Medicine to Françoise Barré-Sinoussi and Luc Montagnier "for their discovery of human immunodeficiency virus." In his introductory statement before the awardees presented their lectures, Björn Vennström, a member of the Nobel Committee for Physiology or Medicine, cited the first isolation of the virus, the recognition that it killed its host cells, and the electron micrograph image that suggested its distinctiveness as the basis for the award. The work by Robert Gallo's laboratory demonstrating that the virus caused AIDS was apparently viewed as less important by the prize committee.[69] Gallo's group was pointedly left out of the prize.

Almost immediately, many members of the American scientific community expressed outrage that the papers providing the convincing evidence of HIV as the AIDS virus were discounted and Robert Gallo and his colleagues effectively snubbed. They concluded that the Nobel committee suffered "Eurobias"; as in 1901, the committee had chosen to honor European scientists and exclude those from other continents.[70] The omission of Jean-Claude Chermann, head of the retrovirology section in Montagnier's group, also led French scientists to demand that he be recognized.[71] Both Gallo and Chermann had received numerous honors for their work, honors that included prize award amounts equal to or even greater than what they might have received from one-third of the Nobel prize. In 1986, for example, the Lasker Foundation awarded its prize for clinical medical research, sometimes known as the "American Nobel," to Gallo, Montagnier, and Max Essex for contributions to research on AIDS. Essex, the award stated, had not only proposed the idea that a retrovirus might cause AIDS but also explored the molecular biology of the AIDS virus and defined its most important antigen, gp120. Montagnier was recognized for "detecting a retrovirus later identified as the cause of AIDS," and Gallo was credited with "determining that the retrovirus now known as HIV-1 is the cause of AIDS."[72] The Nobel committee made no such fine distinctions.

The Nobel's status as the oldest major prize created to honor research in scientific medicine, however, lent it a special prestige coveted by scientists around the world. Like all the categorical prizes, the physiology or medicine prize could be split by no more than three people, and it was not awarded post-humously. In many years, because of controversies over priority, individual scientists and their supporters contested the award, but the committee's decision always stood. In 2008 Peter Biberfeld, director of the immunopathology laboratory and AIDS specialist at the Karolinska Institute, where the Nobel prizes originated, but who was not on the 2008 physiology or medicine prize committee, stated that the omission of Robert Gallo from the prize for discovery of the AIDS virus was "an enormous mistake that will haunt Karolinska Institute for a long time."[73] In 2009 his colleague Anders Vale of the Clinical Virology and Division of Clinical Microbiology, Karolinska Institute, Stockholm, wrote, "It is evident that Gallo's group was not only first to show that HIV is the cause of AIDS but that the French group had not been able to discover this new virus without the active assistance of, as well as, previous work by Gallo. It will also be evident that Gallo and his associates had no reason to 'steal' any French isolate."[74]

French partisans and those who believe that Gallo and his colleagues acted unethically or illegally, despite what two official bodies concluded, will remain convinced that the Nobel committee made the correct decision (the inquiry into Gallo's work will be discussed in chapter 6). Gallo's supporters will continue to dispute the award. Minds are not likely to be changed among contemporaries of the two researchers. From a longer historical perspective, as with the laboratories of Pasteur and Koch, the teams of researchers headed by Montagnier and Gallo will both be viewed as essential players in finding the cause of AIDS.

3

Clinical Research, Epidemic of Fear, and AIDS in the Worldwide Blood Supply

"It is an indescribable experience knowing that what you are doing will have an impact on the lives of tens, if not hundreds, of millions of people. That gives you a lot of energy to do what you are doing."

—ANTHONY S. FAUCI[1]

Beginning in the summer of 1981, physicians in hospitals around the world attempted to ease the suffering of AIDS patients and to understand what was going wrong in their bodies so as to provide more effective therapies. Each hospital that addressed AIDS no doubt experienced examples of heroic staff efforts on behalf of patients but also fear among some staff of becoming ill themselves if they came too close to this unknown disease.[2] This chapter will focus on the efforts of the medical research community in the laboratories and clinics of the nation's premier biomedical research agency, the National Institutes of Health, to understand what was happening to the bodies of people suffering from AIDS and to treat the symptoms from which they suffered. This clinical research was conducted against the background of public fear of the unknown disease, a fear that affected the actions of not only some health care providers but also dentists, first responders, morticians, restaurant workers, and cosmetologists—anyone who chanced to come into contact with another person's blood during the course of work-related activities. It also paralleled the tragedy of hemophiliacs infected with AIDS through blood products that were essential to their being able to live a normal life and its outcome in blood-banking policy, monetary damages to the families of those affected, and even criminal charges filed against physicians and policymakers in some countries.

Early Clinical Research on AIDS at the National Institutes of Health

The NIH Clinical Center is not a general hospital. It is exclusively a research hospital. This means that patients must be participating in a research *protocol*, a detailed research plan designed to increase knowledge about a specific medical problem. Patients must be screened so that other conditions they might have will not compromise the results learned through the protocol. One AIDS patient was treated at the Clinical Center in 1981, and more arrived in the following years. The first young man, who was referred by his physician, was admitted to a protocol conducted by investigators in the Metabolism Branch of the NCI, headed by distinguished immunologist Thomas Waldmann. The "omnibus Metabolism Branch immunodeficiency disease protocol, 77-C-66" supported "studies on the blood and relatively simple immunological tests on individuals, ...who...have evidence of an immunodeficiency state." Waldmann catalogued that first patient's condition upon admission: "[He] began having lassitude and weakness in February 1981. Weight loss and fever ensued, and he was admitted in April 1981 to the Hartford [Connecticut] Hospital where he had *Pneumocystis carinii* pneumonia, lymphocytopenia, cytomegalovirus in the blood and urine, herpes simplex II perianaly, *Candida* esophagitis, and *Mycobacterium avium* tuberculosis of the lung, bone marrow, and esophagus. Initially, he was not as ill as you might have suspected from this history."[3]

Waldmann and his colleagues were stunned at the profound inability of the patient's body to respond to any sort of infection. "We were all groping, trying to understand what was going on," he stated. He called upon his NIH colleagues who were expert in many different specialties to study the unusual infections, especially in the patient's eyes and brain. "In that era," he noted, "one couldn't be fatalistic, even when someone was in an apparently irreversible state. One had to assume that somehow one might be able to reverse the immunodeficiency." The day-to-day care of this patient was led by Waldmann's postdoctoral fellow, John Mitisi, but all efforts proved futile. Throughout the fall, the patient spiraled downward. His neurological abnormalities rendered him less and less able to deal with things rationally. Finally, on October 28, 1981, he died "of hypotension and respiratory failure, with multisystem involvement," that is, of low blood pressure and inability to breathe, along with failure of other organ systems. Waldmann's group conducted an autopsy in which they found "massive necrosis, encephalitis, and degeneration of the brain." Thus was the devastation of AIDS first revealed to the physicians and scientists of the United States' premier medical research agency.[4]

Waldmann also noted another aspect of AIDS embodied by this patient. His family had not been aware that he was homosexual, and the revelation proved to be "a very serious blow" to his relationship with his family. Family members did not abandon him, but neither did they stay continuously by his bedside. His former partner and friends, in contrast, did abandon him. None of them visited, even though he was "in a critical and life-threatening condition, throughout his whole four-month stay."[5]

No other AIDS patients came to the NIH Clinical Center until January 15, 1982. During a snowstorm that shut down the federal government, the director of NIAID, Richard Krause, fielded a phone call from a Pennsylvania physician who had a patient very ill with *Pneumocystis* pneumonia. Krause arranged for the patient to be admitted to the intensive care unit at the NIH Clinical Center in the protocol on human immune problems investigated by Anthony S. Fauci, chief of the NIAID Laboratory of Immunoregulation.[6] For this man and later patients, Fauci and his postdoctoral fellow H. Clifford (Cliff) Lane launched their study of the pathogenesis of AIDS—the step-by-step process that caused the disease symptoms—as they cared for him (figure 3.1).

Anthony S. (Tony) Fauci was intrigued by the challenge a new disease of the immune system posed. The Brooklyn native had excelled at Cornell University Medical College and in 1968 came to the NIH as a clinical associate for three years of postgraduate training as a member of the U.S. Public Health Service. This appointment was highly competitive because it satisfied the clinical associate's military obligation at a time when any new physician's alternative was to be drafted and sent to Vietnam to care for wounded soldiers.[7] Fauci joined the Laboratory of Clinical Investigation, NIAID, whose chief was Sheldon M. Wolff, a physician interested in fever, its causes, its effects on the human host, and its role in infectious, inflammatory, and immunologic disorders.[8] Fauci initiated a study of patients with one subset of immunologic disorders, those causing inflammation of the blood vessels, or vasculitis. Wegener's granulomatosis, one particular type of vasculitis, almost always proved fatal. Interested in how

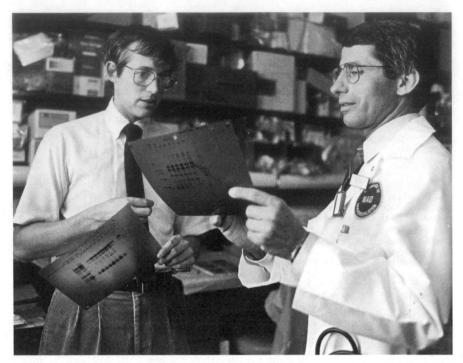

Figure 3.1. H. Clifford Lane (L) and Anthony Fauci (R), 1987. *Courtesy of U.S. National Institute of Allergy and Infectious Diseases.*

the immune system is regulated, Fauci decided to try very low doses of cyclophosphamide, a drug normally used in high doses as part of chemotherapy regimens in cancer patients. The drug also markedly suppressed the immune system. His goal was to reduce the hyperactivity of the immune system that resulted in Wegener's without completely destroying the immune system. His work reduced the death rate in Wegener's from 100 percent to only 7 percent, essentially curing the disease. This work cemented Fauci's reputation and revealed his focus as a research physician:

> It was gratifying not only because I could do some good but because I actually saved the lives of some people. That is the epitome of what you want to do in medicine. I've always wanted to be involved with diseases that were very, very serious. I would rather be involved with patients who have fatal diseases than those with diseases that are just an annoyance. That just happened to be my bent. I wanted to be where the action was.[9]

When AIDS appeared, Fauci stood at a career inflection point, where he could continue his work in basic immunology or embrace this new problem. He decided to redirect the work of his laboratory completely. He recalled, "Some people, I remember, were a little—I would say—concerned about me. They said, 'He has been so successful in what he is doing with fundamental immunology and the hypersensitivity diseases. Why does he want to switch over to an area where we do not have any idea what the disease is and in which he is not an expert?' But the fact was, nobody was an expert yet."[10] By June 1982 Fauci and Lane had treated five AIDS patients. Two had already died, and the other three were not doing well.

One of the three surviving patients, Ron Resio, had a healthy identical twin. Ron, a federal physical scientist in Alexandria, Virginia, who was homosexual, had a heterosexual twin, Don, an environmental scientist who lived in Mississippi and also worked for the federal government. Don made two-night trips to Bethesda every six weeks between the summers of 1982 and 1983, when Ron finally succumbed to AIDS.[11] The Fauci-Lane team at the NIH Clinical Center began by infusing Ron with healthy lymphocytes from Don. Ron's strength returned for a short period, only to decline rapidly. His lymphocyte status was measured via a skin-response test like those used to determine allergies. The larger the weal when the skin was injected with a suspect protein, the greater the immunological response. As Ron's strength declined, the skin tests clearly showed a declining immune response. Next, the researchers tried a bone-marrow transplant, hoping that Don's healthy marrow would produce healthy lymphocytes for Ron. Again, Ron improved for a period but then declined once again, suggesting that the causative factor in AIDS was not corrected but rather remained to infect and destroy the transplanted cells.[12]

From the point of view of the research physician, what was happening in Ron's body was confusing. According to careful, tedious sorting of the various immunological cells in Ron's blood, only the helper T cells seemed depleted. Why the B cells failed to make antibodies to microbes like *Candidiasis* or *Pneumocystis,* organisms to which almost everyone is exposed by the time he or she becomes an adult, was a mystery. For a time, researchers also believed that there might be too many suppressor T cells or that the suppressors were overreacting in AIDS patients, but their careful studies showed that this was not the case.

What they learned, but did not know initially, was that the helper T cell is the "master" cell of the immune system. It secretes substances that trigger all the other immune cells to activate as needed. The AIDS pathogen selectively destroyed helper T cells with the result that patients' immune systems were essentially helpless to respond (see figures 1.1 and 1.2 for diagrams of the humoral and cellular immune-system process).[13] The frustrating efforts to understand and help Ron Resio were summarized by Cliff Lane:

> With this patient, I spent hours every day in his room explaining what we had done that day, what the lymphocytes were doing. I gave him the skin test myself because I wanted to be sure it was given the same way. I would give him the skin test, read the skin test, talk about something new, whatever. I would just spend hours and hours. Then, it was horrible—he started to develop CMV retinitis. That is a progressive, destructive disease of the retina where you go blind.[14]

As his vision deteriorated, Ron became more angry and depressed. In an effort to help their patient, Lane and Fauci enlisted Robert B. Nussenblatt, Alan Palestine, and other investigators in the National Eye Institute to search for a drug that would control CMV, an opportunistic herpes virus. The first drug tried was then known as dihydroxyphenylglycol (DHPG) and is now called ganciclovir. It was chemically similar to acyclovir, a drug that had recently been found effective against other herpes virus infections.[15] Ganciclovir and foscarnet, a later therapy studied by NEI, became the drugs of choice against cytomegalovirus infections in AIDS, but not before Ron Resio died in August 1983.[16]

Fauci and Lane also attempted the reconstitution of Ron's immune system, utilizing interferon and interleukin-2. Interferon is a protein released by cells of the immune system when they sense pathogens. It "interferes" with infection by triggering action by the immune system. Interleukin-2 is another protein that recognizes the presence of infection in the body and signals the immune system to ramp up production of T cells that will kill the invading organism. Neither of these immune-system proteins halted the relentless progress of Ron's infection. His twin Don noted that the staff at the NIH Clinical Center also attempted to help Ron deal with the existential question, "Why is this happening to me?"

but that neither NIH researchers nor any other physicians in 1983 knew how to restore him to health, and in that sense, all the medical efforts were failures.[17] By volunteering as a research subject, however, Ron Resio helped to advance knowledge about exactly how AIDS destroyed the immune system.

In treating other AIDS patients at the NIH Clinical Center, investigators in the National Institute of Neurological and Communicative Disorders and Stroke (NINCDS), including Nobel laureate D. Carleton Gajdusek, also joined the intramural clinical consultation to study neurological complications of AIDS.[18] Scientists in the National Institute of Dental Research (NIDR) addressed the problems of AIDS patients who suffered candidiasis and Kaposi's sarcoma in their mouths and throats.[19] Phillip Smith and Sharon Wahl of NIDR also demonstrated that AIDS debilitated another immune response, the ability of immune system scavenger cells called macrophages and monocytes to engulf and destroy foreign bacteria that had infected the body.[20] Brick by brick, knowledge about how AIDS affected the human body, what therapies would help, and what still needed to be learned was amassed and published by investigators at research facilities around the world so that physicians everywhere could benefit from one another's observations.

Epidemic of Fear

Patient-care staff at hospitals and hospices caring for AIDS patients, including the NIH Clinical Center—nurses, phlebotomists, nutritionists, social workers, clerks, maintenance personnel, housekeepers, and others—were often afraid that this disease, whose cause was not known, might infect them or be transmitted to their families. Barbara Fabian Baird, a nurse who took care of many of the earliest AIDS patients at NIH, observed that if

> the cleaning people went into a patient's room, they went in gowned from top to bottom or they did not go in. A room would not be cleaned for a week or so before we realized what was going on. The nutrition people would leave the trays outside the patient's door, they would not take them into the room. After much staff education, after the virus was identified, after the CDC and others identified the appropriate precautions, and after many classes for nutrition staff and other personnel, people finally got it right.[21]

David Henderson, the hospital epidemiologist for the Clinical Center, was the person responsible for managing staff fears so that the research programs could continue, and the way he chose to counter fear was with information. Henderson recalled that "fighting the hysteria with fact in the early days was nearly a full-time job for me," and to do this, he cultivated contacts in the print, television, and radio media so that he could know in advance when an AIDS story was about to break. If the news media were planning to broadcast a story that said something like, "Baseball catcher gets AIDS from pitcher's spitball," Henderson would have to assess the actual risk compared with other risks in life and decide how to present the information to the Clinical Center staff before the story became public. He would say, "Here is what it is, here is what it means. This does not change what we already know, or it does change it, or here is how it changes what we know."[22] Once the cause of AIDS had been found, it became easier to say with certainty what precautions different staff members should take when interacting with AIDS patients in different capacities.

Nurse Baird herself became the test case that demonstrated how difficult it was to catch AIDS in comparison with some other infectious diseases. While dealing with one of the first AIDS patients, she was accidentally stuck with a needle contaminated with the patient's blood. When she realized what had happened, she said,

> I gathered my thoughts and saw that the patient was okay. Then I went out into the hallway and I saw the patient's doctor. With tears running from my eyes, I said, "I do not know what I have done to myself, but I think I am scared." . . . I went to employee health and they did not know what to do. But they did know that this patient was hepatitis positive, so they knew they had to protect me against the hepatitis. . . . The nurse at employee health said, "I will give you some immunoglobulin and say some prayers for you."[23]

Baird later tested positive for the hepatitis B infection, which is known to be highly contagious, but she never contracted the AIDS virus, which later tests demonstrated was much more difficult to transmit.

Much has been written about perceived homophobia among physicians, public health officials, and medical researchers. There was indeed homophobia in individual cases, and NIAID's Anthony Fauci testified at a hearing in 1983, "There's no question and no denying that there is a feeling among members of any of a number of professions, or in the general population, that patients with AIDS, many of whom are homosexual, are a little bit different. I think that that has probably, at least early on, led to a little bit of a complacency about the approach towards this disease."[24]

Among the research physicians and scientists at NIH who cared for the early patients and tried to mitigate their suffering, however, the principal reported reaction to learning that nearly all of the earliest AIDS patients in the United States were gay was surprise. Many heterosexual physicians, having grown up in privileged homes and attended rigorous undergraduate, medical, and graduate programs, remarked on their naivete about their patients' lifestyles and their assumed connection with AIDS. For example, Henry Masur, who came to the NIH Clinical Center in 1982 as assistant chief of critical care medicine, described his encounter with AIDS patients at a New York hospital in 1980:

> We didn't know that they were all gay or IV drug abusers. The first evidence we actually had that our initial case was gay came when . . . he suddenly leaned over and said, "Give me a kiss." I just looked at him. In retrospect, it was clear that he was gay: he had a red bandanna in his back pocket and wore an earring, but being naive like most physicians, I hadn't put all that together. Not as many people knew about the gay culture then as they do now. At least, I hadn't read that much. We really didn't know anything about the sexual orientation of the other patients. A couple of them were drug abusers, but a lot of the people who go through the infectious diseases rounds come from hospitals that serve that kind of clientele.

In contrast, some homosexual physicians were unwilling to acknowledge a "gay disease." Ron Resio noted that before coming to NIH, he was under the care of a homosexual physician who simply "refused to believe that there could be a disease that singled out gay men, so he rejected even the concept of AIDS, let alone the notion that Ron had it."[25] Naivete, rigid thinking, and homophobia conspired to frustrate early efforts against AIDS.

Some doctors, nurses, dentists, and first responders refused to participate in the treatment of AIDS patients. Often, the social group surrounding the health care professional exerted pressure against involvement with AIDS. NIH nurse Barbara Baird recounted an interaction she had when she moved into a new home in the 1980s:

> A neighbor came up . . . [and] said, "Welcome to the neighborhood," and that sort of thing and asked what I did. I said, "I'm a nurse. I work at NIH." "Oh, what kind of work you do?" "I work with AIDS research." I thought she was going to kick me out of the neighborhood. She said, "If you do, I am surprised you even tell anybody about it." About the same time, or maybe shortly before that, my dentist and my doctor wrote on my chart, "Works with AIDS patients." . . . It was like I wore a big letter "A." My doctor and my dentist wanted to make sure that, if I was going to pick up AIDS at work and if I was foolish enough to work with these patients, then just because they were giving me care they were not going to be exposed. They were very careful.[26]

NIH nurse Christine Grady, in contrast, enjoyed a more supportive experience as she took care of AIDS patients through three pregnancies. She discussed the danger of HIV to the fetus with as many people at NIH as she could and concluded that, "short of a needle stick or something," neither she nor her babies were at risk of being infected by her AIDS patients. She also understood, however, that any patient infected with CMV posed a threat to a developing fetus. "There were people who advised [me] that there were some invasive kinds of procedures that I should avoid doing with the AIDS patients because they were heavy carriers of CMV, and [I should] use certain precautions, which I did," she said.[27]

Not only were practicing physicians and dentists wary of their patients who cared for people with AIDS during the early 1980s, but some also went overboard in attempts to ensure the safety of their instruments. Lois Salzman, a virologist who worked for both NIAID and the National Institute for Dental Research during the 1980s, recalled conversations with her dentist in the mid-1980s when she was undergoing a root canal procedure.

> He had lots of questions because there was a paucity of information. . . . He told me that he had had a patient who came in and who told him

he had AIDS, and . . . after the patient left, he gathered up the instruments and destroyed them, hundreds of dollars' worth of precision instruments. And I said to him, "That's not necessary. It's a fragile virus. Treat it with 12% Clorox and you'll kill it." So he called me a week later and he said he had had [another AIDS] patient. . . . [He] treated the person, and having listened to me, he thought if 12% was good, he would do even better to sterilize the instruments in 100% Clorox. But that destroyed his instruments, so he lost hundreds more dollars.[28]

Salzman noted that dentists were especially worried about AIDS because so many of them had contracted hepatitis B from their patients, and they knew that AIDS was spread the same way but was much more lethal.

More has been written about first responders, such as firemen and paramedics, who refused to give mouth-to-mouth resuscitation for fear of infection and about restaurant owners who fired gay staff members for fear of driving away patrons. Fear peaked in about 1985, after the causative virus of AIDS had been found but before any therapy had been developed to combat it. One of the most severe embodiments of fear was the harsh treatment of young hemophiliacs infected with AIDS through administration of contaminated clotting factor to control their bleeding. In 1985 Ryan White, a Kokomo, Indiana, public school student, was banned from attending classes with noninfected children. In 1986 in Arcadia, Florida, Ricky, Robert, and Randy Ray, brothers infected with AIDS via infected antihemophilia factor, were similarly banned from attending public school. Courts ultimately ruled that the boys were not a health threat to their schoolmates and should be allowed to attend classes, but the public recoil from AIDS-infected students in both cases was ugly. In Florida, the Rays' home was burned down shortly after the court ruling.[29]

Celebrities and AIDS

In the summer of 1985, the world learned that the actor Rock Hudson had AIDS, and on October 2 he died of the disease. This news bombshell brought AIDS and homosexuality into open public discussion because Hudson had typically been cast as a symbol of heterosexual masculinity. If Hudson was gay and could contract AIDS, perhaps sons and brothers in other families might also be gay and at risk for the disease.

In 1986 popular entertainer and pianist Liberace was rumored to have AIDS. He died in February 1987 without publicly acknowledging his infection, but subsequent biographers have confirmed that the heart attack that killed him was a complication of AIDS.[30] More open about his HIV infection was Olympic diver Greg Louganis, who was diagnosed in 1988. Instead of hiding his condition, Louganis wrote a bestselling book about it, *Breaking the Surface: The Greg Louganis Story,* which was subsequently made into a movie.[31] Similarly, in 1992 tennis champion Arthur Ashe revealed that he had contracted AIDS and became a spokesperson for those suffering from the disease. Before he died in February 1993, he established the Arthur Ashe Institute for Urban Health.[32]

In November 1991 Earvin (Magic) Johnson, one of the greatest basketball players of the late twentieth century, announced that he was infected with HIV and would retire from the sport. This announcement eclipsed even Rock Hudson's stunning acknowledgment in 1985 in terms of press coverage. In 2004 the sports television network ESPN named Magic Johnson's announcement one of the top ten moments in sports during the previous twenty-five years. What made it even more significant was Johnson's admission that he had contracted AIDS through multiple heterosexual encounters, not through homosexual sex. This both raised the level of fear about AIDS and simultaneously confirmed that it was not limited to any particular group of people.[33]

Other high-profile AIDS cases drew attention to the fear and despair that accompanied the early years of the epidemic. Elizabeth Meyer Glaser, wife of actor Paul Michael Glaser, contracted the AIDS virus in an infected blood transfusion when she gave birth in 1981. That child, a daughter, and a subsequent child, a son, both contracted HIV from their mother, although all remained undiagnosed until 1985, when the daughter began suffering from various opportunistic infections. Both Glaser and her daughter died from AIDS; her son lived long enough to benefit from the lifesaving drugs that were developed in the mid-1990s (see chapter 5) and has become a spokesperson for people with HIV. Before she died in 1994, Elizabeth Glaser established a pediatric AIDS foundation that supported research on AIDS drugs for children and mother-to-child transmission of AIDS.[34]

A different sort of high-profile AIDS case emerged in 1990, when a young Florida woman, Kimberly Bergalis, claimed that she had been infected with HIV intentionally by her dentist, David Acer, a homosexual man who died of

AIDS. Bergalis maintained that she was a sexual virgin and had not undergone any blood transfusions. She embodied the bitterness felt by many who believed that they had contracted AIDS as "innocent" victims and that the health care system and government had paid too much attention to the civil rights of people with AIDS and too little to the danger they potentially posed to noninfected people. The *New York Times* quoted her as saying, "Anyone who knew Dr. Acer was infected and had full-blown AIDS and stood by not doing a damn thing about it. You are all just as guilty as he was. You've ruined my life and my family's. If laws are not formed to provide protection, then my suffering and death was in vain."[35]

Before her death in 1991, Bergalis testified before the U.S. Congress in support of a bill to mandate HIV tests for health care workers, but the bill failed to pass. The case became contentious as those infected sued Acer's estate. Although the CDC had conducted tests and had them independently verified showing that Bergalis and other patients were infected with the same strain of HIV as the dentist, representatives of Acer's insurance company challenged these results and supported articles and a *60 Minutes* program suggesting the CDC's work was wrong. Once the cases were settled out of court, however, the brouhaha subsided.[36] Whether Acer infected these six patients intentionally or accidentally has never been established. No other patient of any dentist has become infected as a result of a dental procedure.

AIDS and the Contamination of Blood and Blood Products

Ryan White and the Ray brothers became the most public faces in the United States of a worldwide struggle over responsibility for contamination of blood and blood products with HIV. As noted in chapter 1, the meeting on July 17, 1982, in which blood safety was discussed proved contentious and unproductive. By December 1982, however, the number of transfusion and blood-product related cases of AIDS made it very hard to argue that a blood-borne agent was not the cause of the disease. In evaluating the response to the AIDS threat to international blood supplies, therefore, one can divide decisions made into those before 1982 and those after. Eric A. Feldman and Ronald Bayer, in their book *Blood Feuds: AIDS, Blood, and the Politics of Medical Disaster*, which details the handling of AIDS in the blood supplies of many countries, go further and add 1982–1985 as another critical period to consider, the time when

AIDS was recognized as a danger to the blood supply but before a test based on knowledge of the causative agent was produced to provide a technology to evaluate the safety of blood products.[37] In short, we must look at blood-banking policies in the pre-1982 period, the 1982–1985 period, and the 1985–present period to compare responses around the world.

BEFORE 1982

Before July 1982 there was not sufficient evidence that AIDS was caused by a transmissible virus to suggest any changes regarding new blood-banking policies. Before December 1982 the evidence that AIDS was transmissible in the blood supply was strongly suggestive but not ironclad. Only with the December *MMWR* publication about an infant developing AIDS after being transfused to treat Rh incompatibility with blood from a donor who subsequently died from AIDS did the evidence become incontrovertible. And even then, there was no reliable evidence about what the mortality rate from this new disease would be. Absolutely no one expected a near 100 percent death rate.

In retrospect, it was clear that many hemophiliacs were infected before any action could be taken. During December 1982, for example, a Pennsylvania mother, Priscilla Hitchcock, wrote to her congressman, Don Ritter, a passionate letter of worry about the risk to her eleven-year-old severely hemophiliac son, Heath, of contracting AIDS. His life "means more to me than words can express," she wrote. "This child has suffered enormously in his short existence." Enclosing an article about the potential threat of AIDS to hemophiliacs, she also noted,

> This added threat to my son's life produces the terrifying realization that he might die, despite all my efforts to keep him safe and alive. . . . Now there is a treatment which allows my son to live. I thank God eternally for this treatment, but now it is this very treatment itself which might cause his death. . . . I have talked with other mothers who are as frightened and confused as I am about what we can do to prevent this disease from afflicting our sons. . . . It appears that this disease is now affecting more hemophiliacs, and at a younger and younger age. If you could have witnessed the years of torment we have already faced in trying so desperately to keep

our sons alive, you would understand why it is so devastating to face the possibility of losing them to this.[38]

Ritter forwarded her letter to the NIH, and Robert Gordon, the senior physician-administrator at NIH charged with answering such inquiries, responded, "Your constituent, Mrs. Priscilla Hitchcock, has reason to be concerned about the risk to her son's health. According to reports issued by the Centers for Disease Control (CDC) up to the present time, there appear to have been nine cases of AIDS among hemophiliacs, most probably transmitted through the injections of antihemophiliac globulin that they require to prevent fatal bleeding, and three among persons who received whole blood or blood cells." In response to Ritter's inquiry about what might be holding back AIDS research at NIH, Gordon also noted, "Financial resources are not the limiting factor in research on the putative AIDS virus, a vaccine to protect against it, or treatment for the condition. Rather, what we lack is the basic scientific knowledge—a test for the disease, an animal model with which controlled experiments can be done, and the like. . . . I doubt that there is a need to act to accelerate medical investigations, as they are already at an intense level."[39]

What blood-banking policies were in place in 1982? Most whole blood donations were voluntarily given in each country. Voluntary donations created a sense of security; it was assumed that only healthy people would donate with no expectation of compensation. This "gift relationship," as described by Richard Titmuss in his 1971 book of the same title, led to the assumption in many countries that domestic blood was safe while imported, purchased foreign blood might be contaminated.[40] Blood products, in contrast, were acquired in a completely different manner, via a system that had emerged only since 1965, when physiologist Judith Graham Pool discovered a technique using low temperatures (hence the term for it, "cryoprecipitate") to separate Factor VIII, which hemophiliacs lacked, from the liquid portion of the blood known as plasma.[41] By the early 1980s, the methods in general use to prepare Factor VIII and Factor IX (needed by hemophiliacs with a different form of the disease), required pooling plasma from 2,000 to 22,000 donors. Plasma for this process was generally obtained from centers at which donors were paid.

In this pre-AIDS period, the major concern for people who had contact with the blood or blood products of others on a regular basis—hemophiliacs, surgeons, dentists, nurses, first responders, and morticians—was the risk of contracting hepatitis B. It was not until November 1981, moreover, that convincing scientific proof was published linking the hepatitis B virus with liver cancer, a finding that confirmed the essential need for a vaccine against hepatitis B.[42] Such a vaccine was available in late 1981, but it utilized human serum as a stabilizer and so was possibly subject to contamination itself.[43] Many health care workers chose to wait until 1986, when a recombinant product free of human serum was manufactured, for vaccination. A screening test for hepatitis B was also available for blood products, but the hepatitis B virus was often undetectable by the test when it was present at very low levels. A heat-treated, or pasteurized, product that killed hepatitis B was available, but it was more expensive, and there was some concern that heating the antihemophiliac factor might lower its effectiveness. Most hemophiliacs simply accepted the risk of contracting hepatitis B in order to utilize antihemophiliac factor. When AIDS appeared, the prevailing mindset relating to hepatitis B governed much of the discussion about the danger of blood products for hemophiliacs.[44]

1982–1985

After the contentious July 1982 meeting about blood safety discussed in chapter 1, evidence continued to grow that AIDS was caused by an unknown virus that was transmissible by blood and sex. The December 1982 finding that a baby had developed AIDS after a blood transfusion left virtually no doubt that the world's supply of blood and blood products was in danger.[45] On January 4, 1983, a meeting was convened at the CDC in Atlanta bringing together interested parties with the goal of building consensus on protecting the blood supply. Those present included representatives from the CDC, NIH, and Food and Drug Administration (FDA); from nonprofit, commercial, and academic institutions concerned with blood banking; from the hemophilia community; and from the gay community. The National Hemophilia Foundation wanted blood banks to question potential donors and exclude any who were gay. The gay community noted that blood needed screening, not groups of individuals. They wanted a surrogate marker, such as the test for hepatitis B, used; most AIDS patients were coinfected with hepatitis B.

Blood bankers were also loath to exclude all gay donors because in some cities they made up a large portion of the donor base. Donald C. Drake of the

Philadelphia Inquirer reported that Dr. Aaron Kellner of the New York Blood Center opposed widespread testing by raising a new issue: money. Kellner said it would cost New York City more than $5 million to implement these blood tests. This included the cost of the tests, the cost of the paperwork, and the value of blood discarded in the 5 percent of cases with false-positive test results. "We must be careful not to overreact," Kellner said. "The evidence is tenuous."[46] Even the director of the Coagulation Branch of the Division of Blood and Blood Products of the FDA, David Aronson, argued, "It's not clear at all that there's a new blood-borne virus involved."[47]

The epidemiologists from the CDC, in contrast, were convinced that a blood-borne agent threatened the blood supply. CDC's Donald Francis, representing the most frustrated of the epidemiologists, demanded to know when the blood bankers believed there *would* be enough cases to act upon.[48] The meeting highlighted a clash of medical cultures: those responsible for making sure a sufficient blood supply would be available versus those who believed that the blood supply was already in jeopardy.[49] "I hope we don't become ostriches here," said David Sencer, New York City's health commissioner. . . . We have got to come to grips with this issue and not just stick our heads in the sand."[50]

Despite Sencer's entreaty, the January meeting adjourned with no formal agreement. Consensus builders looked for small steps that could be taken. Various draft forms, similar to the one in figure 3.2, were devised asking potential donors who fell into high-risk groups not to donate blood or to check a box saying that their blood should be used "only for research purposes." The latter option permitted them to donate while not disclosing publicly that they fell into a risk group. Hospitals encouraged patients to consider autologous donation before surgery—that is, storing their own blood in advance in case it was needed. Donations from friends and family were discouraged, however, in case a friend or family member fell into a high-risk group but did not wish to divulge this.

In March, two months after the meeting, the U.S. government decided to issue formal guidelines related to the blood supply. A CDC *MMWR* article signed by the CDC, NIH, and FDA, strongly advised members of high-risk groups not to donate blood. They were also advised to limit their number of sexual partners in order to decrease the probability of developing AIDS.[51] In large part, members of the gay community reluctantly complied, agreeing with James Curran that an unknown deadly disease trumped the civil rights issue for the moment.

HIGH RISK GROUPS

Recently, the medical community has noted the occurrence of a very serious disease known as Acquired Immune Deficiency Syndrome (AIDS). The Center for Disease Control has documented an increasing number of cases of this disease throughout the country.

As the name indicates, the disease seems to disrupt the patient's immune system, that is, impairs their ability to fight off disease. Very little is known about the disease - about its causes - except that it is known to be fatal and that currently specific treatment is unknown.

In the past, you have helped us to help others through your plasma donation efforts. We are now faced with a situation in which only you can help us insure a safe product to those whose lives depend on it. Because of our goal of reducing the possibility that this disease might be transmitted through our products, we are now asking for your commitment also.

Until the cause of this disease is determined, we are asking people TO NOT DONATE BLOOD OR PLASMA who are a part of any of the following groups:

1. Persons with signs and symptoms suggestive of "AIDS"
2. Sexually active homosexual men with multiple partners
3. Sexually active bisexual males (one having sex with both sexes) with multiple partners.
4. Haitian entrants into country last (3) years
5. Present and past abusers of intravenous drugs
6. Sexual partners of individuals at increased risk of "AIDS"

Please inform the medical historian if you are a part of these groups. Our physician is also available to answer any questions which you might have concerning AIDS. Thank you for your cooperation.

I hereby certify that I have read and understand this document and to the best of my knowledge I am not a part of any HIGH RISK GROUP.

29 May 83
DATE

Hinton Wray, MD
WITNESS

Figure 3.2. 1983 voluntary blood-donor disqualification form. *Courtesy of the Office of NIH History, U.S. National Institutes of Health.*

For Haitians, another high-risk group, however, the recommendations were perceived as a national humiliation. They continually fought to have their right to give blood reinstated and, after seven years, were finally successful.[52]

Between March 1983 and the time a blood test for the AIDS virus was developed, the CDC issued additional advisories on protections against AIDS transmission in the workplace. The advice given in November 1985 included precautions for personal service workers such as restaurant workers, barbers, cosmetologists, tattoo artists, acupuncturists, and ear piercers. The risk of casual transmission in schoolrooms and restaurants through contact with bodily fluids such as tears or saliva was emphatically described as nonexistent. Housekeepers were instructed how to sterilize objects such as linens that might become contaminated with blood. Members of professions in which blood might be routinely contacted were advised to become educated about sterilization of instruments, good personal hygiene, and careful cleaning of the work area.[53]

1985–2011

After the retroviral cause of AIDS was established, an assay for detecting the virus in culture could be adapted into a test for the presence of AIDS antibodies. As noted in chapter 2, two different tests were submitted to the U.S. Patent Office in 1984. The Pasteur Institute prepared a test that proposed using the HIV proteins p24 and p25 as the antigen. The test prepared at the National Cancer Institute used gp41 as its antigen. It was not known at that time that p24 and p25 were detectable only very early after a person was infected with HIV but that gp41 was detectable at that time and throughout the incubation period as well as when full-blown AIDS appeared. As a confirmation test to rule out false-positive ELISA readings, moreover, the NCI test introduced the Western blot procedure, a more expensive but sensitive assay normally used only in the basic research laboratory. Its inclusion as a confirmatory test for HIV marked the first time this test had been used for clinical diagnosis.[54]

In 1985 the FDA approved the Gallo laboratory's test and licensed Abbott Laboratories to produce it. It began to be utilized in the United States in March (figure 3.3). In February 1985 Abbott applied for a license to market its test in France, but the Pasteur Institute lobbied successfully to postpone approval of Abbott's test until the test produced by Pasteur Diagnostics, the institute's marketing arm, was available. Health policy researcher Monika Steffen of the University of Grenoble, France, noted that strong lobbying to postpone approval of the Abbott test was made at a meeting called by the French prime minister in May. An original decision to delay implementation of testing in France was changed, however, when Prime Minister Laurent Fabius and his advisers decided that the despite their concern for French industrial interests, it would be more politically beneficial in an election year to begin screening blood earlier than proposed. Thus the Pasteur Diagnostics test was approved in June and the Abbott test a month later, in order to meet the prime minister's announcement that blood would be tested beginning on August 1.[55]

Testing in other countries also began during 1985: Italy in March, Australia in May, Germany and the United Kingdom in October, and Canada in November. Zimbabwe led African countries, requiring testing in July 1985. India and Thailand lagged behind, beginning to test their blood and blood products only in 1987 and 1989. Similarly, heat treatment of blood products commenced once the medical community was in agreement about a viral cause of AIDS. In October 1984 heat treatment of blood products became mandated in the United States. Most of the other industrialized countries followed in 1985.[56]

By the early 1990s public officials began to be called to account for their timid actions between 1983 and 1985. The principal group to claim damages from drug companies was the hemophiliac community. Hemophiliacs had not been socially active in the past. Antihemophiliac factors on which hemophiliacs had depended to live a normal life, however, had infected more than half the hemophiliacs in many countries with AIDS because some 60 percent of all plasma for making Factor VIII and Factor IX was collected from paid donors in the United States. In large part, moreover, the hemophiliacs were infected before AIDS was even recognized as a new disease transmitted by blood and blood products. Nonetheless, as a number of writers have pointed out, in the wake of disasters such as thalidomide, Chernobyl, Agent Orange, Three Mile Island, Bhopal, Love Canal, and mad cow disease, no group that had been harmed on so large a scale was likely to accept their fate as a tragic circumstance. They sought someone to blame and a source for providing damage claims for their suffering. Hemophiliacs and their families were no different.[57] The outcome of cases, however, varied widely. Sherry Gliad, a professor of health policy at Columbia University, has pointed out that liability standards for blood were not

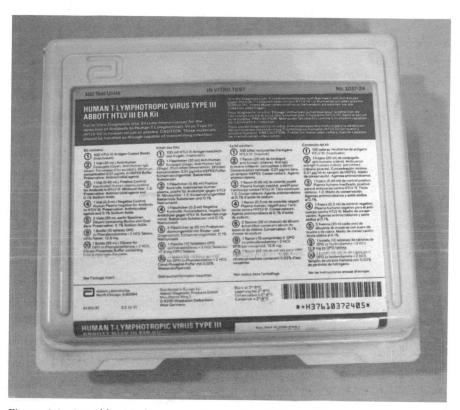

Figure 3.3. An Abbott Laboratories diagnostic AIDS test kit, 1985. *Courtesy of the Stetten Museum, U.S. National Institutes of Health, and U.S. Food and Drug Administration History Office.*

strictly applied in any case brought against blood bankers by people infected with AIDS through blood or blood products.[58]

FRANCE

In France, a fund to compensate people infected with AIDS through blood or blood products, their infected partners, children, and heirs was established in 1991. Criminal accusations were also leveled against physicians in France. The trials and appeals of these men dragged on for more than a decade and raised strong feelings on both sides about the responsibilities and obligations of physicians to protect the public.[59] In 2000 a law that raised the level of proof required to convict individuals for "involuntary crimes" caused the highest appeal court in France to reverse the convictions of the French physicians.[60] Charges against members of the government of Laurent Fabius had also been dismissed in the 1990s. The principal outcome of the *scandale du sang contaminé*, therefore, was a complete reorganization of the national blood system in France. Existing organizations were abolished, and new bodies were created to make the French system more compatible with that of the European Union.[61]

JAPAN

In Japan, compensation for hemophiliacs infected through blood products was forthcoming by 1989, but the Japanese hemophiliac community wanted more than monetary recompense. They wanted public statements of apology from all involved in not warning hemophiliacs about the danger of AIDS or taking active preventive steps in the 1982–1985 period. Eventually, they were successful. Beginning in 1996 the Japanese minister for health and welfare, Kan Naoto, met with two hundred HIV-infected hemophiliacs and their families and said, "Representing the ministry, I make a heartfelt apology for inflicting heavy damage on the innocent patients. I also apologize for the belated recognition of the ministry's responsibility for the case. I understand that the delay has tormented the victims."[62] The five pharmaceutical companies that manufactured the contaminated blood products followed the minister's lead. The presidents and top executives of each company met with representatives of the hemophiliacs to deliver personal apologies for the physical and mental suffering they endured. Eric Feldman of the New York University Institute for Law and Society described the actions of Kawano Takehiko, president of Japan's Green Cross company, which dominated the pharmaceutical industry and had tremendous influence on government: "Kawano then accepted responsibility on behalf of his company, got down on his hands and knees, and bowed so deeply that his forehead touched the floor. It was the defining moment of the conflict."[63]

OTHER INDUSTRIALIZED NATIONS

In the United States, Italy, Germany, Denmark, and Australia, the outcry was at times heated, but the results less dramatic than in France and Japan. Compensation programs in Italy and Denmark, for example, muted subsequent protests.[64] In the United States, the hemophilia community was divided. The National Hemophilia Foundation, which had proceeded cautiously in the 1982–1985 period, became itself the target of some hemophiliac groups seeking redress.

A 1995 report by the Institute of Medicine of the National Academy of Sciences detailed the weaknesses in the U.S. blood system.[65] FDA commissioner David Kessler also issued a stinging indictment of blood safety policies that needed reform.[66] The results, as in most countries, was not only a reform of the bureaucracy but also, perhaps more importantly, a qualitative shift in thinking about the vulnerability of national blood supplies. In 1998 Congress enacted the Ricky Ray Hemophilia Relief Fund Act, which provided compensation payments of $100,000 to hemophiliacs who were treated with HIV contaminated clotting factor products between July 1, 1982, and December 31, 1987. Their spouses, children, and specified family survivors were also eligible for payment. The program ended in November 2003.[67]

CURRENT BLOOD DONOR CONTROVERSY

Some of the blood-banking policies initiated in the mid-1980s continue to be implemented even though they may no longer be necessary. One of these is the restriction in many countries around the world, including the United States, disqualifying men from donating blood if they have had sex with men—even once—since 1977. A few countries have lowered the bar: Israel set the limit at thirty years since last exposure; New Zealand and South Africa, five years since last exposure; Argentina, Australia, Hungary, Japan, and Sweden, one year since last exposure.[68] Italy and Spain use a different definition of risk. Men who have sex with men (MSM, see chapter 7 for the origin of this abbreviation) are not automatically disqualified. The standard followed is sex within the year that poses a risk of sexually transmitted diseases—that is, unsafe sex. In 2006 the FDA approved the use of a nucleic acid donor screening test for HIV that reduced the window period during which a person might be infected but not detectable by any screening system from 15 days to 5.6 days.[69] This technological safety screen has led to renewed calls for discarding the outright ban on blood donations from men who have had sex with men.[70]

Conclusion

The advent of AIDS shattered the complacency of a medical system that believed it had conquered infectious diseases with antibiotics and vaccines. AIDS was not like other infections. Its incubation period was often a decade long, although in some cases much shorter. Its most striking characteristic, which emerged slowly, was that no one who progressed to the symptoms of full-blown AIDS ever recovered. This was in stark contrast to other infectious diseases, for which a mortality rate of 30 percent was considered very high. Between 1981 and 1985 clinicians were able to treat only the symptoms of the opportunistic infections and cancers of their patients, knowing that whatever they did, it would not stop the ultimate progression of AIDS. Early in the epidemic, immunologists recognized that the human immune system had gone awry in people who had AIDS, but in the early 1980s they stood at the beginning of detailed basic knowledge about molecular immunity and, indeed, learned a great deal of basic information through their work with AIDS patients.

The advent of AIDS thus marked a paradigm shift in understanding best practices for blood banking and for professions in which practitioners had contact with patients' blood. Before AIDS, few dentists, morticians, or first responders wore gloves, masks, and eye protectors, even knowing that they were at risk for hepatitis B. Administration of blood and blood products before AIDS similarly emphasized the benefits to patients and minimized the risk of contracting hepatitis B. In the years since AIDS appeared, all these professions teach the wearing of gloves, masks, and eye protectors as best practices. All blood and blood products are tested for HIV, and all blood products are heat treated.[71]

4
AIDS as a Cultural Phenomenon

"We cannot factor a complex social situation into so much biology on one side, and so much culture on the other. We must seek to understand the emergent and irreducible properties arising from an inextricable inter-penetration of genes and environments."

—STEPHEN J. GOULD[1]

What is the meaning of AIDS? Is it simply a neutral infectious disease phe-nomenon like chicken pox, or does it convey something about the people who become infected and the societies in which they live? In the industrialized world, where much of the initial transmission of AIDS was via homosexual sex, conservative political leaders shied away from addressing what they viewed as a distinctly unpleasant, if not abhorrent, subject. In much of the developing world, initial transmission of AIDS was via heterosexual sex. Political leaders in those countries also avoided addressing AIDS, even in the face of data from blood tests showing rising HIV infection. They used as cover the fact that large numbers of people were not yet sick or dying from AIDS and suggested that a problem didn't really exist. Everywhere, the injecting drug users who contract-ed AIDS were viewed by many as "beyond the pale" of any help. In this chapter, we shall look at AIDS in its broader context and attempt to clarify what politi-cal, social, and economic responses to AIDS in various countries tells us about the meaning of AIDS in those societies. This chapter will focus on industrial-ized countries. Chapter 7 will address the meaning of AIDS in underdeveloped countries.

Historian Charles Rosenberg has written a great deal about the meaning of epidemics to the societies that experience them. Traditionally, an epidemic was an event with a clear beginning, middle, and end. We can designate June 1981 as the beginning of the AIDS epidemic, as we are doing when we say the epidemic has approached its thirtieth anniversary. Because of the nature of HIV infection and its end-stage manifestation in opportunistic infections and cancers, often a decade later, there is no obvious middle and end to the spread of HIV infection in any population. It has never "gone away" for significant periods. HIV arrived and has continued to spread in human populations. Infected people who reach the stage of full-blown AIDS do not recover and exhibit immunity to a recurrence of the disease.

The emergence of AIDS, therefore, confounded traditional assumptions about the definition of epidemics. Nonetheless, certain responses characteristic of traditional epidemics have marked the course of AIDS. In 1992 Rosenberg wrote about the public response to epidemic disease: "Recognition implies collective action. One of the defining characteristics of an epidemic is in fact the pressure it generates for decisive and visible community response. . . . In the stress of an epidemic . . . failure to take action constitutes action. An epidemic might in this sense be likened to a trial, with policy choices constituting the possible verdicts."[2] With this in mind, let us look at how AIDS was viewed— "constructed" is the term used in academia—in industrialized societies between 1981 and 1995 and how those views contributed to policy choices made in different countries.

The Medical View: An Infectious Disease

As we saw in chapter 1, epidemiologists who had described and tracked previous epidemic diseases recognized by mid-1982 that AIDS was most likely a disease caused by a microbe that was transmitted by blood and sex. By the end of 1982 their data were sufficient to convince them that contaminated blood and blood products could transmit AIDS, that the AIDS agent—then still unknown—was transmitted sexually, and that mothers could transmit AIDS to their babies, although the mechanism was not yet clear. In the absence of clear proof of causation, medical leaders charged with protecting the public health argued passionately that the most effective course to halt the epidemic would be "harm reduction." Such a program involved educating people about the dangers of unprotected sex and providing condoms to those who requested them, identifying surrogate markers to reduce the chance that contaminated blood would transmit the disease, and attempting to enroll injecting drug users in treatment programs or, at least, providing them with sterile needles. Unfortunately, reducing harm often clashed with other societal values—religious, political, and legal.

The Culture of the 1980s

AIDS was identified as a new disease at a time when conservative ideas were resurgent in industrialized democracies. In a book anticipating the 1980s published by the Hoover Institution, Milton and Rose Friedman predicted:

> The failure of Western governments to achieve their proclaimed objectives has produced a widespread reaction against big government. In Britain, the reaction swept Margaret Thatcher to power in 1979 on a platform pledging her Conservative government to reverse the socialist policies that had been followed by both Labour and earlier Conservative governments ever since the end of World War II. In Sweden in 1976, the reaction led to the defeat of the Social Democratic Party after more than four decades of uninterrupted rule. In France, the reaction led to a dramatic change in policy designed to eliminate government control of prices and wages, and sharply reduce other forms of government intervention. In the United States, the reaction has been manifested most dramatically in the tax revolt that has swept the nation, symbolized by the passage of Proposition 13 in California, and realized in a number of states in constitutional amendments limiting state taxes.[3]

In the United States, these views were further validated in November 1980 when Ronald Reagan was elected president. Reagan conservatives primarily aimed to reduce federal support for domestic social programs. Social conservatism, especially as expressed by fundamentalist religious groups, focused a great deal of effort on opposition to the *Roe v. Wade* decision of 1973 that made abortion legal. The beliefs that underlay the view of abortion as murder were grounded in traditional religious beliefs about the proper roles of men and women, how families should be constituted, and what sexual behaviors were acceptable. Together, these political and social currents clashed with proposed pragmatic public health policies to prevent the spread of AIDS.

Among religious groups whose spokespeople had access to the legislators in Congress and to the White House staff who shaped federal policy, AIDS was often viewed as the punitive consequence of offending biblical prohibitions against behaviors that included homosexual sex, one of the two risk factors first identified with the transmission of AIDS. For all Christian denominations, as well as for Islam and Judaism, AIDS made manifest "a conflict of values surrounding human sexuality." As described by French sociologist and AIDS activist Daniel Defert, all the major monotheistic religions define sexuality not as a "human instinct that must necessarily receive satisfaction or expression" but rather as an act infused with spiritual meaning for one's self through abstinence before marriage and for one's spouse in marriage through fidelity. Religions also assumed a responsibility "to enforce obedience to their rules and commandments." They also emphasized "the importance of charity towards the weak, the poor, the infirm, the sick." Often during the early years of AIDS these two impulses existed side by side, so that religious groups might provide AIDS hospice care but at the same time lobby strongly against condom distribution and inveigh against "the homosexual life style."[4]

To public health officials, for example, condoms represented the most pragmatic and neutral technique available to help stop the spread of AIDS— a simple hygienic approach. For religious groups, however, condoms meant much more—they meant that sex was a pleasurable activity separate from the end of procreation, and to many they symbolized the equality of heterosexual and homosexual practices since they protected both equally from the threat of disease. Especially for the most conservative denominations within each religion, such beliefs made it impossible to consider condoms merely as devices to prevent the spread of a virus; they were threats to a belief system. For people not involved with public health issues daily, AIDS thus became a disease of people who engaged in deviant behavior. It was fully preventable, in this view, if only people would follow the precepts of religious practice.[5]

Response of the U.S. Federal Government

The domestic policy of the Reagan administration, as described by economist Karen Davis, was driven by the larger goal of abating inflation in the general economy.[6] To this end, public health agencies were expected to reduce their expenditures across the board. The system of Public Health Service hospitals around the country, created in 1798 to make medical care available to merchant seamen, was terminated and the hospitals closed. Budgets at the Centers for Disease Control and the Food and Drug Administration were stagnant or reduced, and personnel were slashed while responsibilities increased. Only the budget of the National Institutes of Health, a perennial favorite of Congress, was granted any increase, and that increase did not keep up with inflation. Aside from the blows to agency staff morale, the reduced budgets meant that fewer resources could be mustered to respond to AIDS, just one example of what a student of food and drug law described as a "hollowing" of federal agencies during the decade of the 1980s.[7] Within two months of beginning their work, the members of the task force set up by the Centers for Disease Control to investigate the disease reported that the problem was "big," and that with existing resources, they were "drowning."[8] Margaret Heckler, who in 1983 became Secretary of DHHS, described AIDS as a priority for the White House but urged DHHS agencies to reallocate funds from other projects to AIDS rather than request new monies.

Almost immediately after the first report of unusual opportunistic infections in the June 5, 1981, issue of *MMWR*, groups designated as "task forces" or "working groups" were formed at multiple levels in the health agencies of the DHHS. James Curran led the CDC's task force. Robert Gordon was appointed as head of the group out of the NIH Office of the Director. Both NCI and NIAID established task forces on AIDS soon thereafter. Leaders of the PHS agencies already routinely met with Edward Brandt, the assistant secretary for health (ASH), and in May 1983 a subgroup was formally organized into a PHS AIDS Executive Committee, headed by Jeffrey Koplan of the CDC.

Before May 1984 the glaring omission among the members of the PHS AIDS Executive Committee was the surgeon general of the PHS itself, C. Everett Koop (figure 4.1). Brandt had told Koop that he "would not be assigned to cover AIDS." The reason was never made clear. Some saw pressure from White House political advisers; others believed that there was personal animosity between Brandt and Koop, a charge Koop denied.[9] Since the 1960s the position of surgeon general had been eroded and supplanted in the bureaucracy by the ASH. The surgeon general had become little more than a spokesperson for public health issues.[10] Koop sought to revitalize the PHS Commissioned Corps and use his office as a bully pulpit for highlighting health issues. It seemed extremely odd, therefore, that "the nation's doctor" was muzzled in speaking about the emerging health crisis of AIDS facing the nation. From the political uproar over Koop's confirmation hearings—the fear that his support for anti-abortion groups would pose a threat to the *Roe v. Wade* decision guaranteeing a woman's right to control decisions about terminating her pregnancy—Koop appeared to be as conservative with respect to AIDS policy as any other Reagan administration official.

In 1984, after Brandt left the Reagan administration, the acting ASH, James Mason, added Koop to the renamed PHS Executive Task Force on AIDS, which Mason himself chaired and Gary Noble of the CDC cochaired. He also agreed with Koop that AIDS demanded a clear spokesperson and freed Koop to make any statement he thought appropriate.[11] In 1986 two other committees were established, the Federal Coordinating Committee on AIDS Information, Edu-

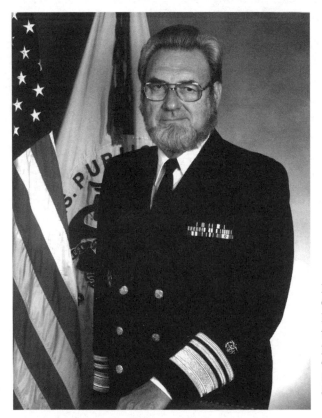

Figure 4.1. Surgeon General C. Everett Koop, who became the U.S. government's principal spokesperson on AIDS. *Courtesy of the U.S. Public Health Service.*

cation, and Risk Reduction and the Intragovernmental Task Force on AIDS Health Care Delivery.[12]

Koop's own analysis of the central tension in the politics of AIDS was that "AIDS pitted the politics of the 'gay revolution' of the seventies against the politics of the Reagan revolution of the eighties."[13] Because the first cases of AIDS appeared in the homosexual communities of large U.S. cities, AIDS was initially stigmatized as a disease that resulted from a lifestyle found abhorrent by people who came into political power via the Reagan revolution. Their reaction to AIDS paralleled their disgust for the homosexual community, and they were often openly hostile to AIDS victims. In 1986 Reagan himself and his secretary of state, George Schultz, made a joke publicly about sending the Libyan leader Muammar al-Qaddafi to San Francisco and giving him AIDS.[14] Such attitudes also predisposed Reaganites to employ euphemistic language such as the "exchange of bodily fluids" instead of more anatomically correct descriptions of sexual acts. In Koop's judgment, this unforgivably slowed down information dissemination to American citizens about how to protect themselves from AIDS.[15]

In February 1986 President Reagan announced in a speech to employees of DHHS that he was asking his surgeon general to prepare a special report on AIDS. According to Koop, he never received a formal request from the White House, but he seized the opportunity and moved forward to produce a document about AIDS. His goals were to allay panic and warn those involved in risky behavior in language understandable to the average citizen. As a Christian, Koop believed in promoting abstinence before marriage and fidelity afterward, but as a physician, he believed in finding a way to help his patients, whether or not they shared his religious views. Thus he was willing to include a recommendation that people use condoms to protect themselves if they engaged in sex outside the parameters he believed best.[16]

Knowing that the Domestic Policy Council in the White House might wish to revise his frank language—and especially that they would most likely want to remove the word "condom" from the report—Koop devised a strategy to gain approval without revisions. He was aware that "these people did not like to spend money," so he had "1,000 copies printed on the best quality glossy stock" that he could find, "in the royal blue of the Public Health Service, with a seal in shining silver, and across the top the title, 'Surgeon General's Report on Acquired Immune Deficiency Syndrome.'" He hoped that the council would realize that to change anything in the report would "cost a fortune," and that would make them have second thoughts about editing. In addition, at the cabinet meeting during which the report was reviewed, he handed out numbered copies of the report and asked to collect them at the end of the meeting to avoid leaks to the press before the document was completed. "I reviewed the report for them, page-by-page, but in a rather superficial manner, and there was very little discussion." Koop was told later that the men in the room did not wish to discuss condoms with ladies present.[17]

On October 22, 1986, Koop held a press conference and released the report. It was mailed to anyone who requested it. Members of Congress sent it to their constituents. The Parent Teacher Association distributed 55,000 copies. Reprints of the text in newspapers reached 2 million people. Koop continued to fend off those, like conservative activist Phyllis Schlafly, who, he said, "would rather have seen promiscuous young people contract and transmit AIDS than expose her own children to the knowledge that there were such things as condoms." Koop also noted that it was not easy for him, as a man about to turn seventy and celebrate his fiftieth wedding anniversary, to be known as the Condom King. He strongly emphasized that he never discussed condoms "without first stressing abstinence for young people and mutually faithful monogamy for older people."[18]

Koop's mailing was followed in 1988 by a report titled *Understanding AIDS* published under the direction of Congress with a special appropriation of nearly $25 million (figure 4.2 shows both reports). The authorizing legislation assigned to the CDC the task of producing and mailing the document to every household in the United States and stipulated that neither the White House nor DHHS would have veto power over the content.[19] James Mason, then-director of the CDC, believed that the report needed a health spokesperson who was nationally recognized and respected. A review of possible candidates produced one name—Surgeon General C. Everett Koop—so Mason invited Koop to be the lead spokesperson for the document. Koop accepted and collaborated on its preparation. Between May 26 and June 15, 1988, 107 million English-language copies were distributed. Four million copies of the Spanish-language version were printed and distributed in Puerto Rico and made available to others on request. This mailing marked the first time the federal government had attempted to contact every citizen with regard to a public health problem. Evaluations of the mailing showed that it was effective in increasing citizen knowledge about behaviors that transmit HIV and about precautions they could take to protect themselves. After reading it, they were also less apprehensive about interacting with family members and others infected with the AIDS virus.[20]

Two years later, in August 1990, the U.S. Congress passed and President George H. W. Bush signed into law the Ryan White Care Act. Named in honor of the teenage hemophiliac infected with HIV whose court case established the right of HIV-infected children to attend school and who died of AIDS in April 1990, the act was the federal government's largest program for people living with AIDS. It was a program of last resort that provided funds to care for AIDS patients when all other resources had been exhausted. The act was repeatedly reauthorized, most recently in 2009 for an additional four years.[21]

At a less public level, DHHS monitored AIDS epidemiology, formulated policy regarding blood and blood products, conducted research on the cause of AIDS, attempted outreach to injecting drug users, and drafted public infor-

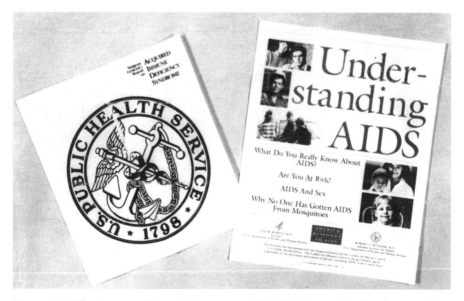

Figure 4.2. The *Surgeon General's Report on AIDS* (1986) was the first large mailing about AIDS produced by the U.S. government. *Understanding AIDS* (1988) was mailed to every household in the United States. *Courtesy of the U.S. National Library of Medicine.*

mation plans. As early as fall 1983 the *AIDS Operational Plan* was issued for the PHS.[22] On paper, the federal response to AIDS was well structured. From 1981 to 1986, however, the central problem with the federal response was the stringent budgetary constraints imposed by the Reagan White House. AIDS was declared the administration's "highest priority" on many occasions, but at the same time, the successive secretaries of DHHS repeatedly instructed their agencies to fight AIDS by transferring monies from their other programs. During the summers of fiscal years 1984 and 1985 (fiscal year 1984 ran from October 1, 1983, through September 30, 1984), Congress provided supplemental appropriations and amended budgets for AIDS projects in addition to the approved budgets for DHHS agencies.

According to James C. Hill, who was appointed as special assistant to the director and AIDS coordinator when Anthony S. Fauci became director of NIAID in 1984, the key event that opened the budgetary gate to increased funding for AIDS was the October 2, 1985, death of actor Rock Hudson. "After Rock Hudson died," he stated,

> we got a signal from the Department [of Health and Human Services] that they would be receptive to a much larger request. We decided that the only way we would make a major push in this area was by going for broke and ask[ing] for so much more money that everybody would know that if they made us take it out of our existing budget, that they would totally destroy our other programs. We were afraid to do that before then, and other institutes were afraid to do it as well. Over one weekend we put together a huge new program. . . . It was a gamble that we took. . . . The NIAID really pushed for a major increase and it worked. Congress appropriated the money.[23]

Hudson's death thus marked the transition point to greatly increased funding for AIDS. By fiscal year 1988, which began on October 1, 1987, the increase was implemented across DHHS agencies. At the NIH, NIAID was able to expand its AIDS research both in Bethesda and across the nation in grants. The NIH Office of AIDS Research (OAR) was created in 1987 as a small office but rapidly expanded to manage all interagency AIDS activities.[24]

Since the White House was occupied by a former actor and actress, Rock Hudson's death also apparently triggered President Reagan's willingness to speak out on AIDS. On September 17, 1985, just before Hudson's death but when the world knew that he was terminally ill, Reagan mentioned AIDS in public for the first time at a press conference in response to a reporter's question about whether children infected with the AIDS virus should be allowed to attend school. His response was still timid: he said that he sympathized with both sides in the issue, even though his own medical experts stated that children infected with AIDS posed no threat to other children in school.

Historian Alan Brandt described an alternative leadership style that "could have changed the meaning of the epidemic in important ways." Brandt referred to the case of hemophiliac brothers infected with AIDS, Ricky, Robert, and Randy Ray.

> In Florida in 1986, when the Ray family's home was burned down because their three sons, who were hemophiliacs, were HIV positive, consider what would have happened if President Reagan had gone on national television that evening. He could have had Nancy sitting in a chair by his side, looking up at him, and he could have said, "What happened in Florida this week was a horrible tragedy. From now on this family will live with Nancy and me in the White House until we find appropriate housing for them. We must begin to recognize the problems raised by this epidemic, and how to address them compassionately.[25]

As Brandt noted, we can never know what would have happened had the Reagan administration assumed such an approach to AIDS, but it is notable that in the absence of such leadership, people infected with HIV were largely blamed for their infections, particularly if they were homosexual men or injecting drug users, the two groups in which most AIDS cases were first diagnosed in the United States. Even the sexual partners and children of injecting drug users did not escape stigmatization. All these affected groups were often blamed for bringing the AIDS virus to "innocent victims" such as hemophiliacs, like the Ray brothers, who themselves were shunned and barred from school and other public places. The phrase "innocent victims" implies that other people who contracted AIDS were "guilty victims." Thus the language of AIDS in its earliest days transformed a biological infection into a moral issue that divided the members of societies into us and them.

Once the causative retrovirus was identified and a blood test for HIV developed, policy decisions regarding testing for HIV infection and the consequences of testing positive arose. In 1987 the CDC added AIDS to a short list of dangerous infections, such as leprosy and tuberculosis, that disqualified individuals from being able to enter the United States, and the Reagan administration began implementing a ban on those who tested positive. In 1991 the CDC revised its position, stating that since HIV was not transmitted casually, admitting people with HIV infection would not seriously imperil the broader population. This decision came after a Dutch person with AIDS, Hans Paul Verhof, was denied entry to speak at a 1989 AIDS meeting in San Francisco, a situation that precipitated a large boycott of the 1990 International AIDS Conference in the same city. Despite strong recommendations from the United Nations and the U.S. National Commission on AIDS, however, in 1993 the U.S. Congress wrote the travel ban into law via the reauthorization act for the National Institutes of Health. It was not repealed until 2009.[26]

Policies in Other Industrialized Nations

David L. Kirp and Ronald Bayer, professors of public policy at the University of California–Berkeley and at Columbia University, respectively, have argued that during the first decade of the AIDS epidemic, "the United States produced the very best policy—and the very worst." The earliest policies of surveillance, testing for the AIDS virus and counseling those found to be infected, screening blood and blood products for the virus, and community-based support and prevention programs were all pioneered in the United States. Banning entry to HIV-positive tourists, opposition to sexually explicit AIDS education literature, condom distribution, and treatment programs or needle exchange for injecting drug users stood at the opposite end of the policy spectrum. As AIDS demanded the development of public policy in other industrialized countries, many embraced the best of U.S. policies but avoided the worst and, indeed, established models that are being embraced in the United States only after three decades of the epidemic.[27]

In the United Kingdom, health policy historian Virginia Berridge wrote, AIDS policies changed from the early 1980s through the mid-1990s as medical professionals learned more about the disease. In the early 1980s AIDS was identified primarily in the male homosexual population. Policymakers largely followed the liberal public health emphasis on protecting individual rights that had developed since World War II. The conservative government of Margaret Thatcher even supported nonpunitive policies of support for gay men and injecting drug users. In 1985, after HIV was identified and a diagnostic test developed, however, the political consensus was strained as it became clear that AIDS might spread into the general (defined as heterosexual) population. In February 1985, for example, Greg Richards, a single man who was chaplain at a prison about thirty-five miles northeast of London, died of AIDS. News of his death caused panic among "respectable ladies who had taken communion wine from the same cup" and those who feared he might have infected prisoners because of his access to them as chaplain. Similarly, kidney patients who had shared a dialysis machine with a person with AIDS were terrified, and just before Americans were informed that Rock Hudson had AIDS, newspapers reported that Lord Avon, son of a former conservative prime minister, had died of AIDS.[28]

Throughout 1985 politicians discussed their responsibilities to protect the larger community while at the same time they attempted to protect individual rights. By the end of the year, a liberal approach was adopted. Berridge summarized the £6.3 million package of AIDS-related policies decided upon by December 1985:

> £2.5 million for a national information campaign to begin the following spring and to run through the whole of 1986. Money was also allocated to the Regional Health Authorities most affected for treatment and counselling; to the PHLS [Public Health Laboratory Service] and to haemophilia reference centres. A separate AIDS Unit was set up in the same month in the DHSS [Department of Health and Social Security] and a telephone advice line opened so that professionals could phone in for advice.[29]

In 1987 political leaders in the United Kingdom transitioned from this intense effort against AIDS—Berridge calls it a "wartime strategy"—to viewing AIDS as a lower priority public health concern. Three factors were responsible for this surprisingly swift shift. First, the licensing of AZT as one therapy for

AIDS promoted the belief that AIDS would be transformed into a chronic disease problem that could be treated, if not cured. Second, AIDS policy was being addressed by the World Health Organization. In 1986 WHO recognized AIDS as a disease threat worthy of its own program. As we shall see in more detail in chapter 7, WHO's director general, Halfdan Mahler, and epidemiologist Jonathan Mann presented a briefing on AIDS to the United Nations General Assembly, the first time that body had ever considered a health issue. As a result, a WHO Special Programme on AIDS was established with Mann as its director. In 1988 it was renamed as the WHO Global Programme on AIDS (GPA).[30] Finally, Berridge argued, the creation of the National AIDS Trust (NAT) signaled that AIDS was becoming "normalized" in the United Kingdom. The lines between voluntary and government support were blurred, and the NAT and other voluntary organizations expanded to include not just HIV-positive people or gay men but others served by mainstream charities.[31]

In the early 1990s, however, challenges to the liberal view of the appropriate U.K. government response to AIDS arose. Social conservatives alleged that there was little risk that AIDS would spread into the heterosexual population and that arguments to the contrary were propaganda being spread by gay organizations to maintain their funding. The publication of Michael Fumento's 1990 book *The Myth of Heterosexual AIDS* fueled this argument.[32] The rise of a challenge to HIV as the cause of AIDS, particularly Peter Duesberg's arguments, which will be discussed in chapter 5, provided fodder for the argument that perhaps AIDS was really caused by multiple factors relating to lifestyle. Finally, a sizable political group believed that a very few AIDS patients were receiving "Rolls Royce" services at the expense of the bulk of the population, which suffered from more widespread but lower-profile illnesses.[33] Although these views seriously challenged harm-reduction policies in the UK, they did not succeed in overturning those policies.

Similar policy debates occurred during the first two decades of AIDS in other European countries, Canada, Australia, and Japan with variations in emphasis. In Spain AIDS appeared primarily among injecting drug users in society's lowest classes; hence the Spanish government could delay the need to act longer than could governments facing organized, middle-class gay men. In Japan, as we saw in chapter 3, AIDS was primarily identified with hemophiliacs, and the major Japanese social response came in acknowledging that the

Japanese blood supply had not been properly protected.[34] In their 1992 book, *AIDS in the Industrialized Democracies: Passions, Politics, and Policies*, Kirp and Bayer noted that AIDS laid bare cultural traditions, policies, and debates about who should pay for the cost of health care; what power public health authorities should have over mandatory procedures such as testing for disease, tracing sexual contacts of infected people, and quarantining the sick; whether or not medical reports on individuals should be treated as confidential materials; whether drug addiction should be addressed as a medical or criminal problem; what status homosexual men and women held in society and what political power they could wield; and which groups should participate in the shaping of public health policy.[35]

U.S. State and Municipal Response

The most successful initial action taken by public health leaders in states and cities across the United States was the establishment of rapid and clear information dissemination mechanisms for affected populations and the physicians who treated them. In February 1982 in New York City, for example, David Sencer, the commissioner of health, inaugurated monthly meetings with physicians in the city who treated AIDS patients. Continued for the next four years, these meetings always included an exchange of information between these two groups. Information exchange also proved important in minimizing irrational fear of infection by health care workers. Especially in the period 1983–87, when public fear and panic were at their most destructive, accurate communications often made the difference between keeping and losing staff at hospitals, firehouses, police departments, and other public service agencies.[36]

A second and more politically vexed public health policy was the decision about whether to close bathhouses in the gay communities of San Francisco, Los Angeles, and New York. The bathhouses represented for many in the gay community a civil rights triumph. After years "in the closet" for fear of losing jobs or being physically attacked, they could openly declare their gay identities and socialize in public at gay bathhouses and bars. Advocates of gay rights vehemently opposed closing the bathhouses. In the years before the AIDS virus was discovered, others in the gay community, bolstered by some public health leaders, believed that the epidemiological findings alone were sufficient to demonstrate sexual transmission, and that since bathhouses were locales in which multiple unprotected sex acts took place, classic public health practice dictated that closing the bathhouses would stop transmission, at least in those locales. Another group argued that bathhouse clients were intelligent enough to begin protecting themselves once informed of the need for safe sex, and that since they were the principal population at risk for AIDS, conducting AIDS prevention education at the bathhouses would lower the rate of transmission of the virus in the entire community. In 1984 the argument was settled in San Francisco when political and public health leaders agreed that the bathhouses should be closed. The next year, Los Angeles and New York City also moved to close bathhouses.[37]

U.S. Presidential and National Commissions on AIDS

In 1986, when the World Health Organization established its Global Programme on AIDS, each country that wished the GPA to mediate assistance efforts between donor countries and those requesting help was asked to create a commission or advisory body to address AIDS. The Institute of Medicine of the U.S. National Academy of Sciences had also strongly urged the creation of such a commission in its 1986 report, *Confronting AIDS*. President Ronald Reagan, who was very slowly beginning to speak about AIDS in the aftermath of Rock Hudson's death, waited until the summer of 1987 to appoint the Presidential Commission on the Human Immunodeficiency Virus Epidemic, and he gave them only one year to conduct hearings and write a report. The members appointed had little knowledge of AIDS, and after three months, the original chair of the commission and another commissioner resigned. Adm. James D. Watkins was named the new chair, and nurse Kristine Gebbie was appointed to replace the member who had resigned. Both Watkins and Gebbie helped the commission pull together and complete its work in the remaining nine months.[38]

The Watkins Commission report, as it was known informally, was surprisingly sweeping in its recommendations, considering the sharply divided philosophical makeup of its members. In its transmittal letter, the commission thanked President Reagan for giving them the opportunity "to view contemporary American society through the lens of HIV." They found that the HIV epidemic was "much more than a medical crisis or public health threat." They saw it as "an opportunity to confront and begin to solve many of the problems our society faces." They presented some six hundred recommendations and listed the top twenty in their executive summary. Among these were dropping the term "AIDS" and replacing it with "HIV infection," greatly expanding access to drug treatment for addicts, increasing scholarship aid to entice nurses to train for service with HIV infected patients, expanding rather than terminating the National Health Service Corps that placed health care professionals in under-served areas, and classifying HIV disease as a disability rather than a disquali-fication for employment.[39]

The Watkins Commission report was largely ignored by the Reagan admin-istration, whose priority was cutting government expenditures, not increasing the scope of government programs. Congress stepped into the void and in 1988 passed legislation sponsored by Congressman Roy Rowland (D-GA), the only physician then serving in Congress, to create a National Commission on AIDS, comprising "individuals with experience and/or expertise pertinent to the AIDS epidemic." The commission was established initially for a two-year term that could be renewed by request of the president. Six members were appointed by Republicans; six by Democrats. The hope was for a nonpartisan context in which they could, as their chair, June Osborn, dean of the School of Public Health at the University of Michigan, stated, "advise both branches of govern-ment, proactively and reactively, as needed, on a broad range of issues arising from the epidemic."[40]

During the commission's four-year life, it produced numerous reports, three of which targeted subjects that were especially difficult to address in American society. First, in a report on the twin epidemics of substance abuse and HIV, the commission reiterated what every public health official since 1983 had recommended: drug treatment programs should be open to all who wanted them. Needle exchange and instruction in using bleach to clean injec-tion "works" should be adopted as short-term techniques for harm reduction.[41] Second, commission members charged that HIV was spreading in prisons be-cause of the "shameful state of health care in prisons and jails."[42] A third subject-focused report was *The Challenge of HIV/AIDS in Communities of Color.* In this report, the commission lamented the mounting disproportion of HIV in minority groups, including African American, Latino, Native American, and Asian/Pacific Islander groups. Utilizing experts from within each community, the commission gave voice to "important concerns and discussion" that were desperately needed.[43] In *AIDS: An Expanding Tragedy* (figure 4.3), its final report as the commission closed down in 1993, members noted that their efforts were like "trying to take a snapshot of a tidal wave: its pace and scope defies capture." They also noted, "The human immunodeficiency virus (HIV) has profoundly changed life on our planet. America has not done well in acknowledging this fact or in mobilizing its vast resources to address it appropriately. Many are suffering profoundly because of that failure, and America is poorer because of this neglect. We are apprehensive because the situation will worsen without immediate action."[44]

Community Responses to AIDS: The AIDS Activists

In the United States during the 1980s, the Reagan administration did not support expanded federal involvement in responding to AIDS; hence caring for suffering people and reducing the spread of the disease fell largely onto community groups. The story of AIDS activism is a story of a marginalized community that organized itself to care for its members when no social safety net was in place and that also took action to force political bodies to address AIDS. Gay communities in large U.S. cities were composed largely of upper-middle-class men, mostly Caucasian, who possessed the skills to achieve their ends. Unlike injecting drug users, gay men as a group were not caught in addiction's web, were not difficult to reach with public health messages, and had become accustomed to demanding civil rights during the 1970s.

As noted in chapter 1, in 1982 members of the gay community in New York organized the Gay Men's Health Crisis to provide information about AIDS prevention, care for people suffering with AIDS-related illnesses, and advocacy at every level of government policy.[45] Similar groups were formed in San Francisco, Los Angeles, and other cities with sizable gay communities. In 1985 five of the earliest community-based organizations—the Gay Men's Health Crisis, AIDS Project Los Angeles, San Francisco AIDS Foundation, Baltimore's Health Education Resource Organization, and Boston's AIDS Action Committee—created the National AIDS Network as a networking and resources center.[46] Paul A. Kawata, who headed the National AIDS Network and later the National Minority AIDS Council, observed in 1989 that these community groups were the "people on the front lines, the people who change the bedpans, who cook the food, who take care of the dying. . . . The greatest challenge that they have

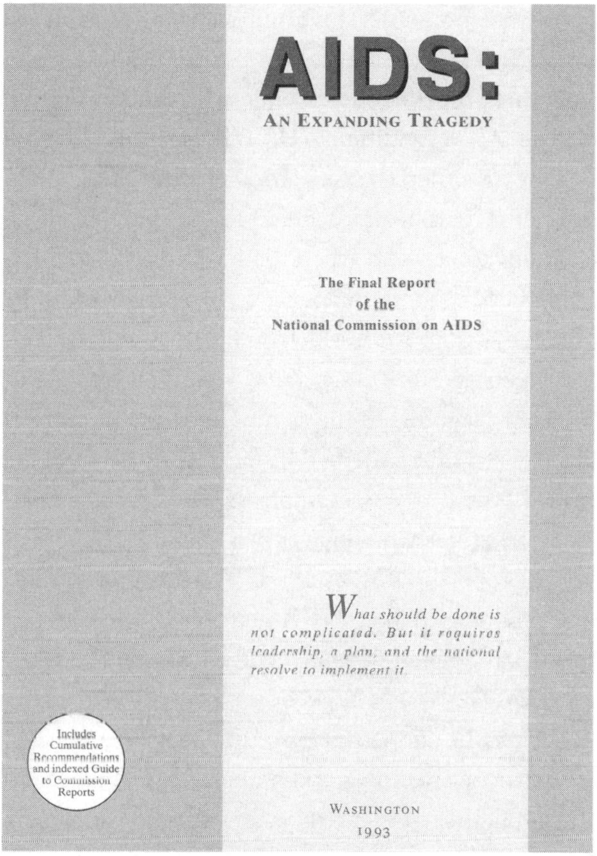

Figure 4.3. *AIDS: An Expanding Tragedy.* The final report of the National Commission on AIDS, 1993.

is to learn how not to cry, because if they took the time to cry every time somebody in their lives died, they would not have time to do their work."[47]

When it came to advocacy, AIDS community organizations had to decide whether to apply pressure as traditional lobbyists within political bureaucracies or to take a more radical approach and seek publicity through public demonstrations. Both methods were employed, often in combination, to achieve particular goals. For example, in 1985 negative media coverage of the bathhouse closure issue spurred a group of New York activists to form the Gay and Lesbian Alliance against Defamation (GLAAD). GLAAD organized peaceful protests and concentrated on insider strategies to achieve political ends. One group of GLAAD members, however, organized the Lavender Hill Mob to utilize street theater tactics. The mob set in motion a tactic known as a "zap" in which a small group of activists would gain access to an event and "directly confront a person, target, or audience at an appropriate moment." This group also pioneered use of the Holocaust metaphor for AIDS.[48]

In 1987 much of the anger that propelled the Lavender Hill Mob was transferred into a new group called the AIDS Coalition to Unleash Power (ACT UP). This group was founded by Larry Kramer, the New York activist who in 1982 had founded the Gay Men's Health Crisis. Kramer preferred strong public demonstrations to pressure politicians to act, and when the leadership of GMHC decided that Kramer would not yield to their preference for working within the system, Kramer resigned from the organization. Much of this story and the subsequent birth of ACT UP was recorded in Kramer's play—the first play about AIDS—*The Normal Heart*. The protagonist of the semi-autobiographical play gave the efforts of American Jews to gain help for European Jews being killed during the Holocaust in World War II as his example of why exerting pressure through existing political structures would never be enough. "The title of Treasury Secretary Morgenthau's report to Roosevelt was 'Acquiescence of This Government in the Murder of the Jews,' which he wrote in 1944," protagonist Ned states in the play. "Dachau was opened in 1933. Where was everybody for eleven years? And then it was too late."[49] The walls of the play's set were covered with statistics about AIDS deaths and examples of the paltry response of government and the press to a disease affecting gays compared with their rapid and fulsome responses to Legionnaires' disease and toxic-shock syndrome a few years earlier, both of which were less deadly and affected far fewer people. For example, although some twelve thousand cases of AIDS had been reported in the United States by 1985, the *New York Times* had written only forty-one articles about the disease; during the 1982 Tylenol scare, which produced only seven deaths, the *Times* wrote about the problem fifty-four times.[50]

On March 10, 1987, when *The Normal Heart* opened in Houston, Texas, Kramer spoke to assembled members of the Houston gay community. He challenged them to take their outrage to the streets to demand more drugs to treat the dying, more services to care for the ill, and more research to find therapies and preventatives for AIDS. Two nights later, 350 people came together in New York to form ACT UP. The first action taken by the new organization came on March 24, when demonstrators hung Frank Young, the commissioner of the FDA, in effigy and chanted, "Ronald Reagan, your son is gay. Put him in charge of the FDA!" Kramer acknowledged that what he sought through this demonstration was media attention, and he was successful. All three television networks covered the story, a photograph appeared in the *New York Times*, and the next day Phil Donahue's television show included footage from the demonstration. Soon thereafter, the FDA announced that it would shorten its drug approval process by two years.[51] (Figures 4.4 and 4.5 picture an ACT UP demonstration,"Storm the NIH," on May 21, 1990.)

AIDS activism began in the United States, but it soon spread around the world. In 1983 the Terrence Higgins Trust was founded in the United Kingdom. The next year AIDES was founded in France. In 1983 Brazilian AIDS activists successfully pressured the Brazilian government to adopt an AIDS program in the state of São Paulo.[52]

Injecting Drug Users and Needle-Exchange Programs

Injecting drug users, their sexual partners, and their children made up another category of people with AIDS. Notoriously unreliable because of the hold drugs had on them, injecting drug users were wary of government officials, especially those in law enforcement. Attempts to reduce the likelihood that members of this group would become infected with HIV fell to advocacy groups often staffed with former addicts or family members of addicts and to public health officials. Early in the epidemic, public health officials suggested that expanding drug treatment programs and making clean needles and syringes available to addicts would slow the spread of AIDS. In the United States, such proposals met with rejection from law enforcement agencies as well as from political conservatives who would have to vote for funds to finance the programs. Politicians and law enforcement instead supported a "war on drugs" in which the law made injecting drug users felons and aimed to stop the importation and distribution of illegal drugs. Law enforcement officials did not believe that addicts would be sufficiently responsible to stay in drug treatment programs, and they viewed the proposals to exchange used needles for clean ones or even to instruct addicts on how to sterilize their works with bleach as government endorsement of the use of illegal drugs. The most extreme viewed death of addicts and homosexuals by AIDS as ridding the world of despicable people.

Informal experiments with needle exchange in the United States originated in the 1970s in California as a way to reduce the incidence of hepatitis B in injecting drug users. In 1984, after HIV had been identified as the cause of AIDS,

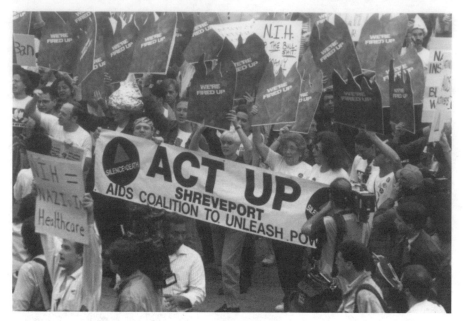

Figure 4.4. ACT UP protest "Storm the NIH," May 21, 1990. *Courtesy of the U.S. National Institutes of Health.*

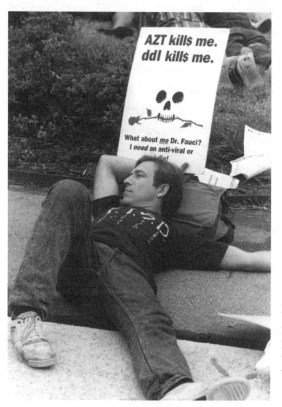

Figure 4.5. Protester targets NIH AIDS spokesperson Anthony Fauci, "Storm the NIH" protest, May 21, 1990. *Courtesy of the U.S. National Institutes of Health.*

a drug users' advocacy group in Amsterdam, the Netherlands, began a syringe and needle exchange as an anonymous, accessible service to reduce harm among addicts at risk for HIV. Evaluations of the program were positive and widely discussed in the United States, but no official action appeared possible. Two years later, however, a former injecting drug user, Jon Parker, motivated by a remark that addicts would never change their behavior and so should not be a focus of HIV prevention efforts, began meeting with addicts and distributing clean needles in New Haven, Connecticut, and Boston, Massachusetts. Parker expanded his efforts and was arrested numerous times as he challenged laws prohibiting the purchase of needles and syringes without a prescription.[53]

In 1988 another drug rehabilitation activist, Dave Purchase, set up a table in downtown Tacoma, Washington, at which he exchanged clean needles and syringes for used ones. Purchase informed local officials, who let the program continue as an informal effort. In time this privately organized program grew into the Point Defiance AIDS Project, which operated under a contract with the local health department. (Figure 4.6 pictures a 2007 needle exchange in Seattle, Washington.) Later in 1988, a needle-exchange program was also established in San Francisco. The San Francisco effort, called Prevention Point, was tolerated even though under California law it was illegal to purchase needles and syringes without a prescription. In 1993 Mayor Frank Jordon declared a state of public health emergency in San Francisco, a move that gave him the power to legalize the needle exchange program. It has continued to operate since that time. In 2009 the program, maintained by the San Francisco AIDS Foundation, operated eleven needle-exchange sites each week, exchanged more than 2.3 million needles each year, and was administered by more than eighty volunteers.[54]

Also in 1988, New York City established a needle-exchange program as an experiment, but the outcome was much different from that on the West Coast. Physician-historian Warwick Anderson has described the stalemate that developed between public health officials and the law enforcement and religious communities who viewed needle exchanges as endorsements by the government of illegal drug use.[55] In New York City, Commissioner of Health Sencer testified at hearings on AIDS in 1983 that it was "a tragedy that the programs for drug abuse that could obviate the need for dirty needles are at this point in time being cut back when a new and deadly health problem is moving through this population."[56] Sencer and other physicians urged Mayor Koch to imple-

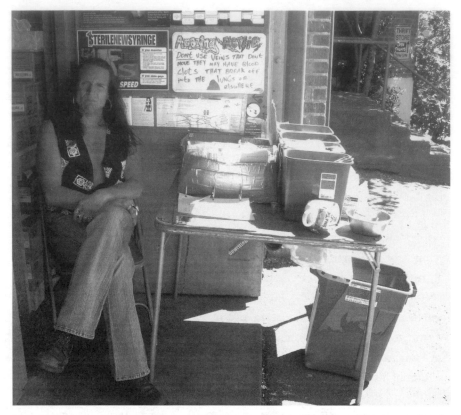

Figure 4.6. Street Outreach Services needle exchange in a back alley of University Methodist Temple, University District, Seattle, Washington, 2007. *Photograph by Joe Mabel, Wikimedia Commons.*

ment a clean-needle program for addicts. They based their arguments on the most pragmatic course to ensure that addicts did not harm themselves or others by contracting and transmitting HIV. Law enforcement officials, in contrast, argued that "addicts were not responsible enough to use clean needles to safeguard their own health: making needles freely available would only encourage young people to try drugs."[57] The Catholic Church also weighed in against any plan to provide clean needles. Cardinal John O'Connor warned New York City against "dragging down the standards of all society." Politicians in the African-American and Hispanic communities in New York City, where addiction rates were the highest, opposed the program, even alleging it amounted to "genocide."[58]

Mervyn Silverman, president of the American Foundation for AIDS Research (amfAR), countered the arguments of law enforcement, saying, "I never

heard of anybody starting drugs because needles were available or stopping because they couldn't find a clean one." National public health leaders, including
James Curran and C. Everett Koop, supported needle exchange as the tactic
most likely to prevent the spread of AIDS among drug addicts and their families. Similarly, a spokesman for a community action group that planned to distribute free needles and syringes in the city in violation of current law stated in
exasperation, "They talk about genocide—this is the real genocide. People can
survive addiction, but they can't survive AIDS."[59] British historian Roy Porter
attributed the stalemate that dragged on throughout the 1980s in New York to
"the mixed blessings of the decentralized state and of City Hall caucus politics."[60] The New York City situation was repeated in almost every other major
city in the United States. It was not until 1992 that a legal needle exchange was
organized in New York City.[61]

African Americans and AIDS

African-American communities suffered especially from denial about AIDS for
two reasons. African-American Christian churches in the United States historically served as the center of community. As such, the church was the principal organization that could speak authoritatively to black communities. The
church also held conservative views regarding homosexuality. Even acknowledging that some men might engage in "down-low" activities, church leaders
were loath to discuss homosexuality in any other context except its sinfulness.
Homosexual black men living outside large cities with coherent homosexual
communities lived closeted lives in order to maintain their relationships with
family and community. Since homosexuality was not a topic most African
Americans were comfortable with, and since AIDS was associated almost exclusively with homosexuality in the 1980s, AIDS was simply not on the agendas
of most churches. Denial of the need for safe-sex instruction sadly paved the
way for HIV to become established in African-American men and, since a sizable proportion of men who had sex with men also had sex with women, in
their female partners.

A second factor promoting denial of the threat of AIDS to African American communities was their historic mistrust of the federal government. This
suspicion can be distilled into one word: "Tuskegee." Between 1932 and 1972,
researchers in the U.S. Public Health Service studied African-American men

infected with syphilis in Tuskegee, Alabama, but left them untreated in order to learn more about the disease's natural history. When penicillin was discovered as a cure for syphilis, these men were not treated while white syphilitic patients received the new drug. When the blatant racism became public in 1972, the African-American community was still fighting for full social acceptance in U.S. society and saw the Tuskegee study as clear evidence that federal health messages were not to be trusted.[62]

Mark D. Smith, president and chief executive officer of the California HealthCare Foundation, who was intensely involved with AIDS issues from the time of his internship in 1983 at San Francisco General Hospital, described other issues that have impeded active preventive work in the African-American community. Suggestions that the AIDS virus originated in Africa, drawn from evidence of cases in Europeans or Africans living in former European colonial areas in Africa, produced a wary response that the disease was being blamed on people of color. Even more important was the inadequacy of the U.S. health care system, which did not have a good track record in caring for poor minority patients with drug abuse and mental health problems even before AIDS appeared.[63]

The AIDS Quilt—The NAMES Project

The most tangible manifestation of the lives lost to AIDS is embodied in the AIDS Quilt, curated by the NAMES Project Foundation. This memorial was conceived by gay rights activist Cleve Jones, who also was a founder of the San Francisco AIDS Foundation. In 1985, for a candlelight march honoring gay San Francisco supervisor Harvey Milk and mayor George Moscone, both of whom had been assassinated in 1978, Jones asked participants to bring placards bearing the names of friends who had died of AIDS. At the end of the march, the names were taped to the San Francisco Federal Building, and the result looked like a patchwork quilt. The image inspired Jones to create a more permanent memorial that would hold a power similar to that of the Vietnam Veterans Memorial Wall in Washington, D.C. In 1986 he made a quilt panel in honor of his friend Marvin Feldman, and in 1987 Jones and others formally organized the NAMES Project Foundation.

In October 1987 the AIDS Quilt was first displayed on the National Mall in Washington, D.C. At that time, it contained 1,920 panels arranged in four-panel blocks. The quilt was displayed in its entirety for the last time in Washington in 1996, when it completely covered the National Mall and contained panels from every state and more than twenty-eight countries. Since that time, it has grown to more than 44,000 panels and is the largest community art project in the world. (Figure 4.7 shows a panel exhibited in Taiwan.) It has been featured in numerous books, scholarly articles, and theatrical and musical performances.[64]

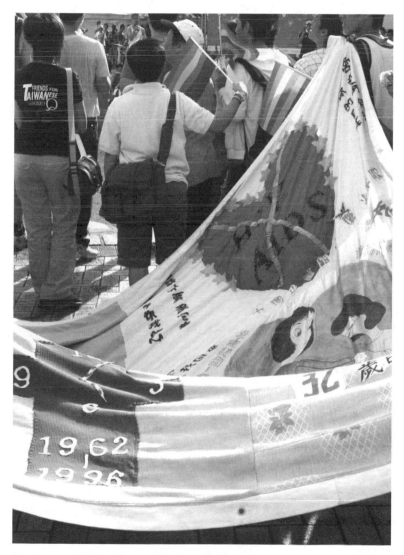

Figure 4.7. AIDS quilt panel displayed before city hall on Taiwan Pride Day, 2005. *Photo by Atinncnu, Wikimedia Commons.*

Celebrity Involvement in AIDS

In addition to community groups involved in patient care and advocacy, physicians and public health officials joined with gay community activists in major cities to form private-sector foundations to raise money for research on AIDS and funding for AIDS care. In April 1983 Mathilde Krim, a researcher at New York's Memorial Sloan-Kettering Cancer Center, and her colleagues formed the AIDS Medical Foundation to raise money for research on AIDS. Two years later, in September 1985, it merged with the newly formed National AIDS Research Foundation to become the American Foundation for AIDS Research.[65] The actress Elizabeth Taylor was closely associated with fund-raising for amfAR. In 1991 she also established her own AIDS charity, the Elizabeth Taylor HIV/AIDS Foundation, with an emphasis on direct care for AIDS patients.[66]

Other celebrities worldwide have become involved in raising money for various aspects of AIDS research and treatment. As noted in chapter 3, actress Elizabeth Glaser established an AIDS charity for children before her death from the disease. In 1991 Magic Johnson, the renowned basketball player, created the Magic Johnson Foundation, which funded a program to make HIV/AIDS services and information available for low-income people in urban communities. In 1992 the English singer-songwriter Elton John created the Elton John AIDS Foundation, which provides grants to community-based AIDS groups. John also collaborated with Dionne Warwick and other artists in 1986 to produce the song "That's What Friends Are For," which raised more than $3 million for amfAR. The French retailer Maison Martin Margiela has since 1994 produced an AIDS T-shirt each year and donated a percentage of the profits to AIDES, the leading French AIDS organization. Similar nongovernmental initiatives exist around the world. In 2010 a group of AIDS organizations from France, Morocco, Mali, Democratic Republic of Congo, Burundi, Burkina Faso, Quebec, and Equador joined together to form PLUS, Coalition Internationale SIDA. All these organizations utilize a variety of fund-raising methods, including AIDS walks and AIDS rides for bicyclists, AIDS marathon training programs, AIDS toy drives, AIDS battles of the bands, direct fund-raising letters, and, recently, fund-raising via social networks on the Internet.[67]

Conclusion

How can we answer the question posed at the beginning of this chapter: what is the meaning of AIDS? Infection with HIV and its ultimate consequence in producing the symptoms of full-blown AIDS is clearly a biological phenomenon. In terms of the human experience of AIDS, however, infection with HIV and its destruction of the immune system, which leads to the many debilitating afflictions of AIDS, this disease has carried much more symbolism. During the three decades that the world has been aware of AIDS, it has elicited extremes in many areas of society from tender care of those afflicted to violent burning of their homes, from political stonewalling to the expansion of public policies to support people with AIDS, and from rejection of groups with which AIDS was identified—homosexual males and injecting drug users—to reconsideration of the meaning and variety of human experience.

In his 1962 book *The Cholera Years,* historian Charles Rosenberg examined the responses of U.S. society to three nineteenth-century epidemics of cholera, in 1832, 1849, and 1866. During the first epidemic, cholera was interpreted not as a specific disease but as an affliction from God on the impious. By 1849 physicians were conceptualizing cholera as a specific disease, but without any means to treat or prevent it, fear of the groups in which it was most common— the poor, often the immigrant poor—led to blaming them for the epidemic. Not until 1866 did public health physicians determine that cholera could be controlled by sanitation methods, especially separating sewage from the public water supply, even though they did not know yet specifically what caused the disease. Medicine's ability to halt cholera epidemics and, indeed, prevent them through public health measures transformed society's view of cholera. It was no longer the wages of sin. Those poor people who suffered most from the disease had not brought the disease on themselves and passed it along to respectable people. Their drinking water was contaminated. When medicine can control a disease, its social, economic, religious, and political meanings diminish.

A rough parallel may be seen in the AIDS epidemic. In 1983 fundamentalist evangelical Baptist minister Jerry Falwell pronounced AIDS a "gay plague." He also opined, "AIDS is not just God's punishment for homosexuals; it is God's punishment for the society that tolerates homosexuals."[68] In 1989 in *AIDS and Its Metaphors,* the writer Susan Sontag observed that even "the disease most fraught with meaning can become just an illness" and cited leprosy, now called Hansen's disease, "as a part of its dedramatization" after Norwegian physician Gerhard Hansen identified its causative bacillus in 1873. Sontag argued that the same thing "was bound to happen with AIDS, when the illness is much better understood and, above all, treatable."[69] During the three decades that AIDS has been recognized as a disease, Sontag's prediction has partly come to pass. Because AIDS can be sexually transmitted, however, it is still imbued with the fear, guilt, and shame that attach to all sexually transmitted diseases. Only if and when AIDS can be prevented by medical intervention will it become "just an illness" from which people used to die.

5

AIDS Therapy

"The field, the whole field, is curing AIDS."
—ROBERT C. GALLO[1]

In Larry Kramer's play *The Normal Heart*, the character Felix asks, "Do you think they'll find a cure before I . . . How strange that sounds when you say it out loud for the first time!"[2] The play debuted in 1985 when no effective therapy of any sort had been discovered to address the underlying immune deficiency caused by infection with HIV. Physicians made heroic efforts to treat symptoms and prolong the lives of AIDS patients, but the eventual outcome was uniformly bleak, the more so because for the first few years of the epidemic, people hoped that a sizable proportion of those with AIDS would recover, as had always been the case in earlier epidemics. But no one with full-blown AIDS survived.

In the search for a cure for AIDS, the story of laboratory research is tightly entwined with social, economic, and political factors. It demonstrates how biomedical research can initially respond to an emergency only to the extent allowed by the level of basic knowledge about the body that exists before the crisis occurs. It also reflects how rapidly deceptive therapies and alternative explanations for disease, fueled by the fear of the sick or their caregivers, arise to claim credence until biomedicine can produce a therapy that puts people back on their feet. This chapter examines both of these aspects of therapies for AIDS and also explores the interaction of AIDS activists with the political issues surrounding AIDS therapy and the economic issues surrounding the patenting and pricing of AIDS drugs.

Basic Science Background to Research on AIDS Therapies

Two lines of basic research converged to provide the context in which research-ers sought a therapy for the immune defect caused by HIV infection. The first was the rise of molecular biology, the study of how the human body works at the level of molecules. Developments in molecular immunology were discussed in chapter 1, but it will be useful to survey the rise of molecular virology over the same period briefly. To devise a therapy that would intervene in AIDS, re-searchers needed to know as much as possible about HIV—how it entered the cells it infected, what happened inside the cell, and how the virus reproduced itself and moved on to infect a new cell. Discoveries in genetics advanced rap-idly in the 1960s after the genetic code was deciphered and led directly to the ability to understand life processes in bacteria and viruses.[3] During the 1970s scientists learned how to cut DNA and to insert new DNA sequences to pro-duce altered, or genetically modified, organisms such as bacteria that could produce insulin for diabetics. Scientists were also aware, of course, that geneti-cally modified organisms might be used for evil purposes or that some sort of accidental release might occur that would threaten human health. Scientists themselves formulated strict guidelines for recombinant DNA research to allay public concerns until many safety tests showed that fear of accidentally releas-ing a new plague was unfounded.[4]

Investigators also created methods to clone (produce multiple copies of a virus's genetic material) and to sequence (determine the genes it contained) DNA. Once the genes were known, scientists described what structure or func-tion in the virus's life cycle each gene coded for, or controlled. For example, one gene might direct the creation of a capsid, or container in which the virus's genetic material is located, while another might code for the enzyme that pulls all the new parts of the virus made in the infected cell together so it can break out of the cell and infect another one.[5] In 1976 scientists published the first complete genome of an organism, a virus whose genetic material was RNA.[6] By the early 1980s, as detailed in chapter 2, when the search for a causative agent for AIDS was under way, molecular virology, like molecular immunology, was making rapid progress but was not yet equipped with the knowledge and tech-niques, such as the polymerase chain reaction (PCR), that have made recent research much easier.

Molecular Virology of the AIDS Virus

During the summer and fall of 1984, the various groups of retrovirologists working on the cause of AIDS utilized molecular technology to clone and sequence the virus each group had isolated and to describe how each gene contributed to the virus's structure or function. They determined that the viruses each group had isolated—then known as LAV, HTLV-III, and ARV—were variants of the same virus, now called HIV, and they began identifying viral genes and their functions. By 1986 *gag*, *pol*, and *env* had been identified as the three major genes of HIV, as they are for all retroviruses. The first, *gag*, coded for the production of HIV's structural proteins, such as the matrix that supports the outer envelope of HIV and the capsid protein, in which the virus's RNA genome is kept (see figure 5.1, a diagram of the HIV virion, or single virus particle). The gene *pol* coded for the critical enzymes reverse transcriptase, protease, and integrase, which directed the reproduction of HIV within a host cell. The gene *env* directed production of the viral envelope proteins that allowed the virus to attach to a targeted cell and fuse with it. Other genes, such as *tat*, *rev*, and *vpr*, were transactivators, which increased the rate of gene expression, while *vif*, *nef*, and *vpu* regulated other aspects of the viral life cycle.[7] Scientists determined that HIV comprises several subgroups with slightly different genes. All, however, replicate rapidly and have an extremely high mutation rate.[8]

All of this technical work enabled the worldwide scientific community to develop a model of the HIV life cycle, the first step in identifying points at which the cycle could possibly be interrupted to stop the damage HIV was doing to the immune system. As figure 5.2 shows, when HIV attacks a T cell, it attaches to the cell surface by fitting one of its envelope proteins like a key into the lock on the cell, the CD4 receptor molecule (cluster of differentiation 4). Once inside the cell, the virus uncoats its genetic material, and its *pol* gene instructs the production of reverse transcriptase, an enzyme that transforms the RNA into a DNA form. Next, the enzyme integrase inserts the viral DNA into the host cell's DNA, where it becomes a part of the host cell and instructs the production of new viral components. At the cell surface, these components assemble, and as they bud out of the cell, the enzyme protease cleaves the components of the forming virion (a single virus), allowing the virus to mature and infect new cells. Each point of this process represents a potential place to intervene.

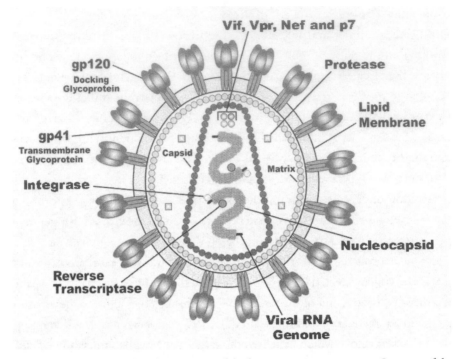

Figure 5.1. HIV virion (single virus particle), showing major structures. *Courtesy of the National Institute of Allergy and Infectious Diseases.*

In 1984, as soon as the life cycle was known, medical researchers had ideas about how to stop HIV at some points in its life cycle but not in others. Until the techniques were available to manipulate the genetic material of viruses, the detailed information that permitted rational drug design instead of a trial-and-error approach simply did not exist. Little work had been done during the previous three decades to develop antiviral drugs because viruses for the most part replicate by using the machinery of the host cell and were viewed as extremely difficult to counter with drugs.

Antiviral Drug Research before AIDS

In 1962 the first two antiviral drugs were introduced. They were idoxuridine, used against herpes keratitis (a viral infection of the eye), and methisazone, used against vaccinia virus (the virus used to give smallpox vaccinations).[9] Two other drugs were subsequently shown to be effective against herpes keratitis, but in addition to these, by 1982 only one additional antiviral drug had been discovered. This was acyclovir, which proved highly effective in the treatment of the two most common herpes virus infections—the common cold sore and genital herpes.[10] When AIDS appeared, therefore, the arsenal of drugs used to treat viral infections was severely limited.

Most of the antiviral drugs initially developed for HIV infection had been studied first for their possible cancer-fighting ability. Samuel Broder, the National Cancer Institute researcher who led the team that first investigated the potential of azidothymidine, better known as AZT, as a therapy for AIDS, observed that rapid research results on a drug to combat AIDS was one more spin-off of investment in cancer research funded by the National Cancer Act of 1971. The program had made the National Cancer Institute "a 'pharmaceutical company' working for the public, in difficult areas where the private sector either could not or would not make a commitment. Ironically, one of the drugs synthesized for the National Cancer Institute was done by Jerome Horowitz under an NCI grant working at what was then called the Detroit Cancer Institute. . . . AZT . . . was initially created and tested as a possible anti-cancer drug."[11]

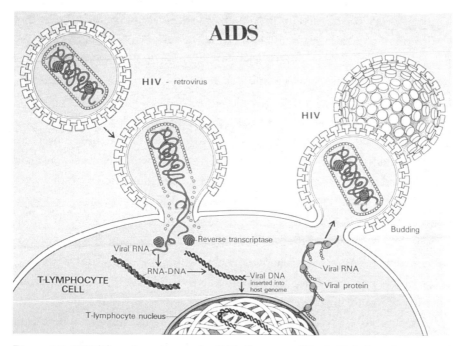

Figure 5.2. HIV life cycle as known in 1987. *Courtesy of Trudy Nicholson for National Cancer Institutes Visuals Online.*

AZT: The First Partially Effective Therapy for Treating AIDS

Before the advent of AIDS, Samuel Broder had spent a sizable portion of his career working on the relationship of immunology to cancer in the laboratory of Thomas Waldmann, chief of the Metabolism Branch. As mentioned in chapter 3, Waldmann treated the first AIDS patient to arrive at the NIH Clinical Center, and Broder was among the physicians who saw firsthand the immune devastation in this young man, even though Broder had already left Waldmann's branch. In an oral history, Broder noted that this patient was "a walking synopsis of what AIDS turned out to be. . . . I remember saying . . . that we had never seen anything like this before, and I hope we never see anything like this again."[12] Of course, that patient was only the first of many that Broder saw.

In 1980 Broder had been promoted to head the Clinical Oncology Program in NCI, and hence he had both a research laboratory and a clinic of patients with whom he worked looking for drugs that could potentially be used to treat cancer. He felt responsible as an NCI physician to observe pathological phenomena in patients and to take that knowledge to the laboratory immediately to attempt to develop therapies to address those problems. At the urging of Vincent T. DeVita, the director of NCI, Broder decided to turn his laboratory's work toward identifying a possible drug therapy for AIDS. At NCI, Broder's principal colleagues in the AIDS drug discovery effort were Robert Yarchoan, who previously had worked as a clinical associate on the humoral immune system in the Metabolism Branch in the laboratory next door to Broder, and Hiroaki "Mitch" Mitsuya, who had been a postdoctoral fellow with Broder and who "could grow anything in tissue culture" (figure 5.3).[13] Yarchoan observed, "Sam often described our group as a SWAT team, by which he meant a small, very focused group of people, rather than a large, bureaucratic program."[14]

In a detailed oral history, Yarchoan described the step-by-step process by which the team brainstormed techniques to determine quantitatively if a drug was actually working and not just toxic to cells. They consulted with other virologists and immunologists about possible candidate drugs and negotiated the legal process to write a protocol, get it approved by an institutional review board (a committee that oversees all human-subject research at a medical center), use established NCI infrastructure to obtain an investigational new drug (IND) approval from the Food and Drug Administration, and initiate the study. The drug they chose initially, suramin, had previously been shown to be a po-

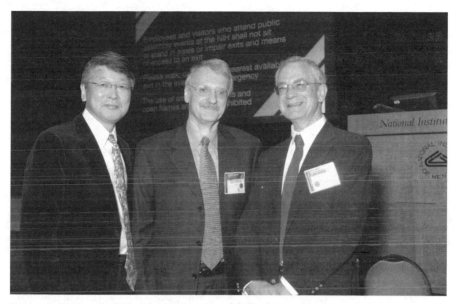

Figure 5.3. Hiroaki "Mitch" Mitsuya, Samuel Broder, and Robert Yarchoan, the team that developed AZT and ddI, at a retrospective symposium on AIDS research at the National Cancer Institute, November 1–2, 2007. *Courtesy of the National Cancer Institute, photograph by Bill Branson.*

tent antiretroviral agent and had already been tested against river blindness in Africa. This meant that they were able to skip the initial in vitro (in a test tube) screening and safety tests in animals because these had already been conducted for the earlier study. Unfortunately, the results from their clinical study showed that suramin simply was not effective against AIDS.[15]

In 1984 the enormity of the threat AIDS posed was brought home to these researchers when they read the results of Robert Gallo's laboratory's first assay for the AIDS virus. Gallo had used serum from a cohort of "relatively monogamous" gay men in the District of Columbia who were being studied by immunologist Gene Shearer to try to figure out how AIDS was destroying the immune system. Some 60 to 70 percent of these men tested positive for antibodies to the AIDS virus. Yarchoan

did a rough mental calculation of the number of gays in the country and the percentage who were likely to be HIV-infected, and estimating that there were half a million to a million people infected with this lethal virus

who did not know it. . . . I could not go out there and give a news conference saying that a lot of people are going to die and that it is a real crisis.
But it was a very weird moment for me, feeling that I was privy to this
information that had not perked through people's consciousness yet.[16]

The burden of this understanding increased the urgency to find some therapy that would slow or halt the disease.

As the drug research work began, Broder asked Mitsuya to develop an assay to show whether or not a drug was working in a test tube—the first stage
in drug research. Mitsuya consulted with Mikulas Popovic in Robert Gallo's
laboratory to learn the difficult techniques of growing T cells in culture. "These
T cells are very difficult to grow," stated Robert Yarchoan. "You almost have to
talk to them."[17] Working after hours so that his colleagues did not have to fear
exposure to the AIDS virus at a time when no one knew exactly how contagious
it might be, Mitsuya developed a highly sensitive cell line that died upon infection with HIV but remained viable if a candidate drug suppressed the virus and
was not toxic to the cells.[18] Broder was interested in establishing a partnership
with a commercial drug company to pursue research on an AIDS therapy. Duke
University virologist Dani Bolognesi arranged a meeting between Broder and
officials of the Burroughs Wellcome Company. Broder said, "I explained what
our capacity was in terms of clinical trials and essentially offered a collaboration with them, with the promise that we would, whatever came up, develop
drugs as fast as we could and that they would get a product out of it. There was
no other way to encourage pharmaceutical companies. They were not the only
company that I visited, but to their credit, they were the first to make a serious
commitment."[19]

In the early 1980s Burroughs Wellcome, which was "heavily involved in
antimicrobial research," decided to review the shelved anticancer drug AZT
for possible use against some bacteria. During the 1970s a German group had
shown AZT to suppress retroviruses that infected murine animals (rodents that
include mice and rats). In February 1985 the NCI-Duke-Wellcome collaboration began, and using Mitsuya's cell line, the investigators were able to demonstrate that AZT had "significant" in vitro activity against the AIDS virus. They
knew that AZT suppressed the function of the enzyme reverse transcriptase in
the HIV life cycle.[20]

With this finding, bringing AZT therapy to AIDS patients took on a sense of urgency never before experienced in the U.S. drug development regimen.[21] Normally, a candidate drug took more than eight years to undergo the clinical testing required to complete FDA review before being approved for marketing (see figure 5.4 for the steps involved). The FDA approved AZT in March 1987, a little over two years after it was first shown to be active in the test tube.[22] At last, after four years of watching patients suffer and die with no effective way to address the underlying immune deficiency, the medical community, not to mention AIDS patients and their supporters, grasped at this first promising drug.

The timetables for advancing AZT through the evaluation process were condensed as much as humanly possible. The in vitro studies were positive in March 1985. On June 15, Burroughs Wellcome, with the collaboration of NCI, presented the necessary animal toxicity data to the FDA along with an application for an IND exemption. The FDA granted the IND seven days later. On July 3, 1985, Yarchoan and Broder administered the first dose of AZT to an AIDS patient on the phase I trial. Phase I trials are used to establish dosage levels, and the thirty-five patients in this trial, which was conducted at the NIH and Duke University Medical Center, were given increasingly potent doses. Although phase I trials are not intended to measure efficacy (how well the drug works), some immunologic and even clinical improvement was noted in patients, as was some toxicity as the dosages increased. Also, physicians observed that AZT crossed the blood-brain barrier, which meant that it might be effective in reversing AIDS-related dementia.[23]

In the fall of 1985 a phase II trial began to evaluate the efficacy and safety of AZT in treating AIDS. Phase II trials enroll more patients in more places to determine whether a drug works and is safe. A somewhat controversial choice was made by Burroughs Wellcome to utilize the most rigorous form of trial: a placebo-controlled, double-blind trial. In such a trial one group of patients is randomly given a placebo, an inert substance such as sugar and often called a sugar pill, while a second group of patients is given the drug under study. The trial is double-blind, meaning that neither the patients nor the medical personnel administering the medications know which patients get the placebo and which get the candidate drug. While the trial was taking place, the Data and Safety Monitoring Board (DSMB), composed of AIDS experts not directly involved in the study, periodically reviewed the patient data being generated "in

Process of Bringing a Drug to Market

1. Laboratory *in vitro* tests and computer modeling.

2. Animal testing (mainly rodents) for toxicity.

3. Trial designed, reviewed, and approved by Institutional Review Board and FDA or other national regulatory body

4. Phase I human test: small number of human volunteers given drug to test for safety and establish proper dosage.

5. Phase II human test: relatively small number of human patients given drug to test for efficacy and toxic side effects.

6. Phase III human test: large number of human patients given drug to establish efficacy in large population and identify potential negative side effects.

7. Drug licensed after data on previous studies reviewed and found acceptable.

8. Phase IV human test: ongoing monitoring of patients taking drug to determine even longer-term efficacy and danger from rare toxic side effects.

Figure 5.4. Process of bringing a drug to market. *Adapted from U.S. National Institutes of Health, "Understanding Clinical Trials," September 20, 2007, http://clinicaltrials.gov/ct2/info/understand.*

order to identify significant trends, good or bad," that would indicate that the study should be stopped or continued. On September 19, 1986, the DSMB stated that those patients receiving AZT "had a significantly higher survival rate" than those receiving a placebo. Only one of the 145 patients receiving AZT had died, compared with 19 of 137 patients on a placebo. Those treated with AZT also had "a decreased number of opportunistic infections and demonstrated weight gain, increased CD4 cell count, and improved immune response." Some patients, however, were not able to receive the full recommended dose because of drug toxicity. Nonetheless, the DSMB recommended that the trial be stopped and all the patients on a placebo be given AZT, because to withhold it in the light of these data would be unethical.[24]

At this point, Burroughs Wellcome, in collaboration with officials at the FDA, NCI, NIAID, CDC, and PHS, developed a protocol to permit patients access to AZT under what is called a treatment IND (treatment investigational new drug). In short order, they developed a plan to administer the treatment IND. They addressed the question of how to get patient-monitoring data from physicians not accustomed to participating in clinical trials as well as the more politically charged question of which patients would get the drug (AZT was in scarce supply). The latter question was decided on the basis of which patients had the greatest need. For enrollees in the trial, Burroughs Wellcome provided AZT free of charge to the patient's pharmacy. The treatment IND, it should be emphasized, was not a clinical trial itself. It was an effort to provide patient access to AZT, and it "represented one of the largest distributions of an unapproved drug ever undertaken."[25]

By December 2, 1986, Burroughs Wellcome had submitted a new drug application to market AZT to the FDA. This was unprecedented, as no phase III, or large-scale, trial had been conducted to provide a reliable base of data on which to conclude that AZT was safe and effective. When toxicities appeared in subsequent years, scientists in the federal government and Burroughs Wellcome as a commercial firm came under fire for marketing it so quickly. But the clarity of hindsight obscured the conviction held by members of the FDA advisory committee who approved the release of AZT that "circumstances surrounding AIDS were unique." By a ten to one vote, the committee recommended that AZT be approved, and the FDA acted on the recommendation on March 19, 1987, releasing it for public sale by Burroughs Wellcome under the trade name Retrovir. By 1989 the results of longer term studies showed that AZT clearly prolonged life for people at all stages of HIV infection, from those showing no symptoms to those with full-blown AIDS. With these findings, the commercial market for AZT mushroomed.

Almost immediately, an outcry erupted when Burroughs Wellcome set the wholesale price of the drug at $188 for a hundred capsules. Patients needed to take two capsules every four hours every day for the rest of their lives, thus a hundred capsules would last seventeen days, and a year's supply of AZT would cost $8,000 to $10,000, depending on the profit margin charged by the dispensing pharmacy. Since Wellcome had provided the drug free of charge during the trial and treatment IND, and since AZT was the only medically approved hope for AIDS patients, AIDS activists protested that Burroughs Wellcome was "profiteering" on the misery and death the disease caused. As economist Peter S. Arno has pointed out, Burroughs Wellcome's strongest justification for the high price was its expectation that other antiviral medications would soon follow, "which meant that the company had a year, two at the most, to recoup its research and development costs."[26] As it happened, however, the next two drugs for AIDS were not approved until 1991 and then used primarily in combination with AZT.

Perhaps the most galling aspect of Burroughs Wellcome's price tag for AZT was that taxpayers had essentially funded development of the drug but had no control over the pricing. Burroughs Wellcome always emphasized its exclusive role in bringing the drug to market and claimed to have incurred substantial research costs in a risky endeavor to develop this drug. In fact, as noted above, AZT had been originally synthesized by an academic researcher funded by an NIH grant; its antiretroviral properties had been first described by German investigators; the assay to identify its activity against HIV was developed at NCI, and it was tested and found active against HIV at NCI; and the initial clinical trial was conducted at the NIH Clinical Center and via an NIH-funded grant at Duke University. In addition, Burroughs Wellcome was given tax breaks when AZT was designated an "orphan drug," meaning that it might be used for only a very small number of patients. The outrage from AIDS activists over the cost of AZT prodded Burroughs Wellcome to reduce the price by 20 percent by the end of 1987.[27]

Very quickly, two lines of attack began to help lower the price further for AIDS patients. First were the political actions taken by ACT UP. On April 25, 1989, nine ACT UP members eluded security at Burroughs Wellcome headquarters in Research Triangle Park, North Carolina, and barricaded themselves into a room on the executive floor. The carefully planned action included cell phones for outside communication, food and water, equipment to chain themselves to a radiator, and supporters alerting the media and helping reporters communicate with the embattled group. The activists demanded that Burroughs Wellcome drop the price of AZT by 25 percent and provide a "genuine" corporate subsidy for those who needed the drug but could not pay for it.[28]

By August, when Burroughs Wellcome had taken no action beyond promising to review costs at some time in the future, ACT UP decided to stage another meticulously plotted political action. On September 14, 1989, ACT UP infiltrated the New York Stock Exchange. After the activists chained themselves to the banister of the VIP landing, they unfurled a banner, "Sell Wellcome," and tossed fake $100 bills stating "We die while you play business" to the traders below. As a result of the intense demonstrations, Burroughs Wellcome further reduced the cost of AZT to approximately $6,500 per year for individuals.[29]

These actions drew media attention to the issue and, as ACT UP had hoped, also boosted legal efforts to challenge the Burroughs Wellcome patent. Samuel Broder at the National Cancer Institute was livid that Wellcome dismissed the contributions of multiple people working for or funded by the U.S. government and claimed sole rights to the patent. Broder convinced the government to probe the AZT patent issue, but since Broder and his colleagues had been involved in development before passage of the 1986 Technology Transfer Act, and because they believed that Burroughs Wellcome was a pharmaceutical "partner" with whom they were developing AZT, they had not filed a patent claim on behalf of the government. Broder later admitted that he had been "somewhat naïve in dealing with Burroughs Wellcome." After the probe, however, the federal government did not follow up and file a lawsuit. No one within the pro-business administration of President George H. W. Bush wished to challenge a corporation in court, and the NIH was not willing to do so without support from the White House.[30]

Eventually, two challenges to the AZT patent were brought to court. The advocacy group Public Citizen made the first. Burroughs Wellcome itself brought the second as a breach of patent suit in response to the announcement by two drug companies, Barr Laboratories of Pomona, New York, and Novo pharm Ltd. of Toronto, Canada, that they would submit applications to the FDA to market generic versions of AZT. The patent challengers argued that NIH scientists should have been named inventors on the patent. NIH was not a party to the suit, although it did agree to license the drug to Barr if the company's lawsuit was successful. Broder, Yarchoan, and Mitsuya were deposed for days by Burroughs Wellcome lawyers who denigrated their efforts repeatedly and maintained the Burroughs Wellcome claim that it alone had a right to the patent. The suit dragged on until November 1994, when the U.S. Court of Appeals for the Federal Circuit ruled in favor of Burroughs Wellcome on all the claims except the ability of AZT to increase CD4 counts. This claim was sent back to the lower court but was not pursued further.[31] The Supreme Court was asked to take the case, but against the advice of NIH, the Justice Department asked that it be dropped. Burroughs Wellcome—which in 2000, through a series of mergers, became GlaxoSmithKline—retained a monopoly on AZT until 2005, when the patent expired.[32]

Treatment for Pediatric and Adolescent AIDS

As with virtually all drugs, initial testing of AZT was conducted on adults, since minor children are considered unable to give informed consent, and research on children must proceed via consent given by their parents or guardians.[33] This means, however, that most new drugs are available for adults well before pediatricians can access them for use in children and adolescents. Since 1982, however, physicians had been diagnosing babies and children with AIDS. By 1986 articles were appearing in journals about the course of AIDS in children and adolescents.[34] In 1987, shortly after the FDA approved AZT for marketing, pediatric oncologist Phillip Pizzo at the National Cancer Institute began a pediatric AIDS program, and pediatric-adolescent physician Karen Hein in New York City launched the first AIDS program focusing on adolescents.[35] Young children and adolescents presented unique problems for physicians treating AIDS patients. For example, the incubation period for infants was much shorter—one to three years—than for adults, and 50 to 90 percent of them presented with disorders in the brain. Pediatric AIDS also raised ethical issues for physicians and the larger society, such as whether children without parents to give consent for them had a right to participate in potentially beneficial clinical trials. Another issue was whether and, if so, how society would care for children with AIDS from the most socially disadvantaged segments of society.[36] In addition to these issues, adolescents who were runaways or homeless were the most vulnerable to becoming infected with HIV and hardest for the medical community to reach.[37]

New Drugs in the AZT Class

After AZT, additional reverse transcriptase inhibitor drugs were developed in the Broder lab, underwent clinical testing at the NIH, and after further testing, were approved by the FDA. Since NIH initially did not have pharmaceutical partners for these drugs, the NIH scientists filed patents on them, and the U.S. government licensed them to pharmaceutical companies. Dideoxycytidine (ddC) and dideoxyinosine (ddI), which also inhibited the reverse transcription activity but at different points in cell division, were two of many drugs eventually developed in this class. With the availability of more than one drug, the NCI scientists were able to start exploring combination regimens. Robert Yarchoan described how he and others on the Broder team at NCI worked out the most effective regimen for using the drugs.

> We found that people did much better combining the two drugs simultaneously at half dose rather than alternating the two at full dose. Over a period of time, people got the same dose of both drugs, but the way that the drugs were given made a big difference. . . . The thymidine-based drugs such as AZT work better in replicating cells because they are better metabolized to the active form. At the same time, ddI works somewhat better in resting cells. If we combined the two of them together, we were hitting both cell populations. And we found some patients that, after over a year on simultaneous AZT and ddI, still had CD4 counts that were higher than when they started. So we had gone from twenty weeks of benefit to well over a year.[38]

In 1989, as Sam Broder and colleagues published the promising results from a phase I trial of ddI, several new approaches to therapeutic AIDS drugs could be seen. First, to avoid the kind of battle over patent rights that AZT had caused, Broder, Mitsuya, and Yarchoan filed government patents for the drug with the three of them as inventors. This, they hoped, would provide them some ethical and legal control over the eventual price set by Bristol-Myers-Squibb, the pharmaceutical company to which the drug was licensed for development. A clause stipulating that ddI be sold at a "reasonable price" was added to the licensing contract. The definition of the term "reasonable price" was not detailed, but the government believed that it provided grounds for revoking the exclusive license if the company tried to set the price too high.

Second, issues surrounding the process for bringing a drug to market were addressed, but not without revealing the tensions always present between bureaucratic agencies in the government and the ethical concerns surrounding access to drugs for severely ill patients. The FDA was charged with ensuring that new drugs sold to the public had been demonstrated safe and effective. A long history of catastrophes had preceded this authority. For example, in 1901, before any regulations existed, a company allowed diphtheria antiserum to be contaminated with tetanus organisms; thirteen children died.[39] In 1937 more than a hundred people, mostly children, died when the new "miracle drug" sulfanilamide, which cured streptococcal infections, was distributed (without any safety testing) dissolved in easy-to-swallow but poisonous liquid diethylene glycol, a chemical relative of antifreeze.[40] In 1962 a huge disaster was barely avoided in the United States when an FDA drug reviewer refused to approve the drug thalidomide, which was widely used in Europe to calm pregnant women and only later shown to be the cause of severe birth defects for their babies.[41] These tragedies spurred the passage of laws that required drug companies to present data showing that their drugs were safe and effective before marketing. The principal mechanism to produce "gold-standard" quality data for drugs, developed in the 1940s and 1950s, was the double-blind, placebo-controlled clinical trial, like the one used initially in AZT research.[42]

The advent of AIDS, however, stressed this system severely because people facing death from AIDS were willing to take a chance on any drug that looked promising. They did not have time to wait for the many years necessary to bring a drug through the FDA review process. From the earliest days of the epidemic, patients and their advocates took whatever steps they could to obtain treatments that might be helpful.[43] In July 1985, for example, Rock Hudson chartered a plane to get to Paris, where the Pasteur Institute was researching a potential AIDS drug called HPA-23, later shown to be ineffective. Activists in California regularly organized trips to Mexico, where the unapproved drugs ribavirin and isoprinosine were sold over the counter. In 1985 a food product called AL-721 became a treatment of interest, only to be shown ineffective against HIV as well. In 1986 activist John S. James launched *AIDS Treatment News* to report on "experimental and standard treatments, especially those available now."[44]

Unproven and Quack Therapies

Chronic diseases and diseases whose cause is unknown are fertile fields for those who would profit from offering unproved therapies. Whether well-meaning or outright quacks, people touting all sorts of therapies for cancer, for degenerative diseases, and certainly for AIDS played on patients' fear of death and willingness to grasp at any possible therapy, however improbable.[45] With AIDS, such treatments appeared almost as soon as the disease was identified and remain widespread today. The antiregulatory political mood of the conservative 1980s fed into mistrust of the FDA's drug approval process, furthermore, and thereby abetted those who purveyed alternative AIDS therapies.

Historian James Harvey Young noted that the earliest deceptive therapies for AIDS were offshoots of questionable cancer therapies. A Dr. Lawrence Burton offered "immunoaugmentative" cancer therapy in the Bahamas, and he soon began to offer the same therapy for AIDS. An unfortunate outcome of Burton's offering was that the blood serum he used for the therapy was infected with the AIDS virus.[46] After a virus that destroyed the immune system was identified as the cause of AIDS, however, most fraudulent therapies turned toward "safeguarding" and "restoring" the immune system to protect or heal people from AIDS. Special diets, intravenous infusions of vitamins, implantation of cells from unborn donor animals, and rectal administration of ozone were a few examples of quack remedies.[47] On the Internet, fraudulent AIDS therapies still advertise while sites about quackery and informational sites about AIDS include articles warning HIV-infected people against fake therapies.[48]

Tensions over FDA Approval of AIDS Drugs

The muddled effort to get approval for ganciclovir as a treatment of an infection that caused blindness in people with AIDS most clearly reveals the stark ethical differences in the FDA's responsibility to ensure safe, efficacious drugs, NIAID's responsibility to organize and conduct rigorous clinical trials to generate the needed data showing that the drug was safe and effective, and activists' demands to gain access to the drug before it had cleared the bureaucracy. In chapter 3, we followed the case of Ron Resio, who participated in one of the earliest AIDS clinical studies at the NIH in Bethesda between 1982 and 1983, as Anthony Fauci and Clifford Lane attempted to understand what was happening in his body and construct intervention strategies to help him. One of the opportunistic infections that struck Resio was CMV retinitis, a disease in which a virus in the herpes family normally kept in check by the immune system attacks and destroys the retina of the eye, rendering its victim blind. Going blind was one of the worst fears that terrorized AIDS patients. Fauci called in Robert B. Nussenblatt and Alan Palestine of the National Eye Institute to consult on the problem, but they were not able to stop or reverse the CMV infection before Resio died.[49]

By 1983 Syntex, the California company that had synthesized ganciclovir in 1980, had concluded that the drug would suppress, though not eliminate, CMV and thereby prevent blindness if used indefinitely. In 1984 Syntex "alerted the FDA to ganciclovir's promise and asked for permission to distribute it without charge until testing and marketing could get under way." Physicians treating AIDS patients rapidly adopted ganciclovir because it worked so well, and confirming the adage that "no good deed goes unpunished," this led to a situation in which it was almost impossible for the FDA to license the drug via its rigorous approval process.[50]

In *Against the Odds: The Story of AIDS Drug Development, Politics, and Profits,* Peter Arno and Karyn Feiden detail the Byzantine twists and turns in the story of bringing ganciclovir to market. The largest hurdle was the FDA's requirement that rigorous clinical trial data be submitted in support of a drug's application. A battle over the patent with Burroughs Wellcome delayed submission of a new drug application until 1987, when Syntex won and Burroughs Wellcome ceased producing its version of the drug. By this time, the drug was in wide use under the compassionate-use distribution system. No physician or patient was willing to participate in a placebo-controlled trial when patients receiving the placebo would go blind and the drug was already available. Syntex thus submitted its application with data collected under the compassionate-use program. These data, however, were not of the rigorous quality the FDA demanded, and an advisory committee voted to reject the application, even as committee members agreed that the drug was effective.

Anthony Fauci summarized the situation: "Those of us who used the drug know it works, that data isn't sufficient to prove it works, you have to do a clinical trial, nobody wants to be on the clinical trial because they know the drug works."[51] Trying to address the classic catch-22 situation, Syntex proposed a compromise trial to obtain rigorous data. Only patients with CMV retinitis on the periphery of the retina, where sight was not yet affected, would be recruited for the trial, and if the disease progressed in the least, those on placebo would be given ganciclovir immediately. This good idea was quickly demolished by three bioethicists, all of whom stated that such a trial was unethical because it put patients at risk when an effective therapy was known.

On October 11, 1988, the fury of AIDS activists boiled over in a demonstration at the Rockville, Maryland, home of FDA offices. More than a thousand protesters chanted, "Shame, shame, shame! No more deaths!" More than 170 people were arrested. ACT UP's members carefully planned their visual aids for TV coverage. Protesters held signs showing bloody handprints saying, "The government has blood on its hands!" They wore black T-shirts bearing the bright pink triangle and words "SILENCE = DEATH," the logo for ACT UP.[52]

The only possible way to obtain the needed data was for Syntex to withdraw ganciclovir from availability until a rigorous trial could be conducted but to allow those patients whose sight was imminently at risk to receive the drug under a treatment IND. Physicians and patients adamantly opposed such a move, however, so Syntex continued its compassionate-use distribution. By this time—1989—ganciclovir had been distributed in the United States for five years and had been approved for marketing in eleven other countries, but it was still not a drug approved for the U.S. market.[53] This untenable situation was eventually sorted out through a discussion between Fauci and Frank Young, the FDA commissioner. Young agreed that the Syntex's NDA could be reconsidered, and at another meeting, the FDA's advisory committee chose to accept data that previously had been considered insufficient. On June 27, 1989, the FDA finally approved ganciclovir for marketing.

The ganciclovir approval debacle illuminated several conundrums facing drug regulation in the United States. At first glance, it would seem to be common sense that a drug so obviously useful as ganciclovir should be approved and licensed despite lack of rigorous clinical trials. Most applications for new drugs, however, are presented on the basis that they appear safe and efficacious, yet neither safety nor efficacy is often proven until long-term trials are conducted. The dire side effects of thalidomide have stood as a cautionary tale for the FDA, which might have approved the drug had it not been for Frances Kelsey's "stubborn" refusal to release it from the bureaucracy because of troubling animal study data. Long-term studies can also show that other drugs, even those long used, do not provide the value promised by their costs. In August 2010, for example, physicians presented data at a heart disease conference in China that some brand-name drugs long used to lower blood pressure provided no effect superior to generic diuretic drugs.[54] From the FDA's standpoint, AIDS drug approval was moving faster than approval of drugs for any other disease. From the standpoint of people with AIDS, who were facing death or blindness, long-term studies were a luxury they had no time to indulge.

The second impact of the ganciclovir muddle was the message it sent to drug companies: they should not make drugs available for compassionate use until after clinical trials that would permit the company to apply for FDA approval had been conducted. This message angered AIDS activists, especially over handling of another drug, foscarnet, which showed promise of being effective against CMV retinitis without depressing bone marrow in patients also taking AZT, a major drawback of ganciclovir. A Swedish company, Astra Pharmaceutical Products, held the patent on foscarnet, and it planned to avoid Syntex's problem with ganciclovir by constructing a trial that would produce "pure" data on foscarnet's effectiveness. The trial's protocol thus stipulated that no one who had ever taken ganciclovir could join the trial of foscarnet. Such a rule was unnecessary, since ganciclovir is completely eliminated from the body within twenty-four hours of taking it, but Astra decided to study only a population who had never taken any drug for CMV retinitis before foscarnet.[55]

Terry Sutton, a San Francisco AIDS activist and person with AIDS, fell into the group excluded from foscarnet trials, and he decided to protest. Sutton had taken himself off AZT in order to take ganciclovir to stave off blindness from CMV retinitis but desperately wanted to participate in a foscarnet trial so that he might resume taking AZT. To draw attention to what he and other AIDS activists perceived as callus disregard of patient needs, Sutton led a group of activists in a sit-in at San Francisco General Hospital, blocking access to the pharmacy and demanding access to the drug. Subsequently, the activists staged a protest that shut down the Golden Gate Bridge at the height of rush hour. These actions garnered media attention but failed to move Astra Pharmaceuticals. On April 11, 1989, Sutton died, and his death, followed by more ACT UP demonstrations in his honor, won FDA support to pressure Astra to make foscarnet more available via a treatment IND. The company grudgingly complied but made the eligibility requirements so strict—for example, physicians were required to complete a seventy-six-page report form for each patient—that few patients were still able to obtain the drug. An NDA was submitted to FDA and approved on September 27, 1991. Patients could then buy the drug legally at a cost of $21,000 per year.[56]

Parallel Track

In 1989, as the ganciclovir debacle was coming to a close and the foscarnet trials were beginning, Anthony Fauci, who had been designated as the major spokesperson on AIDS within the U.S. government, met with ACT UP activists in New York City. He listened to the activists' concerns about better access to promising drugs, especially an idea supported by ACT UP's Jim Eigo and Project Inform's Martin Delaney called the "parallel track." At the June 1989 International AIDS Conference in Montreal, Fauci discussed the proposal with ACT UP's Larry Kramer. Kramer, the most angry and outspoken of AIDS activists, had called Fauci an "incompetent idiot" in a newspaper article, but he was pleased to learn about Fauci's endorsement of the parallel-track concept. Parallel track differed from the existing FDA treatment IND in that drugs that would be made available via parallel track were those specifically for HIV/AIDS. They would also be made available earlier in the process.

Implementing the parallel track caused some heated discussion between the FDA, which believed that its treatment INDs fulfilled the activists' needs, and NIAID, which was focused on ensuring that patients entered clinical trials so that reliable data would be generated for making decisions on new drugs. As it turned out, only one drug, another reverse transcriptase inhibitor called d4T and marketed as stavudine, was ever made available via the parallel-track mechanism. The more important aspect of the program, however, was the bridge built between AIDS activists and Anthony Fauci's NIAID. FDA officials had also met with activists but had been less successful in gaining their trust and cooperation, largely because the FDA was legally obliged to follow the law and regulations pertaining to drugs being reviewed and thus had no flexibility in the face of activist demands that they move faster. Fauci's initiative resulted in the activists' coming to believe that federal government officials would listen, make them a part of the process of looking for solutions to AIDS, and take steps to provide compassionate access for patients with no other options.[57]

The AIDS Denialists

In the midst of protests about the cost of AZT and the growing evidence that the drug worked for only a short time and had toxic side effects, a distinguished molecular virologist published a theory that HIV was not the cause of AIDS.[58] Peter Duesberg earned his PhD in chemistry at the University of Frankfurt and

garnered scientific acclaim in the 1970s through his work identifying and mapping the first true oncogene, *src*, from the genetic material of the Rous sarcoma
virus, a retrovirus that caused cancer in chickens.[59] In 1986 he was elected to the
National Academy of Sciences.

The following year Duesberg published his original criticism of HIV in
a paper titled "Retroviruses as Carcinogens and Pathogens: Expectations and
Reality." The title itself indicates that Duesberg's arguments were not limited to
the AIDS agent but encompassed all retroviruses that do not possess transforming *onc*, or cancer-causing, genes. "Retroviruses without *onc* genes," Duesberg
wrote, are "the most common and benign passenger viruses of healthy animals
and humans."[60] He argued that HIV is likely such a passenger virus with no
significant pathological effect.

Duesberg elaborated his arguments in a second paper published in the *Proceedings of the National Academy of Sciences of the United States of America*, and
in 1988 the journal *Science* published a policy forum in which Duesberg and his
critics summarized their arguments.[61] In 1997 Duesberg also published a book,
Inventing the AIDS Virus, explaining his arguments in a public forum.[62] Despite
all of his strongly worded assertion that HIV did not cause AIDS, Duesberg had
never conducted research on AIDS. He was not a physician, so he never treated
an AIDS patient or gathered epidemiological data from patients.

It seems highly unusual that a distinguished bench scientist would wade
into the world of human disease and make claims that stood to affect life and
death for AIDS patients with no more experience than Duesberg had with the
disease. It should be noted, however, that AIDS was not the only field of science
about which Duesberg had made unusual claims. Shortly after his pioneering
work on retroviral oncogenes was recognized, Duesberg declared that retroviruses did not cause cancer after all. Instead, he began to conduct research on
an older theory, aneuploidy, based on an abnormality in chromosomes, as the
cause of cancer.[63]

A major element in Duesberg's objection to HIV as the cause of AIDS was
that the virus, in his judgment, failed to satisfy Koch's postulates (see chapter
2, figure 2.7, for statement of Koch's postulates). Duesberg argued that HIV is
in violation of Koch's postulate stating that the virus must be found in all cases
of the disease because it was not possible to detect free virus, provirus, or viral
RNA in all cases of AIDS. HIV also failed to meet a second postulate, he said,

because it could not be isolated from 20 to 50 percent of AIDS cases. Countering his arguments in the *Science* policy forum were William Blattner and Robert Gallo of the U.S. National Cancer Institute and Howard Temin of the University of Wisconsin–Madison—all three distinguished investigators.

Representing the large number of mainstream scientists who rebutted Duesberg's arguments, Blattner, Gallo, and Temin responded that both detection and isolation of the virus were hampered by the limitations from 1984 to 1988 of existing laboratory methods and that increasingly sensitive tests showed HIV infection "in essentially all AIDS patients."[64]

Duesberg also contended that HIV was in violation of Koch's postulate requiring the reproduction of disease in an animal model because "pure HIV does not reproduce AIDS when inoculated into chimpanzees or accidentally into healthy humans." The opposing scientists easily rebutted the chimpanzee portion of this argument, noting that "most viruses are species-specific in host range and in capacity to produce disease." They contended, furthermore, that HIV "does indeed cause AIDS when inoculated into humans" who have no underlying medical condition that might also account for the resulting immunodeficiency. "Accidental needlestick injuries with HIV-contaminated needles," they stated, "have resulted in HIV seroconversion and then clinical AIDS." This is true, but Duesberg's assertion that not every needlestick resulted in seroconversion is also true. In medicine, however, it is well known that host defense mechanisms vary—that is, that some people have strong immune systems that can fend off infections while others have weakened immune systems and get sick when they encounter a virus. No disease organism produces frank infection in every contact with every potential host.

In addition to the arguments based on Koch's postulates, Duesberg stated that it is paradoxical for HIV to cause AIDS only after the immune system has mounted a response to the infection, arguing that all other viruses are most pathogenic before an immune response is detected. He also asserted that the long incubation period, up to eight years or more, is bizarre for a virus that replicates in one or two days. In this argument, Duesberg appeared to be suggesting that HIV and other new retroviruses follow a specifically defined, disease-inducing process. Blattner, Gallo, and Temin countered with the observation that many viruses are pathogenic after immunity appears, and many have long and variable latent periods.

Mainstream scientists bolstered their case for HIV as the cause of AIDS in this *Science* policy forum with epidemiological evidence gained since the 1984 papers from Gallo's laboratory that convinced the scientific community that HIV caused AIDS. They noted that in every group studied prospectively, positive seroconversion was followed by progressive immunodeficiency and clinical AIDS "in a predictable sequence." Finally, they argued that interruption of HIV transmission by screening donated blood for HIV antibodies halted the further incidence of AIDS in blood transfusion recipients. "Scientists conclude," they state, "that a virus causes a disease if the virus is consistently associated with the disease and if disruption of transmission of the virus prevents occurrence of the disease." In logical terms: without HIV there is no AIDS.

Because of the status Duesberg enjoyed as a member of the National Academy of Sciences, he drew support for his theory from many people with AIDS and their supporters who were disenchanted with AZT therapy because of its toxicity, its cost, or its inability to cure patients outright. In addition, as we shall see in chapter 6, some journalists and scholars viewed mainstream scientists as a cabal intent on retaining power over research funds at the expense of anyone who dared to disagree with them.

In the 2009 book *Denying AIDS: Conspiracy Theories, Pseudoscience, and Human Tragedy,* psychologist Seth Kalichman described the characteristics AIDS denialists hold in common with other denialist groups, such as Holocaust deniers and climate-change denialists.[65] A dogmatic and religious rigidity about their beliefs and paranoia that others are out to deny them freedom of speech lead them to continue repeating their arguments no matter how many times they have been refuted. AIDS denialists also desire to undermine public belief in mainstream science. As we shall see in chapter 8, in cultures where their views have gained currency, the death toll from AIDS has been enormous.

The most impressive support for Duesberg's ideas came from a number of prominent scientists, most of whom, however, were not trained in medicine. Nobel laureate Kary Mullis, a chemist and inventor of the polymerase chain reaction, supported Duesberg's HIV denialism as well as his own climate-change denialism and belief in astrology.[66] Robert Root-Bernstein, a physiologist and MacArthur Fellowship winner, also questioned the HIV-AIDS link.[67] New York physician Joseph Sonnabend, who treated many of the earliest cases of AIDS and strongly propounded the "safe sex" message, was pulled into the Duesberg camp because of his concern over the toxicity of AZT. He preferred the idea of a multifactorial cause of AIDS.[68] A full list of those supporting Duesberg was posted on the website Virusmyth. The most striking thing about the people and their writings in support of AIDS denialism on this website is that virtually all predate 1996.

Highly Active Antiretroviral Therapy

What happened in 1996 that made many former supporters stop considering the Duesberg hypothesis as plausible and made even those luminaries like Mullis, Root-Bernstein, and Sonnabend distance themselves from the anti-HIV thesis? The answer closely mirrors the public response to the first use of diphtheria antitoxin in 1891. Emil von Behring's use of diphtheria antitoxin converted skeptics of the germ theory of infectious diseases to believers when they saw dying patients recover before their eyes. In 1996 development of a new class of drugs allowed the creation of a highly active combination AIDS therapy that similarly enabled people with the disease to resume normal lives. Nothing convinces people that a disease theory is correct like the living proof offered by an effective therapy: thousands of people who were dying are once again on their feet, going to work, and living normal lives.

Although highly active antiretroviral therapy (HAART) seemed to burst upon the scene in 1996, the development of the new drug class that made it possible began about 1986, when AZT was just being introduced to combat AIDS.[69] One of the major problems with AZT or even two-drug therapy was that it could not completely suppress HIV replication. As the virus continued to replicate in the drugs' presence, it developed resistance to them. To prevent this, it was necessary to find a more effective way to suppress HIV. This became possible with the development of protease inhibitors and their combination with previously developed drugs in the AZT class.[70]

In 1986 two pharmaceutical companies, Merck Research Laboratories and Hoffmann–La Roche, launched plans to develop a new class of drugs to fight HIV, based on inhibiting the action of the virus's protease enzyme (see figure 5.2). The following year, Terry D. Copeland and Stephen Oroszlan in the Laboratory of Molecular Biology and Carcinogenesis at the National Cancer Institute filed a patent for the use of HIV protease inhibitors on behalf of the federal government. In 1988 they synthesized HIV protease, permitting the production of sufficient quantities of the enzyme to enable Merck scientists to determine its three-dimensional structure—the first step toward rational drug design, the process of searching for a drug whose molecular structure would block the action of HIV protease.[71]

In addition to Merck and Hoffmann–La Roche, Abbott Laboratories also established a program to identify and produce HIV protease inhibitors.[72] Initial candidate drugs were not hard to produce because these companies had previously worked on other protease enzymes that were similar. As each company's protease inhibitor was produced, the scientists had to decide whether to test it as a monotherapy—a one-drug therapy—against HIV or whether to use it as a combination therapy, often called a drug cocktail, in combination with the AZT class of drugs. Merck's drug, indinavir (sold under the trade name Crixivan), was used in a study that showed the "convincing superiority of the triple combination" therapy (indinavir + AZT + 3TC) over either one drug or a combination of AZT-type drugs alone.[73]

This study, along with another, also demonstrated that the drug cocktail so suppressed HIV that the virus became undetectable in the blood of infected people. This finding was possible only because of the introduction of new tests. The quantitative polymerase chain reaction, or Q-PCR, developed by Hoffmann–La Roche, and the branched-DNA, or b-DNA, test, developed by Chiron, allowed researchers for the first time to measure a person's viral load, or amount of virus in a specific quantity of blood, quickly. Within a two-year period, it became apparent that the new tests provided better predictors of someone's risk of developing full-blown AIDS over a fixed period than did the number of CD4 cells in the blood.[74] In addition, it became evident that with HIV suppressed to such a great extent, viral resistance to the drugs developed only very slowly or even not at all.

Merck's indinavir and Abbott's ritonavir (sold under the trade name Norvir) both proved outstanding in reducing mortality or progression of HIV infection to full-blown AIDS. In the spring of 1996, David Kessler, commissioner of the FDA, met with representatives of both Merck and Abbott and "urged them to submit whatever data they had" for an FDA Antiviral Advisory Committee meeting so that both drugs could be evaluated simultaneously. In December 1995 the FDA had approved the first protease inhibitor, Hoffmann–La Roche's saquinavir (sold under the trade names Invirase and Fortovase), which was weaker than Merck's indinavir or Abbot's ritonavir, and the FDA hoped to get all three drugs on the market because of fears that the weaker drug might induce widespread resistance to all three drugs. The Abbott and Merck drugs were both quickly approved in early March 1996.[75]

Another aspect of HIV disease revealed by the new tests was the exceptionally large amounts of virus produced each day in an infected person. They also showed how dramatically HAART could reduce the heavy viral load. Members of George Shaw's group at the University of Alabama–Birmingham and of David Ho's laboratory at the Aaron Diamond AIDS Research Center of the New York University School of Medicine prepared mathematical models for the decline of HIV to undetectable levels after administration of combination therapy.[76] Ho recommended that, because of this, combination therapy should be initiated as soon as infection was diagnosed.[77] In early 1996 Ho also utilized these models to predict that combination therapy would be able to eradicate HIV from an infected person's body and to predict how long this would take.[78]

The suggestion that HIV might be "eradicated" sent hope soaring for people with AIDS and their families and friends. David Ho became an overnight media star and was named *Time* magazine's "Person of the Year" for 1996. Others in the AIDS communities counseled caution, noting that studies needed to be done to see whether HIV could be undetectable yet hiding in the body, ready to come back if therapy was stopped. Within a year, scientists at NIAID and Johns Hopkins University School of Medicine reported the results of studies that clearly showed how HIV remained in lymph nodes and other sites in the body, where it would remain held in check until HAART therapy was discontinued. At that point, HIV would rapidly begin reproducing once again and resume its destruction of the immune system.[79] This meant that people infected with HIV, much like diabetics who needed insulin every day, would need to take HAART drugs for the rest of their lives. Even so, as long as they took their drugs, AIDS patients could usually keep HIV in check. Thus fifteen years after AIDS was recognized—what seemed like a lifetime to anyone infected but what was actually an amazingly short time in terms of the history of disease—HIV-positive people could actually plan for an active future rather than get their affairs in order before they died.

New York Times reporter David Dunlop captured some of the reaction of people with AIDS who were preparing to die, only to receive the sudden reprieve of HAART drugs. San Franciscan Greg George, who led a peer-support group for people with AIDS, reported that a common reaction in his group could be interpreted as whining: "I'm going to live, but now I've got to figure out how to feed myself or pay the mortgage. It's mind-bending to have these dilemmas," George said, "but I'm as grateful as I can be to be struggling with this one." Zahra Abdur-Rahman, a forty-six-year-old woman from the Bronx, New York, hoped to see her sixteen-year-old daughter graduate from high school. She also hoped to live to be fifty. "But I'll be grateful to see forty-seven," she said, "because I didn't expect to see that."[80]

Chemokines and Second Receptors

At the same time that combination therapies were being introduced, two additional discoveries about how HIV destroys the immune system produced new targets for therapeutic drugs. One of these was the discovery of the second receptor on cells necessary for HIV to infect the cell. In 1984, shortly after HIV had been identified as the cause of AIDS, scientists in Robin Weiss's laboratory in England and in Luc Montagnier's laboratory in Paris identified the CD4 molecule as the principal receptor for HIV, allowing the virus to infect T cells and macrophages.[81] Researchers knew, however, that mice also have cells with CD4 receptors, but mice do not become infected with HIV. This strongly suggested that there must be a second receptor on human T cells and macrophages that worked with the CD4 receptor to permit HIV entry into human cells.[82] Several laboratories worked actively to identify the second receptor, but for a decade, no candidate molecule could be demonstrated as the elusive receptor.

In 1996 Edward A. Berger and colleagues at NIAID finally identified one molecule that served as the second receptor for HIV on T cells. They named the molecule "fusion" to reflect its role in helping HIV fuse with a T cell, but in accordance with standard terminology, it was called CXCR-4.[83] The second receptor for HIV on macrophages was named CCR-5. This receptor was identified in 1996 as an outgrowth of work by other investigators researching chemokine factors (proteins secreted by cells) that suppressed the activity of HIV but did not kill it outright. (See figure 5.5 for the revised HIV life-cycle diagram introduced after these discoveries.)

Jay Levy and colleagues at the University of California–San Francisco had observed the existence of such factors as early as 1986, but until assays were developed to study the factors that were suspected of being at work, nothing further could be learned.[84] The breakthrough came with the development of two novel cell lines in Robert Gallo's laboratory at NCI. Using these cell lines, Gallo and colleagues identified the chemokines RANTES (regulated-upon-activation, normal T expressed and secreted), MIP-1ά (macrophage inflammatory protein-1α), and MIP-1β (macrophage inflammatory protein-1β) as the major HIV-1 inhibitors.[85] This work suggested strongly that the second recep-

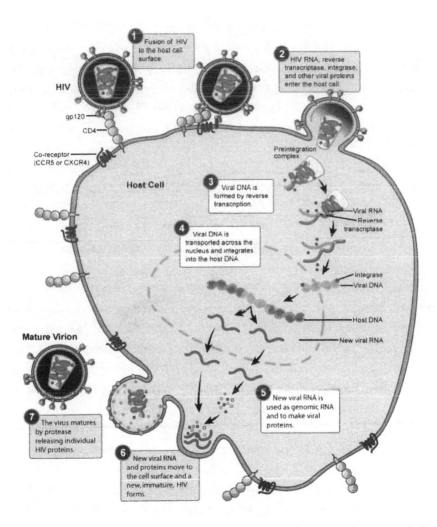

Figure 5.5. HIV life cycle as known in 2009. *Courtesy of the National Institute of Allergy and Infectious Diseases.*

tor used by HIV to enter macrophages might be a chemokine receptor that was sensitive to these chemokines.

In April 1996 investigators in Marc Parmentier's group at the Université Libre de Bruxelles reported the cloning, sequencing, and functional characterization of a chemokine receptor that responded to MIP-1á, MIP-1β, and RANTES; they named it CCR-5.[86] This coincidental finding—they were not looking for a second HIV-1 receptor—spurred the field considerably in conjunction with the Gallo group's observation. Starting with these two pieces of the puzzle, five different groups soon published studies describing CCR-5 as the second receptor on macrophages. Each group used a slightly different strategy in addressing the problem, and this made their cumulative evidence very convincing. The laboratories contributing were headed by Edward Berger and Philip Murphy at NIAID; Jay Levy at UCSF; David Ho at the Aaron Diamond AIDS Research Center; Dan R. Littman at the Skirball Institute of Biomolecular Medicine, New York University School of Medicine, and the Howard Hughes Medical Institute and Nathaniel R. Landau at Aaron Diamond; Robert Doms at the University of Pennsylvania; and Joseph Sodroski of the Dana-Farber Cancer Institute in Boston, Massachusetts.[87]

Apparently Immune Individuals and Long-Term Nonprogressors

One of the most important results of the discovery of second receptors offered an explanation for why some individuals remained uninfected even after being exposed multiple times to HIV through unprotected sex with HIV-positive people. Other unusual cases are those few people who test positive for HIV but do not progress to full-blown AIDS (long-term nonprogressors). Investigators proposed that a genetic variation in the CCR-5 receptor might offer an explanation for both of these conditions, and in fact, this variation has since been identified.[88] Officials at NIH, the principal funder of AIDS research, were pleased to see new avenues of research open up with these findings. William Paul, head of the NIH's Office of AIDS Research, said, "Once you have something like this in science, the dam breaks, and the problem is not to entice people to do the experiments, but to keep out of their way." Anthony Fauci, however, cautioned that the recent findings led many "to think that everything is falling into place and that's the end of the story. But we have been in it long enough to know that it is very unlikely that this is the end of the story."[89] Both officials, however, were

encouraged by the possible new methods of blocking HIV entry that these findings suggested.

Since that time, the entry of HIV into cells has become a target for a drug
called enfuvirtide and marketed in 2003 as Fuzeon by Hoffmann–La Roche
and Trimeris. In 2007 Pfizer began selling maraviroc as a CCR-5 coreceptor
antagonist trade-named Selzentry. That same year, another target in HIV's life
cycle—the process by which the genetic material of the virus is integrated into
the host cell's genome—was attacked by raltegravir, a drug developed by Merck
and sold as Isentress.[90]

More recently, a singular therapy for a San Franciscan AIDS patient with
leukemia has raised hopes for another approach to exploiting cells with the mutation that disables CCR-5 receptors. Timothy Brown learned he was HIV positive shortly before HAART was introduced. In 2006, after ten years on drugs and
then living in Berlin, Germany, he developed leukemia. When chemotherapy
failed to control the cancer, Brown's only hope was a stem-cell transplant from
a bone marrow donor. Brown's oncologist, Gero Hütter, realized that he had
an opportunity possibly to cure both the leukemia and the HIV infection if he
could give Brown stem cells from a bone marrow donor with the mutated CCR-
5 receptor. He identified one such donor among possible matches for Brown
and in February 2007 performed the transplant. Initially, Brown recovered well,
but then he relapsed; Hütter tried a second transplant from the same donor,
which finally succeeded in controlling the cancer. In the intervening four years,
Brown has been not only cancer free but also HIV free. He has taken no HIV
drugs since the transplant. Sensitive tests can find no trace of HIV in his body,
and even if some virus remained hidden, the mutated CCR-5 receptors would
protect him from new infection. This single apparent cure of a person with HIV
infection is not an approach that can easily be adapted to the 33 million people
living with AIDS around the world. The success of using stem cells with variant
CCR-5 receptors in Brown's case provides impetus to the line of research on
therapies utilizing such cells effectively without requiring that a patient's immune system be shut down and a risky bone marrow transplant performed.[91]

AIDS Therapies after Thirty Years

Several themes emerge from the story of the search for AIDS therapies. First,
the success of HAART therapy has been so complete that the terminology has

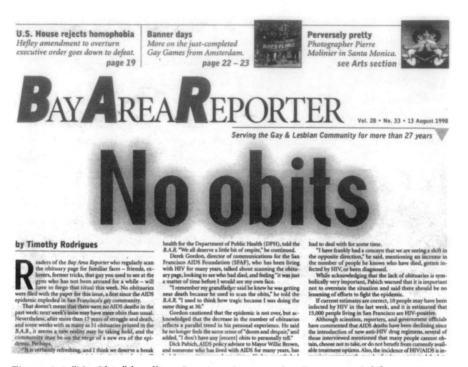

Figure 5.6. "No Obits" headline, *Bay Area Reporter*, San Francisco, California, August 13, 1998. This date marked the first time since 1981 that the newspaper had received no AIDS deaths to report. *Courtesy of the* Bay Area Reporter.

changed simply to ART, antiretroviral therapy. Second, rapid identification of the life cycle of HIV laid the groundwork for thinking about how to proceed in stopping the devastation the virus caused. Third, no single laboratory can be identified as the one above all others that should be recognized for contributions to developments in therapy. Fourth, collaboration among investigators in government, academia, and industry made possible the rapid advances in AIDS therapy. Fifth, charlatans and well-meaning but misguided individuals will always attempt to profit from unproved therapies for any disease and to challenge the authority of scientific medicine. Finally, the tensions between the sick who demand therapies and various bureaucratic agencies established to ensure the safety and efficacy of drugs can be creative or destructive. The history of developing AIDS drugs highlights both outcomes.

The work of producing AIDS therapies that have permitted those infected with HIV to resume normal living, however, stands as a tribute to all who contributed to the process. Journalist Laura Douglas-Brown, who began her career in 1995, just before the FDA approved HAART, expressed the human impact. By 1997, she noted, the death rate from AIDS dropped 47 percent. "I found myself at the very cusp of the generation that did not witness mass death and devastation from the disease. Now . . . I know countless people living with HIV, but I can count on one hand the people I have known who have died from it." The most joyous news to the gay community in the United States, in which AIDS had first been identified, was the 1998 bright red banner headline in the *Bay Area Reporter*, San Francisco's lesbian-gay-bisexual-transgender newspaper: "No Obits" (see figure 5.6). This marked the first time since 1981 that the newspaper had received no AIDS deaths to report.[92]

6

Communicating AIDS

"It takes a thousand voices to tell a single story."
—NATIVE AMERICAN PROVERB

During the thirty years that AIDS has been known, all sorts of people have communicated ideas about AIDS, via medical articles, public health posters, popular and scholarly articles and books, Internet postings, reference materials for people with AIDS and their families, Broadway plays, television, and other media. The sheer volume of communications related to AIDS sets it apart from writings about historic epidemics. Early in the epidemic, historians worried that much of this documentation would be lost as those involved in the early years aged and died.[1] Almost everyone involved with AIDS, however—patients and caregivers, community organizations, AIDS activists, health care personnel, public-health officials, medical researchers, news media, and academic scholars—realized that AIDS was a new disease and that documentation about how people in our time responded to it should be archived. Many groups thus took steps to save documents, photos, artifacts, and oral histories. This chapter will examine media related to the epidemic—including writings of various sorts, as well as audio, video, and Internet communications—and suggest how they have shaped our understanding of AIDS. I will not try to be comprehensive but will suggest certain themes that have characterized segments of the literature relating to AIDS.

Medical Writing

Much of this book has been concerned with the biomedical writings about AIDS that document what science and medicine can say about the disease. In the nineteenth century, the English scientist William Thompson, Lord Kelvin, articulated the scientific approach to the study of nature: "When you can measure what you are speaking about, and express it in numbers, you know something about it."[2] Most writing of this sort, therefore, is highly technical, because the basis of scientific argument is presenting measurable data and drawing tentative conclusions as to what those data mean. The scientific process is based on rational thought by human beings, not on emotion or faith in religious deities. Individual scientists may or may not hold personal religious beliefs, but they never expect their colleagues to judge their scientific claims on any basis except those of rational analysis of observable data. Similarly, they may hold varying political and economic beliefs, and may exhibit any number of human failings. When they put on their "scientist" hats, however, they must collect data measurements and interpret them as rationally as possible and be ready for other scientists to challenge their methods and interpretations.

Scientific observations must also be reproducible—that is, able to be repeated in other laboratories by other scientists who, if they observe the same outcomes of the experiments, will be more likely to be persuaded that the original interpretation of the data is correct. Should scientists attempting to reproduce experiments find errors in the experimental method, obtain different outcomes in their experiments, or believe the data indicate an entirely different conclusion, they will also make their findings known via scientific publications. Other scientists may tackle the problem to see for themselves what the data suggest. The reason scientists have such faith in the scientific method is that it is always open to reexamination and reinterpretation if new data appear. "Science is self-correcting" is the underlying belief on which science operates—that is, that each scientist is free to reexamine data and put forth his or her own interpretation for the larger community to consider and accept or reject. Biologist Stephen J. Gould has noted, "The only universal attribute of scientific statements resides in their potential fallibility. If a claim cannot be disproven, it does not belong to the enterprise of science."[3] No scientific claim can be based on a religious faith that is not subject to challenge.

Utilizing the scientific method does not mean, however, that biomedical scientists are paralyzed by constant uncertainty. When multiple scientists come to the same conclusion about the meaning of observable data, they agree to call the interpretation the "best fit," in philosophical terminology. Especially in situations of medical crisis, such as the AIDS epidemic, these agreed-upon meanings are considered "facts" and are used to build plans for therapeutic intervention in or prevention of the disease process.

As we saw in chapter 1, the first medical articles about AIDS were reports published in the CDC's *Mortality and Morbidity Weekly Reports*, a weekly newsletter sponsored by the U.S. government that surveys disease reports in the United States. (Figure 6.1 reproduces the first paragraphs of the initial June 5, 1981, paper.) The *MMWR* continued to be the principal source of information about the epidemic through the summer and most of the fall of 1981, until the first peer-reviewed publications appeared in major medical journals such as the *New England Journal of Medicine, JAMA: The Journal of the American Medical Association, Science, Nature,* the *Lancet,* and other medical and scientific journals around the world. The process used by these prestigious journals to determine which papers on AIDS were accepted and which rejected reveals much about the larger scientific community in the early 1980s.

Ruth M. Kulstad, an editor who handled AIDS papers at the journal *Science* during this period, described the way papers were chosen for publication during her tenure, a story that, with modifications, reflects the policies of most major scientific journals. She pointed out that there was "a perennial shortage of space in the journal for reports of original research" and that editors had to balance the subject matter of submitted papers since *Science* is an interdisciplinary journal. In addition, the journal submitted all except the most inappropriate papers for outside peer review, and the identification of appropriate reviewers was a "crude" system in the early 1980s, based on a precomputer punch-card database and editors' idiosyncratic organization systems.[4]

"There was no shortage of ideas on the cause, or causes," of AIDS, Kulstad noted, and the editors attempted to assess the validity of data presented in deciding which to publish. Primarily, etiological theories could be divided into those that believed AIDS was the result of multiple factors and those that supported the idea of a single cause. In the latter group, she described a number of newly identified diseases in animals—including feline leukemia virus, canine

1981 June 5;30:250—2

Pneumocystis Pneumonia — Los Angeles

In the period October 1980-May 1981, 5 young men, all active homosexuals, were treated for biopsy-confirmed *Pneumocystis carinii* pneumonia at 3 different hospitals in Los Angeles, California. Two of the patients died. All 5 patients had laboratory-confirmed previous or current cytomegalovirus (CMV) infection and candidal mucosal infection. Case reports of these patients follow.

Patient 1: A previously healthy 33-year-old man developed *P. carinii* pneumonia and oral mucosal candidiasis in March 1981 after a 2-month history of fever associated with elevated liver enzymes, leukopenia, and CMV viruria. The serum complement-fixation CMV titer in October 1980 was 256; in May 1981 it was 32.* The patient's condition deteriorated despite courses of treatment with trimethoprim-sulfamethoxazole (TMP/SMX), pentamidine, and acyclovir. He died May 3, and postmortem examination showed residual *P. carinii* and CMV pneumonia, but no evidence of neoplasia.

Patient 2: A previously healthy 30-year-old man developed *P. carinii* pneumonia in April 1981 after a 5-month history of fever each day and of elevated liver-function tests, CMV viruria, and documented seroconversion to CMV, i.e., an acute-phase titer of 16 and a convalescent-phase titer of 28* in anticomplement immunofluorescence tests. Other features of his illness included leukopenia and mucosal candidiasis. His pneumonia responded to a course of intravenous TMP/SMX, but, as of the latest reports, he continues to have a fever each day.

Patient 3: A 30-year-old man was well until January 1981 when he developed esophageal and oral candidiasis that responded to Amphotericin B treatment. He was hospitalized in February 1981 for *P. carinii* pneumonia that responded to oral TMP/SMX. His esophageal candidiasis recurred after the pneumonia was diagnosed, and he was again given Amphotericin B. The CMV complement-fixation titer in March 1981 was 8. Material from an esophageal biopsy was positive for CMV.

Figure 6.1. "*Pneumocystis* Pneumonia—Los Angeles," *Morbidity and Mortality Weekly Report,* June 5, 1981, 250–52. This was the first medical article describing an apparently new disease entity that came to be known as AIDS. *Courtesy of the U.S. Centers for Disease Control and Prevention.*

parvovirus, and Potomac horse fever—and the currency given to ideas that the causative agents for these diseases might also be the cause of AIDS.[5]

The key decision editors made was choosing reviewers for submitted papers. All editors were aware that some reviewers tended to reject most papers while others "liked everything." In fields such as human retrovirology, a tiny number of investigators were qualified to assess papers, and it is a tribute to the process that scientists were generally able to restrain personal, political, or social biases in assessing the work of their colleagues. Kulstad summarized her view of the process: "Editors can make mistakes, and so can reviewers. What is important, for the progress of science, is that good work gets published somewhere, preferably with little delay, and that poor work, if it does get published, is shown to be poor, also with little delay."[6]

The editors of all major journals were neither passive conduits for articles from particular laboratories nor unaware of the political issues raised by some articles and the ethical issues posed by embargoes on stories of great public health significance. In 1983 and 1984, before the AIDS virus was discovered, *Science* published articles reporting the appearance of proteins of the human T-cell leukemia virus in blood samples from hemophiliacs and transfusion-associated AIDS patients and donors. The authors of the papers were scientists at the Harvard School of Public Health and the CDC, and their concern was to alert the public that the blood supply might be tainted with the unknown AIDS virus. The American Association of Blood Banks opposed this position, but the editors of *Science* believed the papers to be rigorous and so went ahead with publication. "Was *Science* being used for political purposes?" Kulstad asked. "Undoubtedly," she concluded, but because of the soundness of the scientific evidence, it was appropriate for *Science* to publish the data and let the readers judge the interpretation for themselves.[7]

Similarly, all journal editors discussed issues raised by the so-called Ingelfinger rule and embargoes. Named after Franz J. Ingelfinger, a former editor of the *New England Journal of Medicine*, the Ingelfinger rule was promulgated in 1969. It prohibited authors from presenting the results of their research in public—both in print and at scientific meetings—before a manuscript had been published in the journal. Similarly, journals embargoed the content of their issues until shortly before the articles were publicly published and released just enough in advance to enable reporters to contact authors for comments to be published approximately simultaneously with the journal. Other prestigious journals soon adopted the same rules, which in practice meant that dissemination of new findings might be delayed for many months because of space considerations in a journal. At issue was the ethics of withholding information of potential medical or public health significance. In 1985 Arthur S. Relman, then editor of the *New England Journal*, included this subject in a special report from the Hastings Center discussing ethical dilemmas related to AIDS.[8]

Because of these restrictions Michael Gottlieb and colleagues chose to make their findings about *Pneumocystis* pneumonia available in the CDC's *MMWR*. This federal government publication was responsible for getting information out to physicians quickly without a conflicting imperative to promote its own standing in the world of academic medicine. Over the next three years, academic journals also worked to fast-track AIDS papers because of its public health urgency. The discovery of the etiological agent of AIDS marked the end of one period of publication about AIDS, a milestone represented by compilations of AIDS papers by major journals. In 1986 the American Association for the Advancement of Science published *AIDS: Papers from Science, 1982–1985*, and the *Journal of the American Medical Association* published *AIDS from the Beginning*, a compilation primarily of *JAMA* articles but also including introductory essays and reproductions of the *MMWR* reports on AIDS.[9]

Physicians and scientists involved with AIDS quickly had to learn to be careful in choosing words when they gave interviews to journalists covering the epidemic. The classic case of miscommunication occurred early in the epidemic, when the *Journal of the American Medical Association* published an article by James Oleske, a New Jersey pediatrician who treated AIDS in babies. His report stated, "Sexual contact, drug abuse or exposure to blood products is not necessary for disease transmission."[10] Because the article appeared in *JAMA*, reporters failed to consult with other physicians and jumped to the conclusion that AIDS was transmissible by "routine close contact," a sufficiently ambiguous description to cover workplaces, families, schools, restaurants, movie theaters, and the like. Eventually, the correct conclusion from Oleske's article was reported: the babies contracted AIDS before or during birth, not from simply living with infected people. The false information, however, seriously escalated public fear of associating with people who might be infected. Demands that restaurants fire waiters who "looked gay," for example, brought the worst fears of the gay community about civil rights abuses into the public square.[11]

Journalism

Printed news media served as a primary source of knowledge about AIDS, especially during the 1980s and early 1990s, since television was slow to cover the epidemic and the Internet was not yet commonplace. Journalists are a large group in the United States, their activities protected by the first amendment to the U.S. Constitution guaranteeing freedom of the press, and they have developed various codes of ethics with respect to their responsibilities. The Society of Professional Journalists summarizes its ethical code under the headings "Seek Truth and Report It, Minimize Harm, Act Independently, and Be Accountable."[12] The American Society of Newspaper Editors "Statement of Principles" was first formulated in 1922, and in its current form states, "The primary purpose of gathering and distributing news and opinion is to serve the general welfare by informing the people and enabling them to make judgments on the issues of the time."[13]

Academic analyses of the role of journalism view news stories as a "cultural product that reflects the ideological beliefs and practices of those who operate news-making mechanisms."[14] Journalists not only tell the public what to think about but also how to think about it.[15] For writing about the AIDS epidemic, this has meant an evolving emphasis from a focus on those afflicted in the early 1980s to the biomedical and political policy issues of the 1990s and 2000s. Initially, the AIDS story was about "innocent" and "not-so-innocent" victims. Then it became a story about "finding a cure" for a viral infection. A cure or preventive vaccine would give the AIDS narrative the ending that news stories seem to need. Finally, because no wholesale cure or vaccine has been developed, AIDS became a story of public policy and efforts by foundations to alleviate suffering as the disease declined in interest for the public and press. Nilanjana Bardhan of the Department of Speech Communication at Southern Illinois University at Carbondale conducted a transnational study of AIDS news narratives and found that across the globe, this pattern was followed.[16]

Two issues that go to the heart of journalism's role in communicating about medicine and science reveal the difficulties of turning broad statements of purpose into published stories. First is the issue of how journalists determine truth when different groups put forth competing versions. The simple answer is to "present both sides of the issue," but in many cases, rigorous adherence to all views in play serves to elevate tiny fringe groups out of proportion. Sometimes, this matters little, but in the case of epidemic diseases, where human life is at stake, the press must decide what emphasis to give differing claims. Second is the extent to which investigative journalism in science is similar to, and different from, such inquiry in politics. Issues of unequal access to documentary evidence, assumptions about scientific process and scientific bureaucracy, and both personal and nationalistic interests contributed to some of the ways AIDS has been presented in newspapers, magazines, and books.

In 1989 James Kinsella published a book reviewing media coverage of AIDS during the 1980s, *Covering the Plague: AIDS and the American Media*. He noted the reluctance of mainstream newspapers, news magazines, and television networks to cover AIDS before 1985 because of a shared skittishness about discussing homosexuality and, especially, the sexual acts that were involved in transmitting the AIDS virus. The openly gay editor of the alternative newspaper the *Village Voice* expressed a different reason for avoiding AIDS coverage: fear of alienating its readership in the New York gay community. Pointing out the danger in sexual activities that were associated with AIDS might offend some of the *Voice*'s gay readers who practiced them, reasoned the paper's "ultraliberal staff."[17] The *New York Times*, under the editorship of Abe Rosenthal, at first confined AIDS stories by its medical reporter, Lawrence Altman, to the inside pages. The first Altman article for the *Times* on AIDS, "Rare Cancer Seen in 41 Homosexuals," was published in August 1981 but buried on page twenty of the first section. It was not until May 25, 1983, that AIDS made the front page of the *Times,* and then only because the U.S. federal government had announced that AIDS was its "no. 1 health priority."[18] These explanations for why editors were slow to publish AIDS articles fed into a near media silence in early years of the epidemic.

The AIDS epidemic changed a number of journalistic conventions, for newspapers, news magazines, wire services, and television. One change was press usage of the term "gay" as a noun. The term "homosexuals" had been the preferred way to describe this population. It was acceptable in some writing to speak of the "gay community," but to write about "gays" as a group was generally prohibited. As the epidemic grew larger and showed no indication of fading away, the mainstream media finally adopted "gays" as a noun, much like its adoption of "blacks" instead of "Negroes" during the civil rights movement as the term preferred by the group itself. The double edge of this change in language, as Kinsella points out, was that journalists tended to report on the epidemic as almost exclusively a gay community phenomenon. The affected gay males tended to be educated, articulate, and willing to be interviewed, while IV drug abusers and their sexual partners and children often lived in unpleasant parts of the city. They were not so easily located and did not make for appealing copy.[19]

After the AIDS virus was identified, another language usage challenged journalists in all media: how to describe how the virus was transmitted. Most television anchors in the United States, for example, were concerned that their broadcasts reached the American public during the dinner hour, when children were likely present. Producers feared that frank language would cause viewers to turn off the television. "Contact between bodily fluids" was about as close as most television anchors would get to a description of viral transmission. In 1985 George Strait, ABC's science reporter, found a way around the language barrier by asking Anthony S. Fauci from NIH to use the term "anal sex" in an interview so that Strait as reporter would not have to speak the words. All three major networks avoided stories about AIDS in the early years because of squeamishness about sexual transmission and the fact that the disease was largely evident in the homosexual community. Only the then-new cable network, CNN, which needed to fill its twenty-four-hour news day, picked up the AIDS story in July 1981 and continued to cover it. CNN's location in Atlanta, Georgia, also gave it easy access to the CDC's epidemiologists for technical expertise.[20]

For all mainstream news outlets, the announcement in 1985 that Rock Hudson had AIDS served as the trigger to more comprehensive coverage of the epidemic, just as it had triggered greater funding from Congress. Kinsella noted, "Hudson's passing made for the perfect TV death. As the eulogies spilled across the screen, featuring the face of the quintessential all-American male, the media across the nation convulsed in one final sigh of belated coverage."[21] If AIDS could strike such a celebrated actor as Hudson, it could threaten us all. For those who decried homosexuality as wrong and the Hollywood lifestyle as decadent, Hudson's death was a cautionary tale.

The one New York paper that took the lead in reporting on AIDS was the *New York Native,* which reported in May 1981 on rumors of a "gay cancer" in New York.[22] The *Native* was, as Kinsella described it, "a product of both the visions and whims of Chuck Ortleb, its editor and publisher."[23] It enjoyed the services of a part-time reporter who was trained as a physician, Larry Mass, and took the lead in publishing information from the CDC and other public health offices about high-risk behavior and the possibility of a virus as the cause of AIDS. These articles were published alongside the more usual fare of the paper, including a provocative first-person story about an experience of sadomasochism.[24]

Ortleb watched his readership fall victim to the new disease throughout 1982, and he railed at the government for being homophobic and for purposely not producing a cure because most AIDS patients were gay. Reporter Mass became "exhausted and depressed" as a result of covering the seemingly unendingly negative stories relating to the epidemic. In March 1983 Larry Kramer (see figure 6.2) published his famous front-page article, "1,112 and Counting," demanding that members of the gay community change their multipartner sexual lifestyles and organize a massive lobbying effort to urge government at every level to respond to the epidemic more strongly. In May, the *Native* published a new theory about the cause of AIDS, that it was caused by the African swine fever virus (ASFV). Ortleb had been intrigued by an article in the *Lancet* raising this possibility. The article had been written by a postdoctoral researcher at Harvard doing work not on AIDS and not trained in medicine but interested in parallels she saw between the two diseases. With this article, the *Native* turned its focus to promoting ASFV as the cause of AIDS and was not deterred by the findings in Paris or Bethesda laboratories that a retrovirus was the etiological agent. In the mid-1980s, Kramer's activist group ACT UP boycotted the *Native*, whose circulation had reached a high of twenty thousand in 1985. In 1987 Ortleb also took up the cause of Peter Duesberg's challenge to HIV as the cause of AIDS. The *Native* continued to support the Duesberg hypothesis until 1996, when HAART allowed people with AIDS to recover their hope for a normal life. By that time, the paper's circulation had fallen to eight thousand, and it went out of business in January 1997.[25]

Aside from the *Native*, the gay press in the United States gave much more coverage to AIDS than did mainstream papers, with one notable exception. In San Francisco, the gay community had been a major political force since the election of Harvey Milk in 1977 to the Board of Supervisors. The *San Francisco Chronicle* was the only daily newspaper in a major city with a reporter assigned to a "gay beat."[26] That reporter was Randy Shilts, who joined the *Chronicle* in August 1981.

Books about AIDS
In 1987 Shilts pulled together many of his stories and published *And the Band Played On: Politics, People, and the AIDS Epidemic,* the first major book about the disease. In his acknowledgments, Shilts thanked his editor at St. Martin's Press for having faith in the book when others had not believed that AIDS would prove serious enough to merit a book-length study.[27] As noted in chapter 1, the book was a cry of despair from the gay community, which was seeing its members sicken and die within a decade after the group as a whole had begun

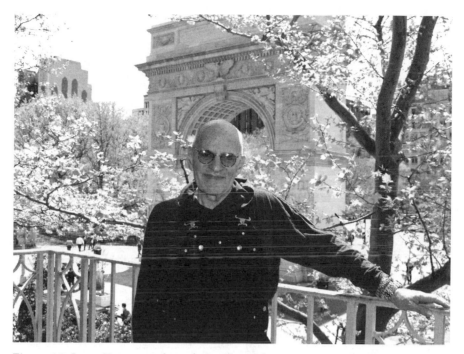

Figure 6.2. Larry Kramer, author, playwright, and AIDS activist; founder of Gay Men's Health Crisis and ACT UP. *Photograph by David Shankbone, Wikimedia Commons.*

to overcome systemic discrimination. Shilts lashed out at everyone—the gay community was not exempt, nor were religions and local, state, and federal officials. It seemed to Shilts that quicker action by public health authorities might have halted the epidemic in its tracks but that they were thwarted by antigay politicians and their religious supporters on the political right.[28]

The book had an outsized impact on many areas of society. Politically, it spurred further action at a moment when the U.S. Congress was poised to move forward with expanded funding for AIDS research. Socially, it highlighted the dedication of many in the gay community to organizing to raise money to help people with AIDS, working directly with sick people, and engaging in political action. An impact of less importance but no less permanent was the concept of a "patient zero" in the AIDS epidemic. Shilts used the epidemiological shorthand of an index case in an outbreak to explain how widely one person could spread the disease. The person he chose as patient zero in the book was a gay Canadian airline steward, Gaetan Dugas, who traveled worldwide and continued to have sex even after he began having symptoms of AIDS. Dugas may well have spread the disease far and wide, but he was not the one person who started the AIDS epidemic—there was no single person who "started" AIDS. To this day, however, many people believe that this one man is the reason AIDS was brought to the United States.

Another impact of the Shilts book, and especially the movie that HBO made based on it, was the launching of the character assassination of AIDS scientist Robert C. Gallo. One of Shilts's scientific sources and a major adviser for the movie was Donald Francis, the CDC epidemiologist who wanted to play a more important role in AIDS research than he was able to, given the resource limitations at the CDC. Francis had incurred Gallo's wrath on more than one occasion, and his role as adviser to Shilts and HBO provided an opportunity to settle a score. Shilts cast Francis as the lone epidemiologist hero of the AIDS epidemic. Shilts, and especially HBO, made Gallo a grasping, ugly scientific character interested only in gaining recognition for himself, caring nothing for AIDS patients. In the movie, actor Alan Alda played Gallo consummately in this mold, and HBO chose to make the movie a story of good versus evil, one of several story lines they were thinking of using. Moreover, in the film the Pasteur Institute's group of scientists were presented in soft focus, conveying through images that their aim was only to help save lives with their science, while Gallo's laboratory was pictured as a huge, industrialized affair with a remote boss who preferred playing tennis to doing science but still wanted all the glory to be had.[29]

AIDS activist Martin Delaney, head of Project Inform, believed that the movie was unfair to the Gallo laboratory. He contacted HBO with a list of errors the writers had made in presenting the story of AIDS research. Some of his recommended changes were incorporated, but the story line did not change. The movie became the sole source of knowledge about the epidemic for many people. In their minds, Robert Gallo became an evil scientist whose actions delayed help for suffering people and Donald Francis became the hero that everyone should have listened to from the beginning. Even twenty-five years later, Gallo received hate e-mails every time the movie aired.[30]

In the early 1990s, the period when AZT-type drugs with all their limitations seemed to promise no more than a prolonged period of dying for AIDS patients, a number of books and articles appeared charging misconduct in biomedical research as well as in politics. The striking characteristic of these books was their lopsided attacks on scientists and agencies in the U.S. federal government. From reading these books, one might conclude that scientists everywhere except those employed by the U.S. government kept impeccable scientific notebooks and records, never raised their voices in frustration, worked only to benefit mankind, and had no personal ambitions for recognition. In contrast, U.S. federal scientists were mediocre, failed to keep proper records, and spent their days slavishly seeking advancement from their superiors, wanting only self-glorification even though their output was poor. These attacks could be made because, as federal officials, scientists, especially those who had risen to the status of "public figure," had no legal protection from any public accusation or inquiry. In addition, authors could obtain copies of any records produced by federal scientists through the U.S. Freedom of Information Act (FOIA) whereas they were not able to obtain similar documentation from other scientific laboratories.[31]

A 1990 example of such writing was Bruce Nussbaum's book, *Good Intentions: How Big Business and the Medical Establishment Are Corrupting the Fight against AIDS*. The author, formerly a business journalist, believed that medical scientists, especially those in the federal government, operated with no accountability and actively sought to suppress the courageous alternative medicine community that wanted to speed access to unproven AIDS drugs. Nussbaum chose to focus on scientists in the National Cancer Institute, and he presented their efforts to develop an AIDS therapy as nothing more than support for Robert Gallo's "glorious scientific battle with the French." Nussbaum spoke of Samuel Broder as someone who wanted to "curry Gallo's favor" and who was motivated only by his belief that association with Gallo would advance his career. The most offensive characterizations of Broder, Gallo, and other Jewish and Italian scientists at NIH were Nussbaum's assertion that one often heard "'guinea' and 'Jewboys' tossed about in casual conversations at NIH." Having introduced this libel in readers' minds, he quickly backed away from it by stating, "Usually it's within the context of friendly scientific competition. Often it's in terms of admiration. But not always."[32] In a review of the book, Roger Lewin argued that Nussbaum fell victim to a conspiracy theory that NIH scientists, the Burroughs Wellcome Pharmaceutical Company, and the FDA worked to ensure that AZT and only AZT would be approved as a treatment for AIDS. By choosing the route of accusation and blame, Nussbaum ignored the complexity of the biomedical process but managed to produce a book aimed at undermining the scientific establishment.[33]

More destructive was John Crewdson's decade-long crusade to discredit Robert Gallo, an effort based largely on documents retrieved via FOIA. As a reporter for the *Chicago Tribune,* Crewdson had begun his career working on the Watergate scandal during Richard Nixon's presidential administration. At a 1988 World Health Organization meeting in Sweden, he was urged "by some people" who remained unnamed to investigate Gallo. His work was encouraged by at least two scientists who had "uncomfortable relationships" with Gallo, Jay Levy and Donald Francis. According to journalist Jon Cohen, writing in *Science* in 1991, Francis told Crewdson that "[Gallo's] done so much damage by dividing the world into for and against Gallo that he should be punished."[34] Gallo and his supporters believe that Francis's personal antagonism motivated him to promote Crewdson's efforts.[35] Crewdson himself seems to have been motivated by a desire to demonstrate that science was no different an undertaking than politics and that Gallo was as crooked a scientist as Richard Nixon had been as a politician.

In 1989, after bombarding the NIH with more than a hundred FOIA requests, many of them specifically for materials from the Gallo laboratory, Crewdson published a fifty-thousand-word, sixteen-page special section to the *Tribune* called "The Great AIDS Quest." From the first paragraph, it was clear that Crewdson was not attempting any sort of objective analysis in his account. On page one, he set out his conclusion: "On the afternoon of the day before his 50th birthday, the American scientist Robert C. Gallo sat down at a small desk in a hotel room in Germany. In the chair next to his was Luc Montagnier, one of the French researchers from whom Gallo had been trying for nearly three years to steal the credit for discovering the cause of AIDS."[36]

Gallo and his colleagues protested about the tremendous amount of time away from research they were required to spend in locating documents to comply with all the FOIA requests. The major problem with Crewdson's use of FOIA in these investigations was that similar data from nonfederal scientists was never available, so there could be no parity of analysis. When Crewdson visited the Pasteur Institute, for example, he initially asked about access to files relating to the history of the institute, and he received permission from Director Maxime Schwartz for research. When he arrived at the Institute Archives, however, he asked to see the AIDS files and cited Schwartz's approval. The chief of archives called Schwartz to verify this, however, and Crewdson's deception so angered Schwartz that the Pasteur Institute refused to show Crewdson any documents.[37]

Crewdson's article triggered two special investigations at NIH and another by Congressman John Dingell, chair of the Committee on Energy and Commerce of the U.S. House of Representatives and its powerful Subcommittee on Oversight and Investigations. Staff involved in the Dingell investigation and its associated bureaucratic inquiries at NIH demanded not only laboratory notebooks and correspondence from the Gallo laboratory but also personal medical information and personnel information. Similar information from other laboratories conducting research on the cause of AIDS was not sought. With no chance to present a rebuttal, Gallo and a key colleague, Mikulas Popovic, were found guilty of scientific misconduct. Only in 1996, when the conviction was appealed and due process permitted to Gallo and Popovic, did the appeals board exonerate Popovic completely and drop all charges against Gallo.[38] In its ruling, the board wrote, "One might anticipate that from all this evidence, after all the sound and fury, there will be at least a residue of palpable wrongdoing. That is not the case."[39]

Crewdson, however, was not finished with his crusade to discredit Gallo. He had moved to Bethesda, Maryland, to be near Gallo's laboratory and continued to submit FOIA requests to NIH even though Gallo left NCI in 1996 to found the Institute for Human Virology at the University of Maryland School of Medicine in Baltimore. In 2002 Crewdson published *Science Fictions: A Scientific Mystery, A Massive Coverup, and the Dark Legacy of Robert Gallo.* Reviewers of the book either praised Crewdson for exposing Gallo's "dark legacy" or observed that Crewdson had built an overwhelmingly biased case that sought to destroy one of the world's leading AIDS researchers. Christopher Martyn's critique for *British Medical Journal* represents a typical review in the scientific community:

Despite the weight of information Crewdson amasses, it's ultimately unconvincing. One has no way of knowing whether it has been presented in a fair-minded way. There's a strong sense of only hearing the case for the prosecution. . . . The author's shock at discovering that scientists are not always honourable in their dealings must surely be simulated. It's a commonplace observation that important discoveries are made by unpleasant people. . . . And the phrase in the subtitle, the dark legacy of Robert Gallo, which implies that lasting harm was done and which, I guess, Crewdson must need to believe to justify writing the book, is never supported by argument or facts. It's far from clear that progress in understanding the causation of AIDS was slowed up by anything Gallo did. Indeed, the reverse might well be true.[40]

Daniel S. Greenberg, a science policy journalist, wrote in *New Scientist* that Crewdson had undertaken his task "with the ardour of Captain Ahab and Inspector Javert. . . . This is an awesomely documented prosecutorial brief," he continued, "that concedes no credit to its target and yields him no doubts. If the Gallo camp has a rebuttal, let's hear it."[41] In 2006 that rebuttal appeared in *Dissecting a Discovery: The Real Story of How the Race to Uncover the Cause of AIDS Turned Scientists against Disease, Politics against Science, Nation against Nation.* It was written by Nikolas Kontaratos, a retired policeman whose father had been in NCI management and who was using the research for a PhD dissertation. The book does not read as fluently as Crewdson's writing, but it presents detailed counterarguments and is as strongly biased toward Gallo's laboratory as Crewdson's work is against it. It also makes available a number of documents not previously published that will be useful to future scholars.

Theater, Television, and Movies

As noted in chapter 4, Larry Kramer's 1985 play, *The Normal Heart,* was the first play to take AIDS as its subject. In 1993 his follow-up play, *The Destiny of Me,* was produced. The plays were spare in wording and self-consciously activist in seeking outrage to fuel political action to hasten the day when a cure for AIDS might be found. Another AIDS playwright, Tony Kushner, wrote in a foreword for a printing of the plays in book form in 2000, "Together the plays constitute an American epic."[42] Aside from Kramer, however, no other playwright wrote about AIDS in the 1980s for live theater.

As Kramer's *The Normal Heart* was to the 1980s, Tony Kushner's 1992 play, *Angels in America,* was to the 1990s. The *New York Times* reviewed its premiere with astonishment:

As a political statement, "Angels in America," a two-part, seven-hour epic subtitled "A Gay Fantasia on National Themes," is nothing less than a fierce call for gay Americans to seize the strings of power in the war for tolerance and against AIDS. But this play, by turns searing and comic and elegiac, is no earthbound ideological harangue. Though set largely in New York and Washington during the Reagan-Bush 80's, "Angels in America" sweeps through locales as varied as Salt Lake City and the Kremlin, and through high-flying styles ranging from piquant camp humor to religious hallucination to the ornate poetic rage of classic drama.[43]

In 2003 HBO produced *Angels in America*, which had been directed for television by Mike Nichols. It received even more glowing reviews. John Leonard of *New York* magazine lauded it as "not only the best television of the year but, hands down, the best movie, period."[44] In a review for National Public Radio, David Bianculli called it a "masterpiece" and described praise for it as "the highest I can bestow."[45]

Film critic John Hartl observed that television played a larger role initially in bringing AIDS to the public because the epidemic "fit into the 'disease of the week' movie format." He added that independent filmmakers produced the first films about AIDS because "the subject clearly meant so much to them."[46] In 1985, the year Rock Hudson died of AIDS, the first feature-length television film about AIDS made its debut. *An Early Frost*, directed by John Erman and broadcast on NBC, told the story of a successful young lawyer who lived a double life until diagnosed with AIDS. It is the story of a family's reaction to the announcement that their son is gay and also infected with the deadly disease. Winner of a Golden Globe, *An Early Frost* portrayed the range of emotion within the family, from the supportive mother to the father who has great trouble accepting his son's homosexuality. Also in 1985, independent filmmaker Arthur J. Bressan Jr. made the first dramatic feature film about AIDS. *Buddies* told the story of a gay man who became a buddy for another who was dying of AIDS. The low-budget film was written in two weeks, and after the actors' preparation in collaboration with the Gay Men's Health Crisis, filming was finished in nine days. Bressan died of AIDS shortly after the movie was released.[47]

Other 1980s movies included the 1986 feature *Parting Glances*, a film by Bill Sherwood about two different ways gay men in New York attempted to deal with partners sick with AIDS, and the 1987 British film by Waris Hussein, *Intimate Contact*, about a hemophiliac boy sickened with AIDS. Another 1987 British TV production by William Nicholson was *Sweet As You Are*, about a heterosexual couple who are devastated by the news that he's been infected. Celebrities with AIDS, including Liberace, Olympic diver Greg Louganis, and Rock Hudson, all had movies made about their lives. Ryan White, the boy from Indiana who became the face of young hemophiliacs with AIDS, was the subject of a 1989 television film. Also in 1989, *Common Threads: Stories from the Quilt*, profiles of people represented in the NAMES Project's AIDS Memorial Quilt, won the first Oscar for an AIDS film, in the category for best documentary.[48]

In the 1990s similar movies such as *Longtime Companion* and *Absolutely Positive* were made by writers, directors, or producers with AIDS. The first high-profile film addressing AIDS was *Philadelphia*, written by Ron Nyswane, directed by Jonathan Demme, and distributed in 1993. It told the story of a young lawyer, played by Tom Hanks, who was diagnosed with AIDS, only to be fired from a large firm on a trumped-up charge of incompetence. Hanks's character sued the firm over the dismissal, and as his case came to trial, his health was shown deteriorating. The power of the movie, which won two Oscars, came from the portrayal of the range of views in American society about AIDS, especially the fearful view held by members of the protagonist's law firm and the conflicted view—antigay but committed to the best legal representation possible—held by the protagonist's attorney, played by Denzel Washington.[49] Also in 1993 the HBO film *And the Band Played On*, discussed previously in relation to the book on which it was based, appeared.

With the advent of the new millennium, AIDS films began to focus on the disease in Africa and other developing countries. The Paris-based film company Dominant 7 produced documentary films for French and international broadcasters. In 2001 one of Dominant 7's founders, Philip Brooks, produced *6000 a Day: An Account of a Catastrophe Foretold*. Through interviews with leading figures in the effort to respond to AIDS—including Eric Sawyer, a founder of ACT UP New York; Sandra Thurman, President Bill Clinton's AIDS adviser; Mathilde Krim, founder of amfAR; Noerine Kaleeba, founder of The AIDS Support Organization (TASO) in Uganda; France's health minister, Bernard Kouchner; and Peter Piot, director of UNAIDS—the movie documented "the tragic degree of indifference and ignorance with which HIV/AIDS has been dealt" even after twenty years because of indifference or stigma surrounding sexually transmitted diseases.[50] In 2002 Brooks worked with Brian Tilley to produce *It's My Life*, a film about the South African government's decision to withhold ART drugs from public hospitals and clinics because its president, Thabo Mbeki, questioned whether HIV was the cause of AIDS (this will be discussed in detail in chapter 8). The protagonist of the film is the HIV-positive chair of South Africa's Treatment Action Campaign (TAC), Zackie Achmat, who resolved not to take the lifesaving ART drug cocktail until it was made available for everyone in South Africa.[51]

Also in the new millennium, films about AIDS received support from the Bill and Melinda Gates Foundation, which aimed to increase AIDS awareness worldwide. In 2002 at the Fourteenth International AIDS Conference in Barcelona, Spain, the film *Pandemic: Facing AIDS* by Rory Kennedy premiered. According to the press release issued by the Gates Foundation, the film melded "intimate personal stories with a global perspective." It was released on DVD by HBO in English, Hindi, Portuguese, Russian, and Thai.[52] In 2009 the Gates Foundation also funded *AIDS Jaago*, four fifteen-minute films produced and directed by Indian filmmakers and utilizing A-list Indian actors.[53]

More disturbing were films in 2002 and 2003 by filmmaker Louise Hogarth, *Does Anyone Die of AIDS Anymore?* and *The Gift*. Hogarth shined a light on a newly emerged segment of gay culture, promoted primarily on the Internet. Proponents of this group's thinking suggested that HIV infection is not dangerous and promoted "barebacking" parties in which young men might receive "the gift" of AIDS. Hogarth contrasted this reckless lifestyle with stories from men who were accidentally infected with AIDS and had been living with life-sparing drugs. These men made clear that the drugs are not without side effects, especially on their hearts, livers, and kidneys, and that seeking intentional infection with HIV carried grave consequences.[54]

In the new millennium, major philanthropic organizations have partnered with international media companies to bring AIDS education information to a worldwide audience. One survey observed,

In China nearly all households had access to television in 1999, and more than 900 million Chinese are regular viewers of Chinese state television CCTV. India has eighty-six million households with televisions, which means that 43 percent of the country's population views TV. In South Africa more than 90 percent of youth (in a 2001 survey) watch TV or listen to the radio, even in rural areas. In the United States, Kaiser's national surveys have confirmed that the media are one of the most important resources for Americans on HIV/AIDS—the media are named more often than health care providers or schools.[55]

To leverage the impact of educational materials about AIDS, therefore, the Henry J. Kaiser Family Foundation and UNAIDS cosponsored a meeting in January 2004 at the UN with its secretary general, Kofi Annan, and the chief executive officers of media companies around the world. The conference launched the Global Media AIDS Initiative with commitments from participants to raise the level of public awareness about AIDS. Included were Viacom, the British Broadcasting Corporation (BBC), the South African Broadcasting Corporation (SABC), Gazprom-Media (one of Russia's largest private media holdings), and the Star Group Ltd. in India, a company held by Rupert Murdoch. The result was a multiplatform initiative, with specific public service announcements on television supported by radio, print, and online materials, briefings about AIDS to television writers and producers so that they might incorporate the information into the story lines of their series, and funds for special documentary programs. The Bill and Melinda Gates Foundation has also become involved in supporting this effort.[56]

Ephemera about AIDS

From early in the epidemic, when self-help organizations in the gay community such as the Gay Men's Health Crisis first formed, leaders worked to circulate prevention messages about AIDS. These efforts took many forms, from posters to matchbook covers to trading cards, which archivists group together as ephemera because they are characteristically short-lived. (Figure 6.3 provides an example of AIDS trading cards.) During the 1980s medical historian William Helfand collected AIDS posters for the U.S. National Library of Medicine.[57] He noted that the most frequent type of AIDS poster consisted primarily of informative text, such as the Australian poster in figure 6.4, which communicated who gets AIDS, what AIDS is, how one gets AIDS, what activities will *not* result in AIDS, and how one can be safe. Another group of posters sought to allay fears that everyday activities will cause AIDS. In Alaska, a poster campaign showing a huge mosquito stated, "Go Ahead! Spread the Word! You Can't Get AIDS from Alaska's State Bird!" A California group, the Center for Attitudinal Healing, published a poster showing a stick figure of a child in a hospital gown saying, "I Have AIDS. Please Hug Me. I Can't Make You Sick." A poster from the Milwaukee AIDS Project included four photos and the headline, "None of These Will Give You AIDS." The pictures showed two people shaking hands, a restaurant table setting, a toilet, and a doorknob.

To communicate the threat AIDS posed, posters often used striking graphic images. A Mexican poster showed a drawing of feet with a toe tag and a sheet covering what was obviously a dead body. The caption proclaimed that with AIDS, the risk is death. To reach injecting drug abusers, the most difficult audience of all at risk for AIDS, a group called AID Atlanta produced a poster showing the profile of a pregnant woman and a baby in her womb holding a syringe. "Don't Give AIDS to Your Unborn Baby . . . Get the Test Before Having a Baby."[58] One of the most powerful images for inspiring fear is that of a skull. The Nipomo Community Medical Center in California utilized the image of a skull

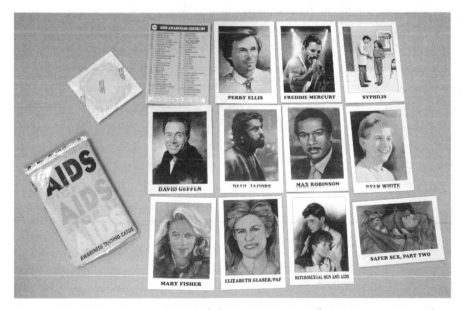

Figure 6.3. AIDS ephemera: "AIDS, fight it, AIDS, stop it," AIDS awareness trading cards, "A Condom in Every Pack." Ansell Incorporated, Dothan, Alabama, June 1992. *Courtesy of the Stetten Museum, U.S. National Institutes of Health.*

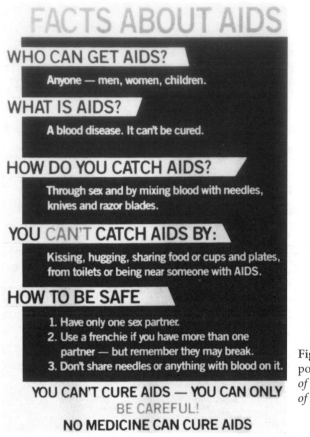

Figure 6.4. Australian AIDS poster from 1980s. *Courtesy of the U.S. National Library of Medicine.*

with a syringe in its mouth to communicate the deadly risk. Another image that conveyed the need for safe sex was based on the Biblical story of the snake and the apple in the Garden of Eden. San Francisco artist David Lance Goines created a graphic of a snake wrapped around an apple nestled in leaves and blossoms for the Student Health Service at the University of California–Berkeley.

One great need was to reach people at risk in particular ethnic groups. Posters with the same copy—"She Has Her Father's Eyes and Her Mother's AIDS"—were printed in different languages and using pictures of people of different ethnicities, such as Caucasian, African American, and Hispanic, in order to reach multiple audiences. Similar efforts resulted in posters promoting safe sex to homosexual men of different ethnicities. A Seattle, Washington, organization called People of Color Against AIDS created a series of posters called "Famous Last Words" and included a poster stating "AIDS Is a White Man's

Disease." In the Philippines, prostitutes were urged to "Be Careful of AIDS. Do Not Agree [to sex] Without a Condom."

Although most poster images have historical antecedents, the grave threat of AIDS has forced discussion of topics not previously considered appropriate in public. The frank admonishment about the necessity of condom use in the Philippine poster aimed at prostitutes reflects this pathbreaking ephemeral form. Helfand noted three Icelandic posters that attempted to demystify condoms by showing ordinary citizens using condoms in unorthodox ways such as playing with one and using another as a head covering. AIDS services in the gay communities of large cities took the lead in producing explicit posters showing the proper way to wear a condom and promoting the erotic possibilities of safe sex, and in developing comic books with stories about gay men and safe sex. A comic strip prepared by the Ministry of Health of Australia and aimed at the aboriginal community told a story titled "You Don't Have to Be a Queenie to Get AIDS." In the story, a man has sex with someone who has AIDS. He goes back to his wife. She gets sick with AIDS. Quickly, everybody gets sick and dies. The message is brief and to the point: condom use saves lives.[59]

Two exceptions to these patterns are notable. First, posters used by the scientific community to announce research seminars or AIDS conferences show a marked preference for using HIV, the AIDS virus, or another scientific drawing as their image. It is almost as if the medical community were posting a "wanted" photograph of the criminal they wish to defeat. Second is the absence of images of AIDS patients. In Helfand's sample of 350 AIDS posters from around the world in the 1980s, not a single one showed a patient with AIDS. In his analysis, Helfand wondered whether viewers would be put off by images of suffering people or whether privacy considerations were involved. This situation changed beginning in the 1990s. With the advent of the World Wide Web mid-decade, multiple organizations began posting posters, photographs, and other AIDS educational materials online that included images of people infected with HIV but not yet sick, people suffering from AIDS, and children who had been orphaned by AIDS.[60]

Alternative Theories, Quackery, and Urban Legends

In chapter 5 we encountered the AIDS denialists and their arguments that HIV does not cause AIDS, assertions they maintain in the face of compelling scientific evidence to the contrary and the demonstration that ART combination therapy enables people infected with HIV to resume a normal life. Their books, articles, and movies have continued to flourish, owing in part to the reach of the Internet. The tenaciousness of the AIDS denialists and those who propose alternative therapies instead of antiretroviral drugs raises the question, what constitutes quackery? Many of the advocates of alternative hypotheses and therapies are sincere in their beliefs to the point of dying or letting their children die from AIDS. Does sincerity protect them from laws requiring proof of safety and efficacy? Do they have the blood of people with AIDS who died believing in their alternative views on their hands? Should the field of AIDS therapies be uncontrolled with only the admonition caveat emptor—let the buyer beware? Here we will briefly survey the broad field of alternative theories about the cause of AIDS and the therapies espoused by proponents.

An AIDS denialist who paid the ultimate price for her beliefs was Christine Maggiore, the founder of an Italian import-export company. After being diagnosed with HIV in 1992, Maggiore became an active denier of HIV as the cause of AIDS, starting a website, Alive and Well: AIDS Alternatives, and publishing a book, *What If Everything You Thought You Knew about AIDS Was Wrong?*[61] She refused antiretroviral drugs during her pregnancy and breast-fed her daughter, who died in 2005, according to an autopsy, of *Pneumocystis* pneumonia with other AIDS-related complications. Maggiore rejected the autopsy's conclusion and continued to maintain that she was healthy. In 2008 she died of apparent AIDS, although no autopsy was permitted.[62]

Nathan Geffen, a leader in the South African Treatment Action Group, has studied AIDS quackery in South Africa for a decade. In a 2007 working paper for the University of Cape Town's Centre for Social Science, he described nutritional remedies for HIV infection that gained the support of the South African government, a situation that will be discussed further in chapter 7. Tine van der Mass, a Dutch nurse living in South Africa, proposed a garlic concoction combined with the extract from an African potato, known as Africa's solution, as a treatment for AIDS. This treatment was broadcast widely in a video, *Power to the People*, endorsed by the South African minister of health. Nozipho Bhengu, daughter of a member of the South African parliament, embraced this treatment for her HIV infection. Tragically, she died of AIDS in 2006.[63]

In 2006 *Harper's* magazine, generally viewed as a respected and carefully edited news journal, published an article by AIDS denialist Celia Farber that repeated Peter Duesberg's claims. Both the *Columbia Journalism Review* and the *New York Times* questioned *Harper's* decision to provide legitimacy to AIDS denialism by publishing Farber's article, calling it "deadly quackery." *The Nation*, another U.S. news magazine, commented in its blog, "It's a shame that a magazine as well respected as *Harper's* has shirked its duty to report on these issues and instead published Farber's article." Despite these and many other protests, *Harper's* refused to withdraw editorial support for the article.[64]

With the rise of the Internet, rumors and urban legends about AIDS spread ever more rapidly, or, to use the conventional biological metaphor, "went viral." The website Snopes.com has chronicled rumors about AIDS since the early 1980s, when a newspaper in India, the *Patriot*, proclaimed that AIDS had been created as a by-product of U.S. germ warfare. The *Patriot* was known as a conduit for disinformation in the Soviet Union, and in 1985 the Soviet newspaper, *Literary Gazette*, printed an article also alleging that AIDS emerged from U.S. germ warfare. The *Literary Gazette's* only source was information that had appeared in the *Patriot*.[65] In addition to Snopes.com, other websites have reported on the legends about AIDS that circulate on the Internet, from stories about either a male or female HIV-infected person who picks up dates in order to infect them intentionally via sex to stealth "pinprick" stories in which unsuspecting victims are targeted in a darkened cinema, public telephone booth, or other anonymous place. These stories are a continuation of the epidemic of fear first discussed in chapter 3 and are a variation on fearmongering about disease that has existed forever in human societies.

Evidence that a dissenting view on HIV and AIDS continues to flourish is clear on the discussion page relating to the "AIDS denialism" article in the free Web encyclopedia Wikipedia. What is also clear from such discussions is that those who take part in the discussion have little or no training in science or medicine and view the issue as rhetorical rather than one with consequences for human life.[66] One of the most recent movies questioning HIV as the cause of AIDS appeared in 2009. *House of Numbers*, according to the *New York Times* review, was cobbled together "from interview fragments with doctors, scientists, journalists and others" to raise questions about the existence of HIV as a virus and thus AIDS as the resulting disease. It argued that the disease was "a pharmaceutical-industry ruse to sell complex drug therapies" and then claimed those therapies were the real cause of the disease. Reviewer Jeannette Catsoulis called the film "a weaselly support pamphlet for AIDS denialists."[67]

Conclusion

In this brief review of the massive literature and other types of communication produced about AIDS, a few themes emerge. The appearance of this new disease changed society's tolerance for public discussion about subjects previously considered off-limits—the terms "condom," "anal sex," and "gay" have become acceptable in written and spoken communications. As we saw in chapter 4, what AIDS means to different people is clearly visible in their communications about it. For practicing physicians and public health officials, communications about AIDS were a means to disseminate information to populations at risk for the disease. For medical scientists, the communication imperative was to obtain data, interpret it, and get it published for other scientists to consider. For the AIDS activist community, communications meant raising awareness about a deadly disease and pressuring civil officials to take action in response to it. For people who harbor a grudge against individuals or governments, books, movies, and other forms of communication permitted them to whet their axes on the AIDS grindstone. For AIDS deniers, communications represented a means to spread their ideas. Finally, the awareness of a new pandemic—an epidemic that affects the entire world—has encouraged those who can recall a pre-AIDS world to make efforts to preserve the memories of those who worked to address the epidemic, those who cared for people with AIDS, those who formulated policy related to AIDS, and indeed, those who suffered from the disease and with the introduction of ART have been able to recover a normal life.

7

The Global Epidemic

"No one could have imagined that a few cases of rare disorders damaging
the immune system would herald a pandemic that has killed more than all
those who died in battle during the whole of the twentieth century."

—*UNAIDS: THE FIRST 10 YEARS*[1]

Decisions and action in the industrialized West dominated the policy and
medical responses to AIDS during the first fifteen years of the epidemic, from
1981, when the first cases were recognized, to 1996, when combination antiretroviral therapy was introduced. During that period, however, the human face
of AIDS was quietly changing to one of poor people in the developing world.
This chapter will focus on the global picture of AIDS, including the early efforts to monitor the epidemic in Haiti and Africa, the difficulty of awaking the
international community to the need for worldwide action against AIDS, and
the strategies that finally put AIDS on a global agenda.

AIDS in Haiti

As we saw in chapter 1, by 1982 Haitians had emerged as a "risk group" for
AIDS, although no one had any idea why this was so. No epidemiologist seriously believed that viruses targeted a single nation-state, so although press
accounts stirred fear of Haitian immigrants among populations not trained in
medicine, the real question to be addressed was, Is the large number of Haitians
with AIDS a fluke, or is the disease widespread in Haiti itself? To answer this

question, U.S. investigators wanted to visit Haiti. At first, however, they were barred because the Haitian government deeply resented what it believed was the scapegoating of Haiti as the source of AIDS. Richard Krause, then-director of NIAID, described the initiative necessary to bridge this diplomatic gap. Karl Western, Krause's special assistant for international health, arranged a meeting between the assistant minister of health for Haiti and the Pan American Health Organization (PAHO), the Western Hemisphere branch of the World Health Organization. Western, who had worked at PAHO before coming to NIAID, knew that PAHO represented neutral ground for the Haitians, and he also knew that the U.S. Public Health Service, NIAID's administrative parent, had long been a principal supporter of PAHO's activities. "We had a good discussion, and they extended an invitation for us to go to Haiti," Krause said.[2]

The team Krause took to Port-au-Prince in the spring of 1983 included epidemiologists and clinical investigators Thomas Quinn and Clifford Lane, both NIAID researchers, and Harry Haverkos of the CDC. The assistant health minister took the group on clinical rounds at Hopital de l'Université d'Etat d'Haiti, and to their surprise, Krause recounted in an oral history, "the first three patients we saw were women, and three or four of the first ten patients had tuberculosis. This was new for us—a large percentage of women and tuberculosis as an opportunistic infection."[3] Thomas Quinn, who had already seen one case of AIDS in a woman in Baltimore, described his thinking as he viewed the patients in Haiti:

> The first thing that we saw were these women, who were just wasted away, coughing, probably having *Pneumocystis* or tuberculosis or whatever, and we were told that they had tuberculosis. . . . But it hit me that there was a comparison with the first woman with the disease that I had seen in Baltimore. . . . It brought home to me that, number one, this disease was not affecting just one gender; it was probably going to hit both. It looked like it was still sexually transmitted because the woman's husband was usually also sick or had died, so I could link it back to that. We asked them lots of questions: Why were these women getting the disease if it was only supposed to be in gay men? . . . As we went around those clinics, it was clear to us that there was evidence of heterosexual spread.[4]

During the ten days the Americans worked in Haiti, the diplomatic tensions eased as common medical interests led to productive discussions. Among the Haitian physicians, Jean Pape, who had trained at Cornell University Medical School in the United States and had worked with NIAID units established at Cornell, took the lead. Having read the early AIDS publications about opportunistic infections and Kaposi's sarcoma, Pape worked with other Haitian physicians who had also recognized the syndrome in Haiti to organize the Haitian Group for the Study of Kaposi's Sarcoma and Opportunistic Infections (GHESKIO). In June 1983 the group challenged publications suggesting that Haiti was the original site of AIDS infections imported to the United States, and in October, the physicians published an epidemiological study of sixty-one Haitian patients whom they had observed over two years.[5]

When the members of the American team returned to the United States, however, they found that the popular press in both the United States and Europe still viewed AIDS as a disease of homosexuals only. "The way it was described by the press," recalled Quinn,

> was that gay men went to Haiti for vacations, and they went to these poor Haitians, who would do anything for some money, and would engage in homosexual acts even though the Haitian men might be heterosexual. Then the Haitian men would go back to their wives and infect them. . . . Women were not spreading it to men. This was solely male to male and male to bisexual male, if you will, who then gave it to the woman. But the woman never gives it to the man.[6]

AIDS in Zaire: Projet SIDA

The evidence being collected in Europe, however, refuted this conclusion. Because of their colonial ties with central Africa, both Belgium and France had established economic relationships with that continent, and physicians in those countries began to see more cases of what they believed to be AIDS in people from Africa who came to Europe for treatment. In Belgium, for example, AIDS was diagnosed in five heterosexuals—three women and two men—from Zaire and Chad. In France, patients with connections to equatorial Africa were identified.[7]

These data and a wave of Haitian immigration to Zaire in the late 1950s and early 1960s strongly suggested that epidemiological studies in central Africa would help clarify the emerging picture of AIDS.[8] In August, Krause, Quinn, and Peter Piot of the Belgian Institute of Tropical Medicine (ITM) met at a café during a professional society meeting in Vienna and discussed how they might organize a study to determine whether AIDS indeed existed in Zaire. Krause agreed to commit NIAID funds toward such a study. Later they met again in Belgium, where they were joined by Joseph McCormick of the CDC, who had experience working in Zaire. By mid-October, Quinn, McCormick, and Piot had arrived in Kinshasa, but as Jon Cohen reported in *Science,* their first problem was "to see whether we were welcome or not."[9] They met with the minister of health, who impressed upon them the many different medical challenges facing his office. He gave permission for them to "go look" but emphasized that this new disease would not take priority over his existing work.[10]

The group met with Bila Kapita, who headed internal medicine at Mama Yemo Hospital, Kinshasa's principal hospital named for the mother of Zaire's president, Mobuto Sese Seko. (Since the 1997 political coup that ousted Mobuto and transformed Zaire into the Democratic Republic of Congo, it has been known as Kinshasa General Hospital.) Like Pape in Haiti, Kapita had already identified many patients whom he believed to have AIDS. The first important finding from a brief three-week study was that the male-to-female ratio of AIDS patients was 1.1 to 1—the disease in Zaire was almost equally split between men and women. In their first joint publication, the Western and African physicians wrote, "Homosexuality, intravenous drug abuse, and blood transfusion did not appear to be risk factors in these patients. The findings of this study strongly argue that the situation in central Africa represents a new epidemiological setting for this worldwide disease—that of significant transmission in a large heterosexual population."[11]

By early spring 1984 Peter Piot had received approval for funding from NIAID to expand the study of AIDS in Zaire only to have the U.S. embassy in Kinshasa block the money for what he believed were political reasons within the U.S. government.[12] The original investigative team members strongly believed, however, that a multilateral research group, including the CDC, NIAID, and ITM, should form a joint research project based in Kinshasa. Curran interviewed and hired an epidemiologist, Jonathan Mann, who was working for CDC in New Mexico, and invited him to direct this new project.

Projet SIDA (AIDS Project, in English translation) began in June 1984 with Mann working with two Zairian physicians, Eugène Nzilamabi Nzila and Bosenga Ngali. By July 1984 NIAID had sent Henry (Skip) Francis and the ITM had sent Robert Colebunders to work on the project. Among the Western physicians, Mann was the overall head and primarily responsible for epidemiology, Francis ran the laboratory for the project, and Colebunders headed the clinical work. For the next six years, the group produced more than a hundred publications that answered basic questions about AIDS in Africa and stimulated other African countries to address their own AIDS epidemics.

A few examples illustrate the breadth of Projet SIDA's study. Among their most important findings were that between 6 and 7 percent of pregnant women at prenatal clinics in Kinshasa were already infected with HIV and that the highest incidence was in women under twenty five years old. They ascertained

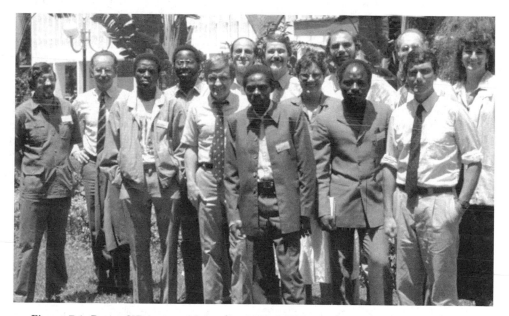

Figure 7.1. Projet SIDA team, November 1986, WHO AIDS meeting, Brazzaville, Republic of Congo. Left to right: Joseph McCormick, Jonathan Mann, Nzila Nzilambi, Henry (Skip) Francis, James Curran, Robert Colebunders, Bila Kapita, Thomas Quinn, Ann Nelson, Peter Piot, Bosenge Ngali, John LaMontagne, Robin Ryder, Stephanie Sagabiel. *Photo courtesy of Ann Marie Nelson, MD.*

the natural history of HIV infection in Zaire. They studied the clinical picture of AIDS in children and adults. They documented the role of female sex workers in transmitting the disease and evidence that the use of condoms reduced infection. They found that children infected with malaria were not at greater risk for HIV infection than uninfected children. In contrast, they found that patients suffering from shingles, a later outbreak of the virus (herpes zoster) that causes chicken pox, were very likely to be infected with HIV. The herpes virus proved to be an opportunistic infection exploiting the reduced immunity HIV caused. Similarly, the tubercle bacillus took advantage of HIV's devastation of the immune system so that AIDS patients could not fend off the ravages of tuberculosis as well as noninfected patients. They evaluated diagnostic technologies for detecting HIV antibodies that were suitable and affordable for use in poor countries. This was important not only for human HIV infection diagnosis but also for screening donated blood.[13]

The problems encountered during Projet SIDA distill the kinds of problems encountered across the developing world in dealing with AIDS. First and most difficult were political problems within Zaire. The Zairian government threatened to jail Bila Kapita for speaking about AIDS in Africa. A high-placed friend intervened, but the Mobutu government banned all talk of AIDS during the 1980s. This led to fear of AIDS among the population expressed as "signs, suspicions, often infantile beliefs" in the absence of any official information.[14] A more fundamental and longer-lasting problem was the tension between what Western nations wanted to learn and could obtain funds for and what African governments desperately needed for their citizens. "Safari research" was the accusation African nations leveled at Western researchers: they would swoop in, bag the data, and leave. Kapita and others complained that the CDC-NIAID-ITM-funded work paid too much attention to epidemiological and immunological research and too little to training Africans to do research or to developing prevention and treatment options. Zairians particularly resented the lack of funding to test the country's blood supply for the AIDS virus, but as James Curran noted, that cost alone would have been equal to the entire Projet SIDA budget. The mandate for funding provided by the legislatures of Western countries was to conduct research, not to fund public health programs or educational programs. This tension has never been completely resolved.[15]

The push and pull between CDC and NIAID investigators complicated these larger issues. CDC's Jonathan Mann wanted to emphasize epidemiology and surveillance within Kinshasa, while NIAID's Skip Francis argued for more virological and immunological studies. Peter Piot and Robert Colebunders of ITM pushed for broader studies outside Kinshasa. It is hardly surprising that personal and institutional antagonisms arose under the trying circumstances in which they worked, and the oral histories of the participants reveal the story from their personal points of view. Curran of CDC, Quinn of NIAID, and Piot of ITM met regularly as the project's institutional overseers. According to all of them, one of their ongoing tasks was to smooth the ruffled feathers of their representatives in Zaire.[16]

Ultimately, political unrest in Zaire forced Western investigators to evacuate. In September 1991 Zairian solders rebelled against Mobutu Sese Seko's government, which was reeling under massive inflation and unable to pay its army. The soldiers' rampage threatened the National Institute of Biomedical Research (INRB), where one part of the Projet SIDA laboratory was located. Fearing that the soldiers would invade and destroy the laboratory, one enterprising American zoologist, Delfi Messinger, "decided to kill a sheep, put its blood in a 50-cc syringe, and squirt 'SIDA' in dripping, meter-high letters on the wall outside the institute. . . . She also put snakes in cages in front of the entrances to all of the institute's buildings and, to 'booby-trap' her car, put a snake in it, too."[17] Messinger's quick thinking saved data and stored samples of the project, but the Western scientists were evacuated shortly thereafter under the protection of Belgian and French forces. Eight months later, both CDC and NIAID cut off funds for Projet SIDA. In 1997 Mobutu was overthrown, and the country was renamed the Democratic Republic of Congo. Congolese scientists who had worked with Projet SIDA continued to conduct studies, but this work was by necessity on a much more limited scale, since funding from United States and European governments had been terminated.[18]

The AIDS Epidemic across Africa: "Slim Disease"

Social, cultural, economic, and political factors in different countries governed the spread of HIV infection across Africa. The disease itself, however, followed a recognizable pattern. In 1984 Ugandan physician Anthony Lwegaba, who worked with David Serwadda in publishing the first description of "Slim" in 1985, described the disease in the city of Rakai in his clinical notes:

> The patient experiences general malaise, and on-and-off "fevers." For which he may be treated "self" or otherwise with Aspirin, chloroquine and chloramphenicol etc. In due course, the patient develops gradual loss of appetite.
>
> In the next six months, diarrhoea appears on-and-off. There is gradual weight loss and the patient is pale. Most patients at this point in time will rely on traditional healers, as the disease to many is attributed to witchcraft.
>
> After one year, the patient develops a skin disease . . . which is very itchy. Apparently it is all over the body. The skin becomes ugly with hyperpigmented scars. There may be a cough usually dry but other times productive.
>
> Earlier on after a year, the patient may be so weak that even when taken to hospital (not much can be done due to late reporting), goes into chronicity and death.[19]

These symptoms were similar to those of many AIDS sufferers in other countries. The main difference was that no Kaposi's sarcoma was recognized at this time in African AIDS patients.

WEST EQUATORIAL AFRICA

Facilitated by longstanding medical relationships dating to the period of European colonial domination in Africa, Projet SIDA and other epidemiological studies in African countries revealed that the pattern of infection and disease varied widely in different regions of Africa according to economic and cultural factors affecting transmission of HIV. In his book *The African AIDS Epidemic: A History*, John Iliffe, University of Cambridge historian of African history, traced the beginning of the African AIDS epidemic to central Africa, where HIV first appeared as a human infection. Retrospective studies of stored sera from central Africa revealed less than a 1 percent incidence of HIV infection in the early 1970s. By the end of that decade and into the 1980s, the incidence rose rapidly to the 3 to 5 percent incidence usually described as the threshold for explosive epidemic growth in the Democratic Republic of Congo (sometimes called Congo Kinshasa), the Republic of Congo (sometimes called Congo Brazzaville), Cameroon, the Central African Republic, Gabon, and Equatorial Guinea. Surprisingly, however, the epidemic appeared to stabilize throughout the 1990s at an incidence level just under 8 percent. Iliffe argued that the epidemic was largely confined to a subset of the population with many ephemeral sexual relationships "in which the men were often significantly older and wealthier than the women." He also observed that "over 90 percent of men in the western equatorial region were circumcised, which probably provided some protection because the foreskin was especially liable to viral penetration," and that other sexually transmitted diseases, especially the genital ulcers caused by herpes simplex virus 2, which facilitated entry of HIV, were relatively rare.[20]

The one exception to this epidemic pattern in west equatorial Africa occurred in the Central African Republic, especially in its main city, Bangui. Apparently, the AIDS epidemic there was fostered by casual sex similar to what occurred in the Democratic Republic of Congo, but through sexual networks of young people about the same age with partners exchanged on average twenty to forty times per year. More than half the women in one study had given birth before they were twenty years old, which also led many of them to rely on sex as a way to provide subsistence for their children. By 1993, 16 percent of women at prenatal clinics were HIV positive. The popularity of injected medications, which averaged eight per year per person in the late 1980s, also contributed to the transmission of AIDS.[21]

EAST AFRICA

To the east of the Democratic Republic of Congo lies the Lake Victoria basin, home to the countries of Rwanda, Burundi, Uganda, western Kenya, and northern Tanzania. This region is densely populated, in contrast to the remainder of east Africa, which lies on the dry Ethiopian plateau and extends to the Indian Ocean. Populations in eastern Kenya, Ethiopia, Eritrea, Djibouti, and Somalia are more scattered. The arrival of AIDS in east Africa was explosive in the Lake Victoria basin and much slower though relentless in the drier countries of the east.[22]

In the overwhelmingly Christian populations of Rwanda and Burundi, sexual behavior among the young was strictly controlled, whereas the sexual activity among the fifteen-to-nineteen-year-old age group in the Democratic Republic of Congo was casual and frequent. The result, according to Iliffe, was an epidemic pattern dominated not by partner exchange but by commercial sex. "On average," he wrote, "men in Kigali made their sexual debut at 18 but married at 24–28; in the meantime, since other young women in this 'austere Catholic town' were carefully protected, they frequented sex workers and often continued to do so after marriage. Circumcision was rare, condoms despised, sexually transmitted diseases widespread, sexual coercion common, and women depended overwhelmingly on a male partner for income."[23] Historian Maryinez Lyons made similar observations about women in Ugandan society, noting that the majority of Ugandan women "live in relation to men as clients." Researchers have found, she stated, that in Uganda, "to be masculine means to provide for and control women. To be feminine is to be pleasing and acceptable to men." Thus in Rwanda, Burundi, and Uganda, a vicious circle ensued. Men patronized sex workers, a high percentage of whom were HIV positive. They transmitted the virus to their wives, who, if their husbands died of AIDS before they did, were often shunned by their birth families and forced into sex work to survive, thereby continuing the chain of transmission of the AIDS virus and reinforcing the myths that women were the source of AIDS and that they maliciously tried to infect men. This belief was clearly reflected in AIDS education posters such as one from Uganda, "I Am Driving Straight Home to My Wife." In the drawing, two female sex workers, assumed to be infected with HIV, try to hail a presumably uninfected male truck driver, who will avoid AIDS by being faithful to his wife.[24]

The truck driver image also pointed to one of three groups of males who were instrumental in spreading AIDS during the 1980s. Long-haul truck drivers on the main routes of the trans-Africa highways infected or were infected by female sex workers in the towns where they stopped overnight and then carried the virus to their sexual partners at their destination. A second, smaller group were the migrant laborers who carried the virus into the rural agricultural communities. A third large, mobile group were soldiers in the military of various countries during the late 1970s and throughout the 1980s. In 1978 Idi Amin, who came to power in 1971 in Uganda, attempted to annex a province of Tanzania, only to precipitate a war that led to his ouster in 1978. As the Tanzanian forces pursued the remnants of Amin's army throughout the 1980s in northern

Uganda, they infected the women with whom they had sex and were probably the source by which HIV spread into southern and middle Sudan along with Ugandan refugees from the conflict.[25]

SOUTH AFRICA

Not surprisingly, the four countries adjacent to equatorial and east Africa— Zambia, Malawi, Zimbabwe, and Botswana—experienced the initial spread of HIV infection in the southern portion of the African continent. Epidemiological factors similar to those in east Africa drove the epidemics in the south. The position of women in society, especially their lack of power in sexual relation-

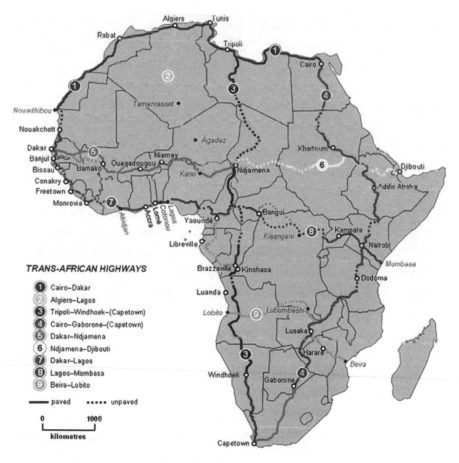

Figure 7.2. Trans-African highways based on 2000–2003 data. *Courtesy of Rex Parry, Wikimedia Commons.*

ships and their need to please men to survive economically, fueled the rising infection rate. The trans-Africa highway system facilitated male mobility between the highly productive economic areas such as copper and diamond mines. Historic cultural patterns of maintaining residences both in the countryside and the city, to which residents had migrated seasonally in the past but cycled between more often with the coming of motorized transportation, helped spread the epidemic from cities to rural areas.

During the 1990s the AIDS epidemic reached maturity in these countries. The most reliable estimates came from blood samples at prenatal clinics, and the infection rate among pregnant women was staggering. Malawi's infection rate peaked at 32.8 percent in 1996, Zambia's at 22–27 percent in 1990–1993, Zimbabwe's at 32 percent in 1995, and Botswana's at 34 percent in 1993, although the incidence continued to grow in Botswana. In 2000 the prenatal infection rate in three Botswana cities was measured at 44, 36, and 50 percent.[26]

The AIDS epidemic in South Africa started later but grew to be the most severe in the world. Iliffe summarized the factors that led to this: "Not only did the socio-economic structures of Apartheid make the country an almost perfect environment for HIV, but the beginning of the epidemic coincided with the township revolt of the mid 1980s and its peak took place a decade later during the transition to majority rule, which compelled ordinary people to concentrate on survival and distracted both the outgoing regime and its nationalist successor from making HIV their chief priority."[27] The most striking aspect of AIDS in South Africa is that no single group such as male migrants or female sex workers can be identified as the core group in the epidemic. Migrants from central Africa who worked in South African mines were one source. South African males who migrated to work along the highways were another. Poverty's encouragement of commercial sex exchanges played a role, as did the desire to be viewed as a "playboy" among young males and a willingness to exchange sex for money or presents among young women who believed that marriage was not viable for their generation. The Zulus' abandonment of male circumcision in the eighteenth century and the increased prevalence of genital ulcers caused by herpes simplex virus 2 also contributed to HIV's spread. At the peak of South Africa's epidemic, between 1993 and 1998, prenatal infection rates rose to between 31 and 39 percent.[28]

West Africa

The AIDS epidemic in West Africa differed from that on the rest of the continent. This was because a second type of HIV had already become established in the human population. Investigators from France and Senegal who were working with Max Essex's laboratory at the Harvard School of Public Health identified the new virus, called HIV-2, in 1985 almost by accident. While studying the natural history of the AIDS virus in Senegal, they found Senegalese infected with a similar but not identical virus. This new virus was about three times more difficult to transmit through sexual intercourse and up to ten times more difficult to transmit from mother to infant. It took longer—up to twenty-five years—to manifest the end-stage symptoms of AIDS; thus mortality from HIV-2 infection was lower than from HIV-1 infection because many infected people died from other causes before they reached end-stage AIDS symptoms.[29]

HIV-1 and HIV-2 met in Abidjan, Côte d'Ivoire, which became the epicenter of HIV infection in West Africa. AIDS spread outward from Abidjan along two routes. First was via female sex workers from Côte d'Ivoire, Ghana, and Nigeria, who sought to establish a small business or fund their siblings' schooling without revealing to those at home how they earned their money. The second avenue of spread was along the routes followed by male migrant labor. Burkina Faso suffered the greatest increase in HIV infection from this source. In Niger and Mali, the same patterns were repeated but at lower levels of infection. The geographical pattern of infection in these countries suggests that the Islamic social order may have exerted a limiting factor on transmission. Women married very young—the median age in Mali was sixteen—and they were often secluded after marriage. Thus, in 1998 only 0.1 percent of women in Niger reported more than one sexual partner within the last year, and most of the 11 percent of men who had experienced extramarital sex were young, unmarried, circumcised men whose partners were sex workers.[30]

In Nigeria and Senegal, the AIDS epidemic was smaller than might have been predicted. Nigeria was a large and diverse country with no major city that served as the conduit to all other sections. Its sex workers were predominately Nigerian and not involved in the larger, mobile West African sex trade. The influence of Islam in the northern part of Nigeria, similar to that in Niger and Mali, also helped to restrain the epidemic. Surprisingly, these social factors seem to have had a larger effect than the state of Nigeria's health system, which was rated by the World Health Organization as one of the worst in the world.[31]

World Health Organization's Global Programme on AIDS

In 1986 Jonathan Mann was approached by the World Health Organization to head up a new program on AIDS. Seeing this as an opportunity to have a greater impact on the rapidly spreading epidemic, he agreed and arrived in Geneva at the moment that WHO's director general, Halfdan Mahler, had reversed course on the threat of AIDS. In 1985 Mahler had urged "that people should keep AIDS in perspective to other diseases." Since that time, reports from around the world convinced him that "everything is getting worse and worse in AIDS and all of us have been underestimating it." With contributions of $5 million from the governments of the United States, Sweden, Norway, and England and with pledges from Switzerland and Denmark, Mahler announced the creation of WHO's Global Programme on AIDS with Jonathan Mann as its director. Its aims would include the following:

> Providing model policies and strategies for combating AIDS, chiefly through educational campaigns, for every country that requests help.
>
> Expanding a global information gathering system to screen and disseminate information to health workers. An effort will be made to help countries benefit from educational programs that have proved effective elsewhere.
>
> Creating an international network among scientists to share information, and a far more aggressive program of research into drugs, vaccines and other therapeutic and preventive health measures.
>
> Tapping the skills of sociologists, behaviorial scientists, communications experts and others outside the traditional boundaries of public health.
>
> Educating health workers about how AIDS spreads and the dangers of repeated use of needles without sterilization between injections, a common practice in third world countries.[32]

This ambitious agenda reflected Mann's strong sense of urgency and understanding that controlling the AIDS epidemic would involve fundamental changes to cultural, religious, and legal aspects of societies. Over the next four years, Mann transformed the Global AIDS Programme from essentially a two-person operation into a 220-person group with a budget of $109 million. Most of the budget did not come from WHO but rather was raised by the program itself through Mann's fund-raising visits to individual countries. This also enabled Mann to enjoy more autonomy than the heads of other WHO programs.[33] "The guy just fizzed with energy," said psychologist David Miller, who worked with Mann to develop counseling and psychosocial training for the Global Programme. "He established AIDS programs in over 100 countries in a remarkably short space of time."[34] Also as a result of Mann's realization that the AIDS epidemic needed as much public exposure as possible, the Global Programme launched World AIDS Day on December 1, 1988. It became a day of observance and reflection that has been ongoing since its inception.[35]

In 1988 Director General Mahler was replaced in the customary rotation of heads of WHO by Hiroshi Nakajima, who arrived to find that the Global Programme on AIDS represented up to one-third of the entire WHO budget. Mann's visibility in the press was very high according to Peter Piot, who had worked with Mann on Projet SIDA. "He actually had become the public face of World Health, and that may not have been appreciated by his bosses. And it was also about control," said Piot.[36] Joseph McCormick of the CDC, who had also been involved early on in Projet SIDA, summarized, "It was pretty clear to all of us that the new director of WHO felt that he was being totally overshadowed by this media superstar. He actually limited Jonathan's travel. There were instances when he wouldn't let him go to a meeting, wouldn't sign off on travel. Whether Jonathan should have stayed and weathered the storm or whether he made the right move—I think that's an arguable point. The fact is, he made that decision to resign."[37] Mann left Geneva and moved to Harvard University, where he continued to advocate for expanded human rights in the AIDS epidemic, eventually crystallizing this vision in two volumes titled *AIDS in the World*.[38] Tragically, on September 3, 1998, he was killed in the crash of Swissair flight 111 off the coast of Nova Scotia in eastern Canada, en route to Geneva.

Director General Nakajima replaced Mann with Michael Merson, another CDC-trained epidemiologist who had previously worked with WHO on cholera in Bangladesh and who had directed the WHO Diarrheal Diseases Control Programme.[39] Walter Dowdle, deputy director at the CDC, was appointed special consultant to the Global Programme. The staff of the Global Programme fell to four, and the organization was transformed into a more typical WHO component.

Merson assumed the directorship as AIDS was being recognized in eastern Europe, the Muslim world, and Asia. Even though little was known about the epidemiology of AIDS in these regions—whether it would be heterosexual sex, homosexual sex, or injecting drug use that would primarily drive the epidemic—the Global Programme faced a $40 million shortfall in its budget for 1991. The United States cut back its contribution to the program from $25 million in fiscal 1989 to $21 million for 1990, and President George H. W. Bush's request was for $19 million in 1991.[40]

AIDS in the Muslim World

As we have seen, the influence of Islam on countries such as Nigeria, Niger, and Mali helped to restrain the spread of HIV. Anthropologist Peter B. Gray at Harvard University has studied how well the aspects of Islamic law as they pertain to sexual behavior have helped to reduce the incidence of HIV transmission in predominately Muslim countries. Islam forbids extramarital sex and homosexual sex and discourages condom use. Muslim men are circumcised, and Islam calls for ritual cleansing after sexual intercourse. These tenets, along with the prohibition on alcohol use, which might facilitate risky sexual behavior, suppress the sexual transmission of HIV. In contrast, Islamic law permitting men to marry up to four wives and divorce easily, along with the discouragement of condom use, means that they may have unprotected sex and multiple sexual partners during their lifetimes, thus promoting the likelihood of HIV transmission.[41] As with other religions, therefore, Islam's tenets regarding sex are a double-edged sword in the AIDS epidemic.

When we expand our gaze from sub-Saharan Africa to the African countries that border the Mediterranean Sea, we begin to see the great expanse of nations that make up *Dar al-Islam*, the "house of Islam." Some fifty countries in the world, reporting 40 percent or more of their population as Muslim, come under this banner. This great expanse stretches across north Africa, through the Middle East and South Asia, and through Indonesia and Malaysia in the Pacific. Most of these countries do not distinguish between the tenets of their faith and laws of their nation-states. They consult the Koran both as a religious text and source of law. The concept of "democracy" as laws embodying the will

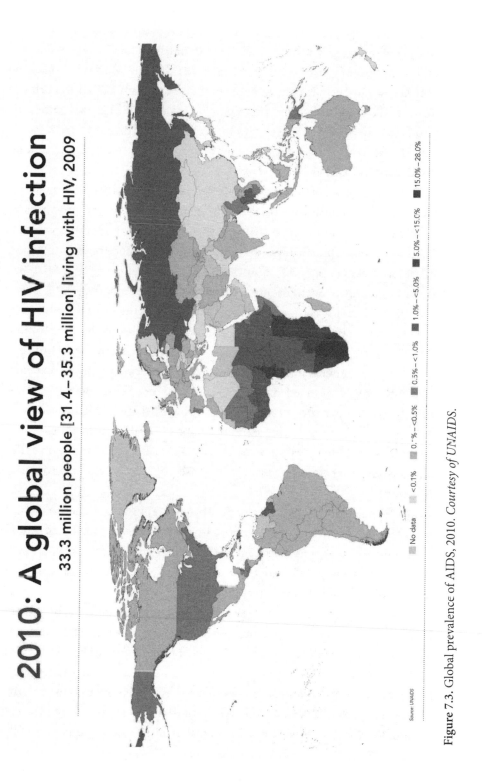

Figure 7.3. Global prevalence of AIDS, 2010. *Courtesy of UNAIDS.*

of the people exists only within the framework of Islam's law. In a report for the National Bureau of Asian Research on HIV/AIDS in the Muslim world, Laura M. Kelley and Nicholas Eberstadt examined how Islam helped to curb the spread of HIV while at the same time encouraging denial of a growing problem that threatened to become a public health crisis. Perhaps the most tragic aspect of this denial was the increasing number of suicides in Islamic nations among individuals diagnosed as HIV positive.[42]

Throughout the 1980s and 1990s, Kelley and Eberstadt argued, religious leaders in these countries asserted that "premarital sex, adultery, prostitution, homosexuality, and intravenous drug use do not occur in the Muslim world."[43] What this meant in practice was that systematic surveillance of HIV infection was "sorely lacking" in these countries. Statistics compiled by UNAIDS are based on these inadequate data and are dependent on reporting by governments that may not wish to publicize bad news. Since there is no tradition of secular democracy in most Muslim countries, mounting public health campaigns that could suggest that citizens are not rigorously following Islamic law is difficult. For example, in 1995 Indonesia's religious leaders "urged that condoms only be sold to married couples—and then only by prescription from a general practitioner" because the leaders believed that religious convictions would stop people from having extramarital sex. Similarly, Islamic clergy in northern Nigeria "urged Muslims to boycott a U.S.-backed seminar on HIV/AIDS, claiming that attendance would increase promiscuity among ordinarily upright believers."[44]

In 1987 the Muslim countries of South Asia—Pakistan, Afghanistan, and Bangladesh—reported zero AIDS cases. In 1988, however, two investigators from the Jinnah Postgraduate Medical Center in Karachi, in collaboration with another at the University of Southern California, examined blood from 230 people who had visited Karachi hospitals and found that the blood of four people, "one male blood donor and three family members of another male, a drug addict," strongly reacted to reagents in two different tests for the presence of HIV. Both infected males among the group that tested positive showed signs of lymphadenopathy (swollen lymph glands), and the child among the four had developmental disorders and neurological manifestations. Since no formal surveillance for AIDS had been conducted in Pakistan, the authors found the existence of these four positive tests and clinical manifestations "staggering."[45] By the mid-1990s, a National AIDS Control Programme in Pakistan was targeting the "most at risk groups," especially truckers, but it was not until 2001, with support from the World Bank, that Pakistan was able to implement an enhanced AIDS control program.[46]

The disparity between reported statistics and actual situation is made clear in Indonesia, where the news agency Antara reported in November 2009 that, although only 11,856 cases of HIV/AIDS had been reported in 2008, the reality was far different. According to Ronald Jonathan, the director of an Indonesian HIV/AIDS organization, these cases represented the tip of an iceberg; Indonesia would suffer some 5 million HIV infections by 2010.[47] The large number of injecting drug users in the country had been the principal point of entry for the virus, but it had spread into the general population via sexual intercourse. In 2009 and 2010, Indonesia's HIV/AIDS epidemic was actually the fastest growing in Asia.[48] Following publication of Antara's story, Indonesia's government launched a safe sex campaign with a National Condom Week. This initiative caused bitter arguments between moderate Muslim leaders, who supported the initiative, and fundamentalist Muslim leaders, who believed that strict enforcement of Islamic law would control the disease. For example, a spokesperson for the Indonesia Mujahiddin Council rejected condom use as a way to protect against AIDS: "We strongly feel that condoms can't prevent people from getting AIDS. The pores of the latex are bigger than the virus itself. . . . AIDS prevention should start by implementing Islamic laws and punishing rule breakers, infidels and those who engage in pre-marital sex. In Islam we normally throw stones at them." In contrast, a moderate Islamic studies lecturer at Indonesia's Muhammadiyah University in Surabaya, East Java, argued, "I'm not against the campaign. I am not against anything that can preserve the life of human beings. There are verses in the Koran that says humans should take good care of their health. It is like a Jihad (holy war) on HIV/AIDS."[49]

AIDS in India

During the last half of the 1980s, physicians reported the first cases of AIDS in Asia. Thomas Quinn, who had participated in the earliest assessments of AIDS in Haiti and Zaire, made a trip to India in 1986. Initially, he reported, "Nothing was happening in Asia. It was very quiet. There was some talk about it [AIDS] going on in the Philippines, but it was the American servicemen in the military that were infected, and there was a concern it might spread. But it was very limited. There just was not much going on."[50]

When virologist T. Jacob John of Vellore, India, asked Quinn to test some blood samples for HIV from sex workers in Mumbai and Chennai, India (cities formerly known as Bombay and Madras, respectively), however, a different finding became evident. Quinn found 11 of 102 to be positive for HIV using the ELISA test. Of those, he confirmed that 10 were positive using the Western blot technique, a more sensitive assay.[51] John and Quinn reported the results to Vulimiri Ramalingaswami, director general of the Indian Council of Medical Research (ICMR), who, in turn, reported the findings to the Indian Parliament. According to Quinn, however, members of Parliament initially rejected the findings: "It can't be. There are no AIDS cases here. How can we have HIV?" Knowing about the long incubation period of HIV, the ICMR took the initiative to create surveillance centers across India, and in 1987 it persuaded the Indian government to launch the National AIDS Control Organization.[52]

As in Africa, the most reliable information about infection rates in India came from blood samples taken at prenatal clinics. These showed that the Indian states in the southern geographical area of the subcontinent had the highest HIV infection rates. Beginning in the southwestern state of Maharashtra, whose capital is Mumbai, and including Andhra Pradesh in the southeast, infection rates among pregnant women rose to more than 1.25 percent in the 1990s. Similar figures were reported in the other southern Indian states—Goa, Karnataka, and Tamil Nadu. The virus was transmitted primarily through female sex workers, men who have sex with men, and injecting drug users.[53]

The far northeastern area of India, attached like a flag to the bulk of the country after Bangladesh was carved out as a separate nation-state, also suffered from higher rates of infection than did northern mainland India. The states of Manipur, Mizoram, and Nagaland border Myanmar (formerly called Burma), a major producer of opium. In the 1980s injecting drug use became popular in this region of India, and HIV infection quickly followed. Infection rates spiked to as high as 70 percent in 1998 among injecting drug users in Mizoram. Since that time, prevention efforts have dropped infection rates to between 3 and 7 percent. Having gained entry to the human population via injecting drug use, HIV was also spread by sexual activity. In recent years, prevention efforts have reduced infection among pregnant women at prenatal clinics to below 1 percent.[54]

The final Indian region to struggle with HIV infection through injecting drug use was Punjab in northwestern India, bordering Pakistan. In 2007 Reuters news agency reported that India needed a "wake-up call" because officials had underestimated the danger of HIV taking hold outside the very large cities of mainland India and the northeastern states bordering Myanmar.[55] In a 2009 report, the Indian National AIDS Control Organization reported that the infection rate among injecting drug users in Punjab continued to be high at 13.8 percent.[56]

By the early 1990s India had created a National AIDS Research Institute in Pune, at which it collaborated internationally with NIAID and Johns Hopkins via Thomas Quinn's network. When asked by Indian government officials to help set up a research program like Projet SIDA in Africa, Quinn contacted a former postdoctoral fellow, Robert Bollinger, who had continued to work at Hopkins and had a strong interest in India. Bollinger went to Pune and worked with institute officials to draft a grant proposal for collaborative AIDS research in India. In the peer review process, that proposal "was ranked number one of all the grants submitted for doing international AIDS research," Quinn stated. Approval and funding of the proposal launched a research collaboration that has continued into 2011.[57]

AIDS in Southeast Asia

The nations of Southeast Asia and the Pacific have suffered from AIDS via the same epidemiological patterns seen in Africa and Asia, with variations according to the cultures of each country. Known as a center for the international sex tourism trade, Bangkok, Thailand, reported its first diagnosed case of AIDS in 1984.[58] As more and more Thai sex workers tested positive for HIV, the Thai government responded with a strong AIDS prevention and education campaign. As reported in *Time*, "Brothels started using condoms. Public-service messages were broadcast on radio and television every two hours. Anti-AIDS messages—often served with a healthy dose of *sanuk*, the Thai sense of playfulness—were spread in schools, hospitals, police stations, and courthouses. After peaking at 143,000 in 1991, the annual number of new cases of HIV infection fell to 19,000 in 2003."[59] By July 2004, however, when the Fifteenth International AIDS Conference was held in Thailand, there was concern that new infections remained high among injecting drug users and some homosexual males and that only 20 percent of sexually active young people used condoms regularly. Thai expenditures for prevention had also fallen to only 8 percent of the total AIDS budget.[60] The Thai situation reflected that of other Southeast Asian countries in that preventing new infections with HIV needed to be a long-term commitment of substantial funds and national will.

Other countries in Southeast Asia experienced the arrival of AIDS in the late 1980s or early 1990s: the Philippines reported its first case in 1985; Singapore and Sri Lanka in 1986; Tonga, French Polynesia, Indonesia, and Malasia in 1987; and others after 1988.[61] According to physician Ofelia T. Monzon, founder of the AIDS Society of the Philippines, doing AIDS outreach in Manila in the late 1980s was a major challenge. "Prostitution was illegal," she noted, "and possession of condoms was evidence of such. In as much as the field workers were distributing condoms and demonstrating their appropriate use, the city police had to be treated to a lecture on AIDS prevention and the need for field workers to carry around condoms."[62]

AIDS in China
In China, the most populous country in the world, the AIDS epidemic followed the same predictable pattern of initial denial followed by attempts to organize prevention campaigns within the strictures of cultural mores. In 1986 the *Weekly Epidemiological Record* of the World Health Organization reported that four hemophiliacs had tested positive for HIV and that one "traveler from abroad" had died in Beijing the previous year.[63] From 1986 to 1988 AIDS was viewed as a threat from abroad. Beginning in 1989 and lasting through 1993, AIDS was known primarily in drug users in China's southwest, the area bordering the Golden Triangle of drug trafficking in Myanmar, Laos, and Vietnam. From 1994 forward, drug users, commercial plasma donors, and, increasingly, individuals who engaged in unsafe sex were diagnosed as HIV positive. By 1998 all thirty-one provinces, autonomous regions, and municipalities reported AIDS cases. This spurred the development of a national surveillance system.[64]

In China, as in many other Asian countries, criminal law was used in an attempt to control injecting drug use, prostitution, and homosexuality. As in the United States, however, incarcerating drug addicts for a period of time stopped their habit only until they were released. Control of prostitution in China was attempted by so-called 100 percent condom use programs, also adopted in Cambodia, Vietnam, Thailand, Mongolia, Laos, and Myanmar. Under this program, the police targeted brothels, nightclubs, and other indoor venues where commercial sex took place. Although the program succeeded in reducing unsafe sex in such establishments, the police were repressive and often abusive to sex workers, who reported that the owners of nightclubs and brothels often forced sex workers to have sex with police in exchange for certification that the institution was compliant with condom use.[65]

In 2002 severe acute respiratory syndrome (SARS) began in China and very quickly spread around the world. Chinese officials acknowledged that a poor public health infrastructure had contributed to the spread of SARS and that a robust public health program, put in place belatedly, had successfully contained the disease—the last Chinese case cleared in 2003. This experience spurred expansion of China's small scale response to AIDS. At the height of the SARS outbreak, Wu Yi, a "respected vice premier," was named acting health minister. The *Wall Street Journal* reported that "Ms. Wu has described AIDS as a 'long-term war' that will be her next focus after SARS and . . . has requested a doubling of the annual AIDS budget from the current $12.5 million."[66]

AIDS in Latin America

In *Science*'s 2006 overview of AIDS in Latin America, Jon Cohen wrote that the AIDS epidemic in South America and the Caribbean had "largely been overshadowed by the more severe problems in sub-Saharan Africa, the vastly larger population of Asia, and the attention that more developed countries have attracted." Yet the area had more than 2 million people living with AIDS, more than the United States, Canada, Western Europe, Australia, and Japan combined.[67] When UNAIDS published its 2010 report on the global AIDS epidemic, the region still had 2 million people living with AIDS. The epidemic had stabilized but was far from contained.[68]

The small nations of Haiti, the Bahamas, Guyana, Belize, and Trinidad and Tobago have the highest incidence of HIV infection in the region—each has more than 2 percent of its population infected. Half the total people infected with HIV live in the four largest countries in the region, Brazil, Mexico, Colombia, and Argentina. Although there is a tendency among North Americans to think of "Latin America" as monolithic, it is instead extraordinarily diverse in ethnicities, cultures, wealth and poverty, patterns of drug use, and sexual mores. This means that no single preventive or therapeutic strategy will work to reduce the epidemic across the region. In addition, weak leadership, homophobia, religious pressures, and stigma for infected people exacerbate the challenges of controlling spread of the disease.[69]

Across Latin America, the AIDS epidemic is fueled primarily by men who have sex with men. Indeed, the term "men who have sex with men," or MSM in shorthand, was coined to describe just the kind of sex that some Latin American men participate in. The machismo culture denigrates any expression of femininity in men, but femininity is defined as passivity. So as long as a male takes the initiative in a sexual relationship, he is not considered homosexual. An example of this is a man having sex with a male transvestite who plays the passive role in the sexual encounter. Meanwhile, women are expected to be subservient to men and thus have little or no leverage in asking their sexual partners, especially their husbands, to use condoms during sex.[70]

Spanish and Portuguese are the predominate languages of Latin American countries, and the Catholic Church is the religious organization principally tying these countries together. As Shawn Smallman, professor of international studies at Oregon State University, pointed out in his 2007 book, *The AIDS Pandemic in Latin America*, the Catholic Church has played a leading role in providing hospice care to persons dying of AIDS. At the same time it has fought HIV education campaigns and refused to mention condoms in any context save the extremely narrow exception provided in November 2010 by Pope Benedict XVI for male prostitutes, for whom contraception is not a central issue. The pope said they were justified in using condoms to prevent infection of their patrons.[71] In May 2011 PBS reporter Ray Suarez reported from an HIV/AIDS conference in Rome that the Vatican "stood firm" against the use of condoms to prevent AIDS.[72]

One Latin American country that has led research on possible preventive efforts against HIV infection is Peru. In Lima and its environs, where 70 percent of infected Peruvians live, two Peruvian scientists—Jorge Sánchez, the former head of Peru's national AIDS program within the Ministry of Health and who now runs the nonprofit Asociación Civil Impacta Salud y Educación (Impacta), and Carlos Cáceres, an epidemiologist at the Universidad Peruana Cayetano

Heredia in Lima—have championed research on AIDS prevention. Both have personal ties to the affected communities. Sánchez is the principal investigator on a clinical trial funded by NIAID and scheduled to end in 2013, testing whether pre-exposure antiviral drugs will protect high-risk individuals from contracting HIV. Even with such leadership in AIDS research, Peru itself has lagged far behind Brazil in providing universal access to antiretroviral drugs for people already suffering from AIDS.[73]

AIDS in Eastern Europe, Russia, and Central Asia

The story of AIDS in Eastern Europe, Russia, and Central Asia—the former Soviet Union and Soviet bloc countries—is depressingly similar to the emergence of the epidemic elsewhere, with only slight variations. As the first infections were reported in the mid-1980s and into the 1990s, when the epidemic was still very small, governments in the region rejected the notion that HIV could possibly take hold. Jon Cohen reported in *Science*, "Many public health officials in the region believed the AIDS epidemic raging elsewhere would make few inroads in their societies. This was a disease spread by gay sex, drug injections, promiscuous heterosexual partnering, and prostitution—behaviors, they thought, their cultures rejected so thoroughly that HIV didn't stand a chance."[74] Alas, as in all other cultures, these activities did indeed exist and brought AIDS along with them.

The driving force behind the spread of HIV infection in this region was and remains injecting drug use, and the single most important inhibitor to effective action to stem the epidemic is government resistance to harm-reduction strategies. Injecting drug users in this region are reviled, hence programs such as methadone maintenance and needle exchanges are not supported. "It's kind of a hopeless situation," said Anya Sarang, a sociologist in Moscow who studies injecting drug users and HIV, "but that's our reality." In addition, surveillance of AIDS in this region is limited to "registered" HIV infections, people who come into the health care system or reside in institutions such as prisons. No attempt is made to survey populations such as homosexual males, and because of discrimination, many people do not come into the health care system until they are in an advanced state of AIDS.[75]

In 2010, at the Eighteenth International AIDS Conference in Vienna, Austria, organizers asked for signatures on a "Vienna Declaration" stating that punitive drug policies fueled the epidemic and calling for "a science-based public health approach to address the individual and community harms stemming from illicit drug use." A brief scan of the list, available on the Internet, of the more than 18,700 people and organizations who have signed the declaration reveals that most are people who have supported this position for many years. Few, if any, representatives of governments that criminalize injecting drug use, including the United States and Russia, have lent their support.[76]

Creation of the Joint United Nations Programme on HIV/AIDS

Between 1990, when Jonathan Mann resigned from the WHO Global Programme on AIDS (GPA), and 1996, when the new Joint United Nations Programme on HIV/AIDS was created, the international response to AIDS was limited by small budgets and WHO politics. Director Michael Merson was able to support diverse AIDS programs in Uganda and Thailand.[77] Nonetheless, GPA was accused of being "too medicalized" and insensitive to the cultural variations of different countries. Other UN agencies, such as the United Nations International Children's Emergency Fund (UNICEF), the United Nations Development Program (UNDP), and the World Bank, fought with GPA about which agency should be in charge of particular programs. In the countries served by GPA, ministries of health were similarly opposed by other ministries that believed they should have greater control over AIDS activities. Donor nations, who were fed up with how these situations stalled effective work in controlling the epidemic, argued for the appointment of an external committee to evaluate the GPA work. Its report, published in 1992, hailed GPA's vision in identifying AIDS as a global problem that required a coordinated international response. It also criticized, however, the "inefficiency of coordination between different UN agencies" that led to duplication of effort. The upshot of this report was the formation of a task force that would restructure the UN collaboration.[78]

In December 1994 Peter Piot, the Belgian physician and microbiologist who had participated in the Projet SIDA investigations in Zaire in 1983, was named director of the new program. In an oral history, Piot noted that before he agreed to take the job, he nailed down two conditions: that he had the power to hire and fire, not just to accept people sent to him from UN agencies; and that the new joint program would have a strong central secretariat with offices in affected countries that would run the actual programs. Like Jonathan

Mann before him, Piot wanted to avoid the usual UN practice of making joint programs accountable to all the different UN agencies because Piot believed this would effectively kill the program's ability to act forcefully. After accepting the position, he retreated with trusted advisers to Belaggio, Italy, for an informal brainstorming session. There the acronym "UNAIDS" was coined for the more unwieldy formal name "Joint United Nations Programme on HIV/AIDS." Piot's sixteen-year-old daughter designed the logo, blending the AIDS red ribbon with the UN logo.[79]

The staff Piot recruited reflected the fact that this program would be a public health implementation effort rather than a medical research or patient care program. His first hires included an experienced UN social worker, Purnima Mane, who had worked for more than a decade on public health and gender-related issues in India; Elisabeth Manipoud Figueroa, a French attorney with experience at UNICEF; Nina Ferencic, a Croatian communications expert with ties to Latin America; and, to be his inaugural director for the country programs initiative, Australian physician Rob Moodie, who had worked with Save the Children Fund, Medicins Sans Frontières, and WHO.[80]

Piot's three initial goals were to put AIDS on the political agendas of the world, to build a large coalition to support UNAIDS's efforts that would be broader than AIDS doctors and AIDS activists, and to mobilize money for work in developing countries. When UNAIDS was launched in 1996, Piot faced an epidemic still uncontrolled by effective drug therapy and for which the quality of surveillance information varied widely. In August 1996, however, at the Eleventh International AIDS Conference in Vancouver, HAART therapy was announced, and people with AIDS suddenly had hope to live normal lives. This proved to be a strong stimulus for the work of UNAIDS, but Piot was also "really concerned that the majority of people who need this [therapy] are in poor countries. Will they have access?"[81] As the 1990s ended, this new global organization to fight AIDS was infused with hope. At the same time, it faced the daunting challenge of a pandemic whose driving forces differed according to culture, politics, and religion in the world's countries. Only during the third decade of the AIDS epidemic was UNAIDS able to make significant advances against the disease while acknowledging that the problem would likely never be completely solved.

8

The Third Decade

"Go and get the word out to voters, to people going through medical schools that should want to get involved more in these world health issues, go to governments in the developing world and talk about how other governments have been doing things right."

—Bill Gates[1]

In June 2001, according to Peter Piot, the world arrived at a defining moment, a tipping point, in its response to HIV/AIDS. The monumental event was a special session of the United Nations General Assembly on AIDS: "A UN General Assembly Special Session (UNGASS), in which the entire UN focuses on one issue, is called to address matters of the greatest global significance. This would be the first time a Special Session addressed a health issue, reflecting a growing consensus in the UN (and beyond) that AIDS was much more than just a health issue, rather a major threat to global human and economic development."[2] Arriving at this point had not been easy for UNAIDS, an organization that had been founded only in 1996. In this chapter, we will examine the step-by-step work of UNAIDS in making the epidemic a topic of worldwide concern. We will also look at the prospects of a vaccine to prevent AIDS and the development of other preventive tools.

Putting AIDS on the International Agenda

For the first twenty years of the epidemic, discussions about the impact of AIDS, outside of the people who suffered from the disease or their caregivers, largely stayed in medical and public health circles and seemed to mean little to world leaders in economic or national security terms. In 1991, for example, two officers in the U.S. Central Intelligence Agency (CIA), Katherine J. Hall and Walter L. Barrows, produced an interagency intelligence memorandum titled "The Global AIDS Disaster," projecting 45 million infections worldwide, largely in Africa, by 2000—an estimate that turned out to be optimistic, as more than 53 million people were actually infected by that date. The reaction of political and military leaders in the U.S. government to this report, however, was indifference. They viewed Africa as having a limitless pool of unemployed young men. "If you have one 18-year-old with a Kalashnikov [rifle] and he dies, you find another 18-year-old," one official reportedly said. They believed that the impact of AIDS on military stability was minimal. Fritz Ermarth, chairman of the intelligence council that approved the study, observed that in 1991, "a critical mass of people that are primed to see a problem like this in strategic terms" simply did not exist.[3]

William H. Webster, director of central intelligence, wanted the report made public but worried that if it came from the CIA, it would lend credence to a Soviet-era disinformation campaign that suggested the AIDS virus had been intentionally created by the CIA as an instrument for germ warfare (this rumor was discussed in chapter 6): "Somebody would try to imply that we're only monitoring our own dastardly deeds." In 1992, therefore, unclassified portions of the report were published by the State Department as a white paper. The public reaction mimicked the response to the classified intelligence report: no one paid attention to it.[4]

Throughout much of the 1990s, even the agencies of the United Nations shied away from tackling AIDS through their budgets. *Washington Post* reporter Barton Gellman noted that from 1992 to 1994 the health division of UNICEF was reluctant to become involved, although its director, James Sherry, tried to expand UNICEF's early childhood mission to include teenagers at risk of a sexually transmitted disease. Sherry's secretary reportedly resigned because he asked her to handle correspondence relating to condoms. UNICEF's child immunization department, moreover, also threatened to resign en masse. "Why are we jeopardizing our relations with the Holy See?" one staff member was quoted as asking. Similarly, the World Health Organization under Director General Hiroshi Nakajima believed that AIDS should not eclipse other global medical problems, especially malaria.[5]

For the wealthy, industrialized countries, AIDS in the developing world was just too expensive to address within foreign aid budgets. Before the advent of effective combination therapy for AIDS, one argument stressed that it would waste resources to offer HIV testing to people who were going to die anyway. In 1998 Duff Gillespie, who headed the programs in population, health, and nutrition for the U.S. Agency for International Development (USAID), stressed that "to save the life of a dehydrating child with diarrheal disease required little more than a foil packet of salts." Tuberculosis could be cured with antibiotics. Programs against these diseases produced results that in congressional testimony strongly supported USAID's effectiveness and efficiency as a steward of federal tax dollars. In contrast, there was no obvious tool for preventing transmission of the AIDS virus, and there was no cure for AIDS. The cost of programs was high, and Gillespie said, the afflicted populations often lacked "an inherently sympathetic 'victim.'"[6]

UNAIDS began its quest to change this situation by addressing the economic impact on the world if rich countries did not help fund treatment of AIDS in the developing world. As a new entity, UNAIDS had to lobby strongly to get Peter Piot on the agenda at the 1996 International AIDS Conference in Vancouver. Most of the press coverage of that meeting focused on the announcement that combination antiviral therapy had been shown highly effective. Of five articles about the conference written by the *New York Times*'s lead medical reporter, Lawrence K. Altman, three focused on the new drugs, and only one covered the growing epidemic in the developing world.

The Vancouver conference adopted the slogan "One World, One Hope" to emphasize the need for people to work together against AIDS. The introduction of ART, however, starkly revealed the existence of two worlds with respect to AIDS: the rich world in which the $20,000 per year price tag for ART was affordable, and the poor world in which treatment of any sort was unavailable for most people. AIDS activists were quick to begin pressuring the major pharmaceutical houses to lower the cost of ART. Jeffrey Sturchio, vice president for external affairs of Merck & Co., recalled, "What I remember about the Vancouver meeting was that at one point the congress hall was full of people throwing fake money printed with the names of pharmaceutical companies to dramatise the point the prices needed to come down."[7] As a result of activists' efforts and UNAIDS's presentation of chilling global AIDS statistics—more than 20 million people worldwide lived with HIV infection, and 94 percent lived in the developing world—for the first time, the developing world was firmly on the agenda of an international AIDS conference.[8]

Two years later, at the Twelfth International AIDS Conference in Geneva, Peter Piot was discouraged. He felt that little progress was being made against AIDS as a global issue, in large part because it was viewed as merely a disease problem for public health leaders that still had little relevancy for world leaders. In an oral history, Piot stated that this led him to understand "that only a political strategy was going to make a difference. I came into this as a scientist," he said. To rethink strategy, he convened an off-the-record meeting in Talloires, France, with members of the AIDS communities and outsiders, such as journalists, who had closely followed the epidemic. About this meeting, he said, "We came up with the conclusion that we needed to go political, to mobilize the top leadership in the world. We needed to bring this to the Security Council because the only two things that matter in national politics are security and the economy. And the rest, as they say in French, is literature. . . . So I became more of a politician than a scientist."[9]

Step by step, Piot and UNAIDS began building political support for action against the spread of AIDS. First, he obtained a call for action on AIDS in Africa as a part of the official statement issued at a 1998 summit meeting of the heads of state of the Organization for African Unity. In May 1999 a meeting of African finance ministers declared that AIDS was "a major threat to economic and social development." Also that month, Ethiopian president Negasso Gidada and His Holiness Abune Paulos, the patriarch of the Ethiopian Orthodox Church, shook hands with HIV-infected Ethiopians publicly for the first time. "This action was highly symbolic for an African country at that time."[10]

In June, Kofi Annan, secretary general of the UN and a native of Ghana, gave the first Diana, Princess of Wales, Memorial Lecture on "The Global Challenge of AIDS." The first of his many public speeches about AIDS, this lecture warned that AIDS was "taking away Africa's future" and was making a "horrific impact" worldwide. Annan's leadership helped increase attention to AIDS in UNAIDS's sibling agencies, such as the World Bank, UNICEF, and the UN Population Fund. When he spoke to the International Partnership against AIDS in Africa, made up of members from the private sector, governments, and nongovernmental organizations, Annan witnessed the response to AIDS move to a higher political level. Louise Fréchette, Annan's deputy secretary general, observed, "When the Secretary-General [makes] AIDS a personal priority, it does reverberate around the world."[11]

In working to put AIDS on the agenda of the UN Security Council, Piot turned to Richard Holbrooke, the U.S. ambassador to the United Nations. Knowing that Holbrooke was traveling to central Africa with other members of the Security Council in the fall of 1999 to investigate the civil wars in the Lake Victoria region, Piot arranged for a different person with HIV to meet him and talk about AIDS at every stop. When he returned from the trip, Holbrooke summoned Piot to discuss what the Security Council might do to help stop the spread of AIDS. Holbrooke noted that the United States was to chair the council in January 2000 and that the country chairing the session set the agenda for the meeting. Exercising his right as session chair, Holbrooke decided to make AIDS the agenda topic. Piot had previously discussed the possibility of such a session with Holbrooke, but he had not anticipated the speed at which Holbrooke could work. Between November 1999 and January 6, 2000, Holbrooke "did all of the political work," including obtaining a commitment from U.S. vice president Al Gore to chair the session. Working through the holiday season, Piot and the UNAIDS staff put together documents providing background, arguments, and evidence.

At the session, Kofi Annan testified that "the impact of AIDS in Africa was no less destructive than that of warfare itself. By overwhelming the continent's health services, by creating millions of orphans, and by decimating the numbers of health workers and teachers, AIDS was causing socioeconomic crises which in turn threatened political stability."[12] Piot observed that the Security Council discussion opened doors for UNAIDS. (Figure 8.1 shows Piot testifying at the Security Council session on AIDS.) "Top leaders told me," he said, that since AIDS "was debated in the Security Council, it must be a serious problem." Piot's decision to make AIDS a political issue with security and economic implications had indeed been a key strategy for making the world aware of the pandemic.[13] Later that year, another Security Council session led to a project to prevent HIV infection in UN peacekeepers and uniformed services. "The military are interesting," Piot stated, "in that once you convince them of something, they don't worry about moral problems of, say, condoms. They say, 'If that's a threat to our combat readiness, you tell me what we've got to do and we'll do it.'"[14]

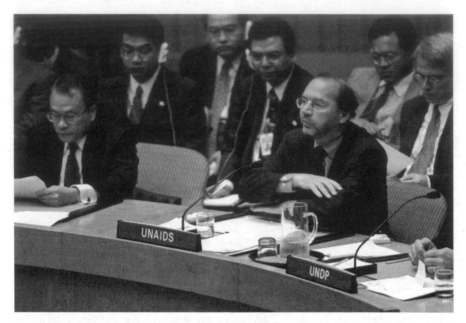

Figure 8.1. Peter Piot, first director of the United Nations Joint Programme on AIDS (UNAIDS), speaking to the United Nations Security Council, January 6, 2000. *Courtesy of UNAIDS.*

After the UN Security Council session, the Ukrainian ambassador to the UN called for a UN General Assembly Special Session on AIDS (UNGASS). Planning for the session, which was held in June 2001, took just more than twelve months, very fast compared with the usual three to four years of preparation involving regional and country consultations. Kathleen Cravero, a career bureaucrat at the UN with a doctorate in political science and a master's in public health, joined UNAIDS in May 2000 as deputy executive director to Piot, with responsibility for planning the UNGASS.

As Cravero worked in Geneva, Piot traveled to Durban, South Africa, in July 2000 for the Thirteenth International AIDS Conference. He called for industrialized countries to shift from donating *millions* for AIDS to donating *billions*. "We can't fight an epidemic of this magnitude with peanuts," he said. He also called upon wealthy countries to cancel the debt of many of the hardest hit African countries. His speech was not well received. The wealthy nations responded that such sums of money would never be forthcoming. Nonetheless, participants in the conference sensed that a line had been crossed in the global response to AIDS: "The alliance of science, people living with AIDS, community groups, the UN, governments and civil society demonstrated just how potent a united stand against HIV/AIDS can be. The conference . . . recognized that AIDS is a crisis of governance. It also recognized that failure to apply the tools and resources available is a political issue. Leadership saves lives."[15]

Also on the fall agenda at the United Nations was the General Assembly's issuance of the "Millennium Declaration" to mark the advent of the new century. This document embodied a statement of faith "in the Organization and its Charter as indispensable foundations of a more peaceful, prosperous and just world." Among the resolutions that embodied specific goals, two addressed HIV/AIDS. By 2015, the declaration stated, the UN aimed to halt and begin to reverse "the spread of HIV/AIDS, the scourge of malaria, and other major diseases that afflict humanity." Second, the UN pledged to provide "special assistance to children orphaned by HIV/AIDS."[16]

Preparations for the UNGASS meeting on June 25–27, 2001, ranged from the media-specific, such as arranging for a neon AIDS red ribbon to be lit every night on the UN building in New York, to the highly delicate, such as negotiations over the wording of the Declaration of Commitment on HIV/AIDS, which all heads of state would be able to sign. (Figure 8.2 shows the UN building in New York with the AIDS red ribbon lit.) Given the various religious and social differences of representatives from member states, issues such as prevention recommendations for sex workers and gay men had to be carefully parsed. Strong feelings also threatened to derail a statement about access to antiretroviral drugs. Brazil had led the way in providing full access to antiretrovirals on demand for its citizens in 1996. The Rio group—comprising representatives from Brazil, Argentina, Bolivia, Chile, Colombia, Ecuador, Mexico, Panama, Paraguay, Peru, Uruguay, and Venezuela—argued with a unified voice for a strong statement advocating access to affordable drugs. For most of the wealthy countries that would be called upon to fund any AIDS initiative, the Rio group's insistence was not acceptable because in 2001 there was no general agreement on how to fund combination antiviral drug therapy for all poor countries. Wealthy nations also believed that emphasizing treatment would reduce funds needed to implement prevention programs.[17]

The final Declaration of Commitment on HIV/AIDS, "Global Crisis— Global Action," posted on the Internet for worldwide distribution, stated that

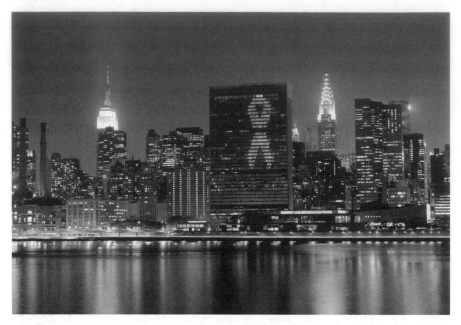

Figure 8.2. United Nations Building with AIDS red ribbon, marking the United Nations General Assembly's Special Session on AIDS, June 25–27, 2001. *Courtesy of UNAIDS.*

the delegates "solemnly declare our commitment to address the HIV/AIDS crisis" by taking defined, measurable action to the extent possible. Leadership, prevention, treatment, human rights, assistance for AIDS orphans, and research and development were some of the areas addressed. Delegates also pledged to "devote sufficient time and at least one full day of the annual General Assembly session to review and debate a report of the Secretary-General on progress achieved in realizing the commitments set out in this Declaration, with a view to identifying problems and constraints and making recommendations on action needed to make further progress."[18]

What was the significance of the UNGASS? Many people, according to Kathleen Cravero, believe that diplomatic meetings such as this are meaningless. Not so, she argued. "UNGASS was an example of UNAIDS at its best—serving its core function well by bringing disparate agencies together to achieve more than any one of them could achieve on its own." For Peter Piot, as noted at the beginning of this chapter, UNGASS represented the turning point after which countries of the world began to fight AIDS in earnest with resources and commitment.[19]

Making AIDS an International Economic Issue

In 1995 Sally Grooms Cowal, a former U.S. ambassador to Trinidad and Tobago, joined the nascent UNAIDS as director of external relations. In 1997
Cowal began working with African business groups, pointing out that HIV-
related absenteeism accounted for significant increases in labor costs. Her goal
was to convince the global business sector that involvement with AIDS prevention and treatment was not just a humanitarian effort but an investment that
would have important consequences for their profitability. In February 1997
Cowal arranged for Nelson Mandela, South Africa's president, and Peter Piot to
participate in the World Economic Forum in Davos, Switzerland. The session
on business in the world of AIDS was completely full, and Mandela impressed
upon the participants that "if you don't do something about AIDS, you can for-
get about development." The outcome of this meeting was the creation later that
year of a global business council to work with UNAIDS. Companies such as
Levi's and MTV joined initially, but little was accomplished before 2001, when
companies began experiencing serious absenteeism as a result of HIV infection
and the international visibility of UNAIDS lent itself more prestige.[20]

Another initiative launched in the fall of 1997 was the UNAIDS HIV Drug
Access Initiative, a collaboration between UNAIDS and major pharmaceutical companies. UNAIDS's involvement was critical, not only because "different companies produced different components of the drug cocktails, but also
because anti-trust laws made discussion of pricing schemes between pharmaceutical companies impossible."[21] The Drug Access Initiative was a pilot project
and included only four countries: Chile, Côte d'Ivoire, Uganda, and Vietnam.
Pharmaceutical companies agreed to drop the price of their drugs by about 40
percent, from $10,000 to $12,000 per year in the developed world to $6,000
to $7,200 per year for the program. Their main concern was whether the in-
frastructure necessary to make use of the drugs appropriately existed in these
countries. UNAIDS again played a critical role by conducting in-depth discussions about implementation with the pilot project countries. All parties also
agreed to the following terms:

> First, there could not be any diversion of discounted products to devel-
> oped country markets. Second, the companies wanted guarantees that the
> drugs would be used in a rational manner, that the treatment programmes

would be structured in such a way that their products would be used for maximum benefit and not lead to waste. Third, UNAIDS had to structure the availability of these products so that any intermediaries in the supply chain could not use the price discounts given by the originator companies to enrich themselves. Last but not least, the companies and the UN agencies agreed on the importance of protecting intellectual property interests, to ensure continued investment in research and development for new HIV medicines.[22]

These stipulations reveal the complexity of the effort to provide antiviral medications to the developing world. It was not simply a matter of making the drugs affordable. Countries differed widely in their control of corruption and abuse of foreign aid of all types. Serving as the liaison between pharmaceutical companies in wealthy countries and the organizations in medium-developed and underdeveloped countries, UNAIDS assumed a daunting task. Although it took a number of years to yield results, the effort demonstrated that, indeed, sophisticated regimes of medication could be implemented successfully in the developing world with only moderate investments in training and laboratory inventory.[23]

Antiretroviral Drugs in South Africa: A Case of AIDS Denialism

Even as UNAIDS was negotiating with pharmaceutical companies to bring down the cost of antiretroviral drugs for the developing world, South African leaders were retreating from ART and embracing alternative AIDS remedies. In 1997 Thabo Mbeki, vice president of South Africa during Nelson Mandela's presidency, and Nkosazane Zuma, minister of health, began a collaboration with scientists in Pretoria who believed they had discovered a new antiviral drug, which was patented as Virodene PO58. In 2007 James Myburgh, editor of the South African online journal *Politicsweb.co.za*, published a five-part series detailing the involvement of Mbeki, Zuma, and other members of the African National Congress (ANC) political party with the promoters of this drug. The enthusiastic patent holders convinced the politicians that Virodene would be an African solution to AIDS controlled and produced in Africa rather than by Western pharmaceutical houses. In addition, they promised the ANC a 6 percent share in the royalties from the drug. The ANC, whose leaders controlled the government, became "deeply emotionally and financially invested in the development of Virodene as an African cure for AIDS," an achievement that would rival the world's first heart transplant, which was performed by a white South African doctor, Christiaan Barnard, in 1967.[24]

Olga Visser, a cardiovascular perfusionist at Pretoria's H. F. Verwoerd Hospital, and her husband, Jacques Siegfried (Zigi) Visser, were the majority stockholders and principal proponents of the drug. Neither had any experience in medical research, and they chafed at the requirements of South Africa's Medicines Control Council (MCC), the regulatory body to which they needed to present laboratory and animal safety and efficacy studies before receiving permission to go forward with human trials of the drug. Instead, they sought Mbeki's and Zuma's political authority to circumvent the regulations, a battle that consumed several years and resulted in the political gutting of the MCC. Ultimately, the replacement appointees also rejected Virodene trials because no safety or efficacy data had been presented. The Vissers then began to search for a site outside South Africa to conduct their clinical studies, and they apparently received funding from the South African government to maintain their patents on the drug while they sought a venue for testing it.

In March 1998 Glaxo Wellcome announced that it would lower the price of AZT in developed countries by three-quarters. This decision came after the CDC, in conjunction with the Thai Ministry of Public Health, conducted a study on the efficacy of a reduced dosage of AZT given late in pregnancy in diminishing mother-to-child transmission of HIV infection. The study had been the subject of vehement debates over the ethics of conducting a trial in a poor country with a reduced, less expensive dosage for a therapy that had been proved to reduce transmission by two-thirds at the higher, more expensive dosage in the industrialized world. The results of the trial, however, demonstrated clearly that the lower dosage reduced HIV transmission to infants by half, and the CDC issued a statement that women receiving a placebo in ongoing prenatal trials would instead begin to receive the efficacious lower dose of AZT.[25]

In July 1998 Rose Smart, who headed the HIV/AIDS and sexually transmitted diseases directorate in South Africa's health department, announced that this treatment would be piloted in Gauteng, the Western Cape, and Kwa-Zulu-Natal. At a cost of just over 300 South African rand (approximately fifty U.S. dollars in 1998) per patient, a lower-dose short course of AZT would be provided for HIV-positive pregnant women. In September, however, the Vissers announced that Virodene would enter a phase I study on "the safety, tolerability and pharmacokinetics of a single dose of Virodene PO58." On October 2 Health Minister Zuma announced that South Africa would not continue with the AZT pilot project for the prevention of mother-to-child transmission.[26]

In response to this stunning decision, AIDS activists in South Africa, led by Zackie Achmat, organized the Treatment Action Campaign and began pressing the government to provide antiretrovirals at least to HIV-positive pregnant women. They led marches for which all participants, whether or not they were infected with HIV, wore brightly colored T-shirts with bold, white, block letters saying, "HIV POSITIVE." The tactic was reportedly inspired by the apocryphal story of the Danish king who wore the yellow star of David that identified Jews during the period of Nazi occupation. In addition, Achmat, who was indeed HIV positive, refused to take antiretroviral medicines until they were available to all South Africans.[27]

Mark Heywood, executive director of the AIDS Law Project in South Africa, observed that Achmat and TAC based their demands on a human rights argument. TAC viewed the HIV/AIDS epidemic as falling especially hard on the poor because of "poverty, inequality, and social injustice" in the larger South African society. The South African constitution written in 1996 when the apartheid system fell articulated the rights of citizens to equality, life, and dignity, and stated, "Everyone has the right to have access to . . . health care services, including reproductive health care."[28] Without knowing of the involvement of Mbeki, Zuma, or the ANC with the Virodene project, TAC trained South African citizens in activism on the "treatment literacy" model pioneered by AIDS activists in the United States. This approach recognized "that in order to fight for rights effectively, people also are required to understand the science of HIV, what it was doing to their body, the medicines that might work against it, the research that was needed, etc."[29] They fought their battles for access to antiretroviral therapy via the South African legal system. In August 2001 TAC filed papers against the government for its refusal to supply antiretroviral drugs to HIV-positive pregnant women.[30]

The government's initial argument for not funding the pilot program with AZT had been that South Africa could not afford it, an argument easily refuted when the cost of a course of prenatal AZT was compared with the cost of caring for a baby with HIV infection. In 1999 Mbeki assumed the presidency of South Africa upon Nelson Mandela's retirement, and Health Minister Zuma was replaced by Manto Tshabalala-Msimang. At that time, Mbeki's ANC party articulated a new argument against funding AZT for HIV-infected pregnant women. In its *Annual Report*, the ANC stated that it "would not be pressurised into this direction, particularly given the unanswered questions regarding the efficacy and toxicity" of AZT.[31] This line of thinking mirrored the embrace by Mbeki and others in the ANC of the AIDS denialists.

Journalist Myburgh strongly believed that Mbeki's shift from acknowledging HIV as the cause of AIDS to embracing denialism was motivated by a deep conflict of interest.[32] Whether it was primarily emotional—his desire to find an African cure for African AIDS—or financial—the provision of a therapy at low cost with his political party profiting—is unclear. In early 1999 the Virodene promoters brought Mbeki's attention to an article by an AIDS dissident, Anthony Brink, titled "AZT: A Medicine from Hell" and a review of the pharmacology literature on AZT that questioned its safety.[33] From this time on, Mbeki began to adopt publicly the arguments of AIDS deniers. In 2000 he asked the South African Health Department to organize an international panel of experts to reassess the science behind the cause of AIDS. This panel included senior international specialists in HIV/AIDS as well as AIDS denialists. The participants' stark disagreement was evident in the recommendations of the report: one set from those who subscribed to HIV as the cause of AIDS and one set from those who denied HIV as the cause of AIDS. President Mbeki and Minister Tshabalala-Msimang chose to follow the recommendations of the AIDS denialists.[34]

In March 2000 the Vissers finally found a country that would permit them to conduct a clinical trial of Virodene without submitting laboratory and animal tests demonstrating its safety and efficacy. Against the wishes of the Tanzanian National Institute for Medical Research, the minister of health in Tanzania approved a placebo-controlled, double-blind trial to determine the "safety, tolerability, pharmacokinetics and efficacy of multiple doses of Virodene PO58 on 64 HIV/AIDS infected male volunteers." The study occurred between September 2000 and March 2002. During this period, Olga Visser pressed Pasteur Institute investigator Luc Montagnier to perform another in vitro test of Virodene and predicted enthusiastically that the clinical trial would show a dramatic drop in viral load and increase in CD4+ cells of the participants. Montagnier replied in a letter that such changes "are generally not observed so quickly with classical antiretroviral therapy."[35]

In December 2001 the Pretoria High Court ruled that the government must provide antiretroviral therapy to prevent transmission of HIV from HIV-infected pregnant women to their children. The Mbeki government immediately appealed the decision, hoping that the time involved in handling the appeal would permit the Virodene study to be completed and the drug validated as an effective African treatment for AIDS. Unfortunately, in early 2002, when the trial results were unblinded and analyzed, the data clearly demonstrated that Virodene had no effect on HIV and only a marginal improvement in the CD4 cell count. In short, Virodene could not cure AIDS, and once again sincere faith in a product by its sponsors could not change the sad fact that it did not do what they had hoped.[36]

On April 17, 2002, the government announced an abrupt reversal of policy. The South African constitution permitted the cabinet to overrule the president, and after the results of the Virodene trial were verified, it issued a statement that "not only would Nevirapine," a drug similar to AZT but found to reduce mother-to-child transmission at the same level with fewer doses and lower cost, "be provided to all pregnant women but also that anti-retroviral treatment would be made available to rape victims," something Mbeki had vigorously opposed. Mark Gevisser, author of a 2007 biography of Mbeki, argued that Mbeki's view of AIDS "was shaped by an obsession with race, the legacy of colonialism and 'sexual shame.'"[37]

In 2003 the Treatment Action Campaign made public a study previously withheld by the South African government showing that 1.7 million lives could be saved by 2010 if antiretroviral drugs were given to everyone needing them in South Africa.[38] Nonetheless, during the next five years of Mbeki's presidency, he and his health minister continued to promote nutritional therapies and to drag their feet on implementation of a national program to distribute antiretroviral drugs. In 2005 Nelson Mandela finally overcame his reluctance as a traditional African elder to speak about sexually transmitted diseases when his son, Makgatho, died of AIDS. With Mandela's support and increasing international criticism of South Africa's policies on AIDS, in 2007 the executive council again went around Mbeki to create the South African National AIDS Council, under the leadership of Deputy President Phumzile Mlambo-Ngcuka and Deputy

Health Minister Nozizwe Madlala-Routledge, with the goals of bringing anti-retroviral therapy to 80 percent of the South African population infected with HIV and reducing the number of new infections by 50 percent.[39] With this initiative, South Africa finally began a program that had been demonstrated effective to save the lives of its citizens. Sadly, a study by Max Essex's group at the Harvard School of Public Health found that some 330,000 lives had been lost unnecessarily in South Africa between 2000 and 2005 because of the government's refusal to implement an antiretroviral drug policy; 35,000 of those lives were babies who had been born unnecessarily infected with HIV.[40]

Access to Antiviral Drugs: AIDS as an Economic Issue
In May 1998 the physician and former Norwegian prime minister Gro Harlem Brundtland became director general of the World Health Organization. One of her principal interests was working with Peter Piot of UNAIDS to make antiretroviral drugs available to developing countries to fight AIDS. Over the next two years, Brundtland and Piot "partly pressured, partly enticed the company leaders towards a much wider use of differential pricing for antiretrovirals."[41] For example, Piot recalled one conversation with Ray Gilmartin, CEO of Merck: "We talked with him about reducing the price, etc., but he said, 'No way, my shareholders won't want it, my board will be against it.' After we left the meeting, Gro and I said, 'We'll try again next year.' But a few weeks later Gilmartin called and said, 'You convinced me, I'm with you.'"[42]

Piot believed that Merck, and soon other pharmaceutical companies as well, not only understood the humanitarian issues involved but also the impact of action or inaction on their reputations. In addition, by participating voluntarily, the pharmaceutical companies could insist on controls to prevent reduced-price drugs from being sold on the black market in developed countries and on protections for intellectual property. In March 2000 they presented a plan to UNAIDS to reduce treatment costs.

Building on the successful pilot Drug Access Initiative, in May 2000 UNAIDS launched the Accelerating Access Initiative, which also included the World Bank, UNICEF, and the UN Population Fund. The effort received a major boost in July 2000 at the Thirteenth International AIDS Conference in Durban, South Africa. Edwin Cameron, a justice of South Africa's Constitutional Court and the first senior South African official to reveal publicly that he was living with HIV/AIDS, made an impassioned speech, decrying the "shocking and monstrous iniquity" in access to treatment and imploring the delegates "to find ways to make accessible for the poor what is within reach of the affluent." While Cameron spoke, members of South Africa's Treatment Access Campaign marched on the conference center, demanding access for all to antiviral therapy.[43]

Under the Accelerating Access Initiative, the price of first-line treatment decreased to about $1,200 per year, and this, in turn, stimulated the development of treatment access plans in thirty-nine countries, each of which negotiated individual pricing agreements with the pharmaceutical companies—a huge bureaucratic effort that slowed implementation.[44] In 2003 fixed-dose combination therapies that reduced the number of pills a person needed to take, from ten to fifteen per day to as few as two per day, were introduced. With the introduction also of generic antiretrovirals, principally by Cipla, an Indian pharmaceutical company, a fixed-dose combination of the drugs stavudine, lamivudine, and nevirapine decreased in price from US$350 annually to as low as US$132 annually in 2005.[45]

Shortly after the Accelerating Access Initiative was organized, Japan hosted the G8 summit, an unofficial annual forum for leaders of the wealthiest world nations: Canada, France, Germany, Italy, Japan, Russia, the United Kingdom, and the United States (with president of the European Commission also included but not raising "G8" to "G9"). For the first time in the group's history, global health was on the agenda. The representatives agreed in principle to establish mechanisms to take action against AIDS and other infectious diseases, especially malaria and tuberculosis. No specific action was mandated at this time, but the recognition by the world's wealthiest countries that disease was an economic issue represented a major step forward toward funding for health programs in the new millennium.[46]

As money became available, a new problem arose for the nations receiving it. Donors often wanted to specify how the funds would be used and required that considerable paperwork be completed for individual projects. Recipient countries, especially in Africa, complained that after meeting bureaucratic requirements, they had no time left to deal with sick people. UNAIDS began working with individual countries to develop a procedure that would be acceptable to both donors and recipients. In 2004 it issued the "Three Ones" principles. For each country receiving donations from various sources there would be:

One agreed HIV/AIDS Action Framework that provides the basis for co-ordinating the work of all partners.

One National AIDS Coordinating Authority, with a broad based multi-sector mandate.

One agreed country level Monitoring and Evaluation System.[47]

With these principles in place, UNAIDS was able to get donors to work together to respond to the needs articulated by the recipient government, not to mandate idiosyncratic programs specified by the donors themselves. Peter Piot observed that the principles worked well in protecting priorities of countries that were relatively strong but not so well in weak countries, where multiple donors continued to organize and insist on multiple programs.[48]

Funding the Global Fight against AIDS in the Third Decade

At the beginning of the new millennium, major donors and countries disagreed about whether it would be better to push for separate funds to fight the most threatening infectious diseases—AIDS, malaria, tuberculosis—or to join forces and create a global fund aimed at reducing these infectious diseases. At two meetings in April 2001, the decision to create a global fund was made. Major donors and UN agencies met in London the same month the Organization for African Unity held a summit on HIV/AIDS, tuberculosis, and other infectious diseases in Abuja, Nigeria. At the meeting in Nigeria, UN Secretary General Kofi Annan called for the creation of the Global Fund, dedicated to battling HIV/AIDS and other infectious diseases. He specified a "war chest" of roughly US$7 to US$10 billion a year from both donor and developing countries. The developing countries at the conference also pledged to devote 15 percent of their national budgets to improve health care.[49] The specific figures were based on a detailed analysis in a *Science* policy forum by epidemiologists from UNAIDS; the London School of Hygiene and Tropical Medicine; the National Institute of Public Health, Cuernavaca, Mexico; and the Futures Group International of Washington, D.C. Their findings represented the first effort to quantify the resources needed to address HIV/AIDS worldwide.[50]

During 2001 the Global Fund began to receive substantial funds from both wealthy and poor governments and from private-sector entities and nongovernmental organizations ranging from the International Olympic Committee to the Bill and Melinda Gates Foundation to the Winterthur Insurance/Credit Suisse Group.[51] In late January 2002 the Global Fund, located in Geneva, became operational. Considerable debate had occurred over who should run the fund, with many private-sector donors strongly opposed to administration by UNAIDS because they believed that any UN effort would be hamstrung by bureaucracy. The donors finally chose as director Richard Feachem, a British physician who had experience as dean of the London School of Hygiene and Tropical Medicine; director of health, nutrition, and population for the World Bank; and founding director of the Institute for Global Health at the University of California–San Francisco and at the University of California–Berkeley.[52]

The Global Fund also resolved to operate as simply a funding agency. It chose not to implement programs with its own staff but rather to work in concert with governments, civil society, the private sector, and affected communities. Grants for education, prevention, treatment, and care were made with as much flexibility as possible so that countries were able to tailor them to their own particular cultures and needs. The fund also instituted a rigorous evaluation process aimed at ensuring accountability. In its online file of pledges through February 2011, the Global Fund listed nearly US$18 billion contributed by more than sixty countries and just under US$1 billion from nongovernmental organizations and private-sector donors.[53]

A second major source of funds to fight AIDS came from the World Bank's Multicountry AIDS Program (MAP). Established in 1999, MAP, like the Global Fund, funded programs run by countries or nongovernmental organizations. Within its overall aim "to dramatically increase" access to prevention, care, and treatment programs, MAP emphasized work with vulnerable groups such as youth, women of childbearing age, sex workers, and men who have sex with men. Initially, Africa was the focus, but later the Caribbean and other global regions were included. Already established partnerships with "countries, UNAIDS, the private sector, and donor agencies" provided the platform from which the bank began to fund programs based on UNAIDS's evaluation of need. In 2005 the bank expanded its commitment to the global AIDS challenge. By January 2010 it reported expenditures (between 1988 and 2010) of more than US$4.2 billion in grants, loans, and credits for programs to fight AIDS. Through the MAP program, it had committed US$1.9 billion in thirty-five African countries, and in the Caribbean, US$153 million for projects in nine countries and one region.[54]

The final major source of funding for addressing the global AIDS epidemic was the U.S. President's Emergency Plan for AIDS Relief (PEPFAR). First enacted under the administration of George W. Bush in 2003 for US$15 billion, the program was reauthorized in 2008 with US$48 billion and an expanded mandate to improve overall global health in addition to addressing HIV/AIDS. Both laws included stipulations that at least one-third of the funds designated for prevention be spent on abstinence-until-marriage programs and that the portion designated to be donated to the Global Fund (up to US$1 billion in 2003, up to US$2 billion in 2008) not exceed one-third of all donations to that fund, a stipulation designed to ensure that other wealthy countries continued to be involved in the Global Fund. Specific items in the 2008 law reflected what had been learned over the first five years of PEPFAR. For example, the later law provided funds to encourage research on a microbicide, a topical gel that would kill HIV and prevent infection. It also identified male circumcision as a prevention method and revised its language to stipulate that both male and female condoms were items eligible for funding.[55] Under the presidential administration of Barack Obama, PEPFAR has been integrated with a new Global Health Initiative. As this book went to press, the president's budget proposal for 2012 included US$6.9 billion for PEPFAR, a 4.8 percent increase over fiscal year 2011 levels, which were funded under a continuing resolution at 2010 levels because Congress had not enacted budget legislation for 2011.[56]

On a lower scale—millions of U.S. dollars annually instead of billions—private philanthropies, led by the Bill and Melinda Gates Foundation, also award grants to address HIV/AIDS, in addition to their contributions to the Global Fund. The tracking group Funders Concerned about AIDS reported that in 2009 they had identified 342 U.S.-based funders, nonprofit and corporate, supporting some 5,500 HIV/AIDS-related grants or projects with approximately US$585 million. In 2009 a similar European group, the European HIV/AIDS Funders Group, tracked thirty-seven European donors who made some 4,080 HIV/AIDS-related grants or projects via a total of €120 million (US$152 million). The reports issued by these groups also indicated that individual donors attempted to coordinate the efforts with one another and with UNAIDS.[57] With the global economic downturn in 2008–2009, philanthropic support in Europe still rose slightly, but in the United States, it diminished by 5 percent, from US$618 million in 2008 to US$585 million in 2009. Funding from the Gates Foundation, which represented 57 percent of all U.S. philanthropic funding, decreased from US$378 million in 2008 to US$334 million in 2009.[58]

Preventing AIDS: The Elusive Search for a Vaccine

Perhaps the most misquoted statement in the history of the AIDS epidemic was attributed to Margaret Heckler, U.S. secretary of health and human services, who during an April 23, 1984, press conference announced that the cause of AIDS had been found. Many accounts reported that she said, "We will have a vaccine against AIDS ready in two years." What she actually said, however, based on the most preliminary knowledge about the AIDS virus and how a vaccine might be made, was, "We hope to have such a vaccine ready for testing in about two years."[59] And, indeed, had HIV been a virus like poliovirus or smallpox virus, such a candidate vaccine might have been produced within two years. Unfortunately, the retrovirus that causes AIDS turned out to be very different from viruses against which vaccines had been successfully made, and at the end of the third decade of the epidemic, medicine seems no closer to producing a vaccine than it was in 1984.

Even though a preventive vaccine against AIDS has been viewed as the holy grail of AIDS research, the one accomplishment that could halt the epidemic by preventing infection, researchers have been stymied in their efforts by both inadequate scientific knowledge and the way vaccine research has proceeded as an organizational process. Making vaccines has never been easy. As we saw in chapter 1, the intellectual foundation for vaccine production historically was based on mimicking the body's immune response to infection. Once a person had recovered from any viral illness, his or her immune system recognized the virus that had caused the illness and increased production of antibodies in the blood to prevent a second infection. The person was said to be "immune" from further bouts with the disease. Vaccines were attempts by medical scientists to stimulate the production of antibodies against a disease-causing virus without requiring the vaccinated individual to suffer the illness.

Historically, vaccines were made by one of two methods. First was the "whole killed-virus" vaccine, made by growing large batches of the disease-causing virus, killing the virus with a chemical, and injecting a measured amount into a healthy person. Influenza vaccine injections and the Salk polio vaccine are examples of killed-virus vaccines. Second was the "attenuated live-virus" vaccine. These vaccines were made by growing batches of a virus in ways that weaken their disease-causing properties. Live-virus vaccines are viewed as being more effective in creating immunity, although some may present hazards of their own if the virus has the ability to revert into a disease-causing state. The Sabin oral polio vaccine and vaccines against measles, mumps, and rubella are examples of attenuated live-virus vaccines.

In 1981, just as AIDS was first identified, a third method of making vaccines was showing great promise. Based on new knowledge about molecular virology and immunology and the ability to manipulate viruses at the molecular level, "subunit" vaccines were being engineered. A subunit vaccine against hepatitis B, consisting of a protein from the surface of the virus, was first introduced in 1981, and human papilloma virus vaccine is also made from a viral protein rather than the whole virus.

Translating these techniques for use against AIDS proved much harder than first realized. By early 1985 researchers at NIH and the Pasteur Institute had sequenced HIV's genetic code and understood that its rate of mutation was much higher than that of the influenza viruses, which mutate so quickly that new vaccines must be made each year. The other biological characteristic of HIV infection that was not at first appreciated, because so little was known about the then-new disease, was that unlike most infectious diseases (from which most people recover spontaneously), no one who developed the opportunistic infections and cancers that characterized end-stage HIV infection, or full-blown AIDS, survived. Thus, the historic understanding that vaccines could mimic the naturally resulting immunity evoked by the body's immune system after infection did not apply to AIDS.

In his history of the search for an AIDS vaccine during the first two decades of the epidemic, *Shots in the Dark,* journalist Jon Cohen identified two approaches to making an AIDS vaccine that emerged in the 1980s. Those researchers whose careers had matured in the 1970s, during the flowering of molecular biology, immediately wanted to pursue a subunit vaccine based on an HIV protein. The most obvious candidate was one of the glycoproteins on the outer coat of the virus, the first proteins that interacted with cells to infect them. The greatest value of such a vaccine was that under no circumstances could it accidentally cause the disease itself. Other scientists, led by Jonas Salk, who had produced the first effective polio vaccine in the 1950s, argued for first trying the proven technique of a killed-virus vaccine. With careful production and monitoring techniques, this group believed that the risk of accidental infection could be essentially eliminated. Cohen described these two groups as "reductionists" and "empiricists," respectively. The reductionists wanted to proceed using a rational approach based on knowledge of the virus and testing of candidate formulations in the laboratory and on animals for safety and strong signs of efficacy before moving into human trials. The empiricists believed that the public health emergency of AIDS called for skipping the longer process and moving promising vaccine candidates quickly into human trials.[60]

In 1986 an empiricist, Moroccan native Daniel Zagury, head of the Department of Cellular Physiology at the Pierre and Marie Curie University in Paris, made the first two candidate vaccines against AIDS. The first vaccine was composed of white blood cells taken from two infected women in Zaire, placed in a test tube, and combined with HIV isolated from the women so that the cells would be infected with the virus, then treated with formaldehyde to kill the HIV. By utilizing whole, infected cells as his vaccine, Zagury hoped to elicit both a humoral immune response in the form of antibodies against the virus, and a cellular immune response in the form of killer cells, specialized T cells that isolated and killed virus-infected cells. This approach, he hoped, would prevent those not already infected from acquiring HIV and also stimulate a therapeutic response for those already ill. Working with Zairian physicians, Zagury injected the vaccine into the women from whom he had harvested the white cells.[61]

Zagury's second vaccine effort utilized a rationalist approach to vaccine design. Using the techniques of recombinant DNA, he inserted a gene for HIV's surface protein gp160 into a vaccinia virus, the virus used in smallpox vaccine. His hope with this candidate vaccine was similar to the first: he believed that when the vaccinia virus infected the body, it would make gp160 appear on the surface of infected cells and stimulate both a cellular and humoral immune response. After testing the safety of this vaccine in monkeys, baboons, and one chimpanzee, he injected himself with the vaccine.[62]

In 1987 and 1988 Zagury and his colleagues published the results of these studies in *Nature*. They were able to say that the vaccines elicited both humoral and cellular immune responses for up to a year after injection, but this said nothing about the vaccine's ability to protect against infection with HIV.[63] Meanwhile, AIDS researchers in the United States and Europe knew very little about Zagury's experiments. In January 1987 Jonathan Mann, who had led Projet SIDA in Zaire before moving to Geneva to head the WHO Global Programme on AIDS, told a U.S. Senate committee hearing focusing on AIDS vaccines that he had no idea whether Zagury's work was well designed or had promise. Anthony Fauci, who had become the designated spokesperson on AIDS at NIH, reported that his institute, NIAID, was coordinating intramural NIH scientists, academic researchers, and industry into teams that would develop and test AIDS vaccines. Called National Cooperative Vaccine Development Groups, they would have use of the facilities of six vaccine evaluation units at universities around the country. NIAID's funding for vaccine development was allocated at 10 percent of its total AIDS budget.[64]

Two issues of particular note arose at this hearing. Fauci was particularly concerned with the need to test candidate vaccines in animals to establish safety and the ability to stimulate an immune response. Chimpanzees could be infected with HIV, but they did not become sick, so a challenge experiment to see if a candidate vaccine would prevent infection might not be directly transferable to humans. David Martin, vice president of the biotechnology firm Genentech, raised the second issue. Industry, he said, was most concerned about two aspects of vaccine production. First was the market—would the government guarantee purchase of the vaccine or mandate that everyone take it? Second was liability. Because some individuals have adverse reactions to any vaccine, manufacturing firms were wary of taking on the potential liability costs that accompanied investment in making vaccines. Martin requested that the government enact tort reform if it wanted the private sector to respond robustly—that is, with significant monetary and staff resources. Developing therapeutic drugs that patients needed to take every day for the rest of their lives was much more profitable than developing a vaccine that an individual would be injected with only once or a few times and that could prompt lawsuits against the manufacturer if adverse reactions ensued.[65]

Cohen argues throughout *Shots in the Dark* that the effort to develop an AIDS vaccine "suffered from disorganization, fractiousness, sleazy politics, sloppy science, a shaky marketplace, greed, unbridled ambition, and leaders with shockingly limited powers."[66] In tracing the details of this damning analysis, Cohen points to a key debate that has characterized the biomedical research enterprise since the end of World War II: is the best strategy to achieve new medical diagnostic tools, therapies, and preventatives to invest primarily in basic research, which is aimed at uncovering new knowledge about the body with no immediate application, or to organize highly directed, targeted, or applied research projects, aimed at a particular medical goal? Since the federal government has been the principal funder of medical research in the United States since 1948, and since the U.S. medical research effort committed by far the largest amount of money to AIDS research, this debate had important consequences for how AIDS vaccine research progressed.

The debate over the proper balance of basic and applied research swung back and forth in scientific and political circles. During the 1950s and the first half of the 1960s, basic research ruled supreme at the NIH. The agency claimed four in-house Nobel laureates by the end of the 1970s and more than fifty Nobel prizes supported by NIH grants.[67] By the mid-1960s pressures from health lobbyists spurred Congress to urge the NIH to focus more strongly on moving research from the laboratory to the patient's bedside. This effort reached a peak in the 1971 National Cancer Act, which provided greatly increased funding to the National Cancer Institute in support of President Richard Nixon's war on cancer. In chapter 2, we saw how the results of the Special Virus Cancer Program, a part of this National Cancer Program, contributed to AIDS research in the 1980s. The effort was not without strong critics, however, and in 1976 the program was shut down. In the 1980s the debate over basic versus applied research centered largely on whether or not the NIH should support the Human Genome Project, a clearly applied effort to map and sequence every gene in the human body. Critics argued that this was not basic research, but Congress supported the project and created a new NIH institute to implement it. More recently, debates over the relative value of expensive, large-scale clinical trials, such as the Women's Health Initiative study of hormone replacement therapy, versus the new knowledge that might emerge from several basic research laboratories for the same money, have embodied the ongoing dynamic between the two points of view.[68]

Those who wanted to organize an efficient search for an AIDS vaccine, such as Maurice Hilliman, the distinguished vaccine researcher who had already developed eight vaccines, recommended that the necessary organizational structure should include "having a central authority guiding research, creating a strategic plan, defining gaps in knowledge, and steering redundancy. The complexity, redundancy, and overinformation in modern molecular biology and immunology has created an immense problem for the vaccinologist to hear the tune amid the static."[69] The model most often cited was that which organized development of a polio vaccine in the 1950s. The National Foundation for Infantile Paralysis, which conducted the annual March of Dimes to raise money for research to develop a polio vaccine, was a private-sector enterprise led by attorney Basil O'Connor, who had wide discretionary powers to choose projects to be supported.[70]

Supporters of this approach often called for a "Manhattan Project for AIDS," recalling the huge, focused, and successful effort by physicists to create an atomic bomb during World War II. Supporters of basic research argued, conversely, that the basic physics were understood before the atomic bomb project began, while the basic biology of HIV infection was not known, hence the analogy was false. Supporters of the empiricist approach pointed out how many times in medical history an advance such as the smallpox vaccine or the use of antibiotics had been discovered before the underlying biological mechanism was known. Reductionists responded, however, that in these examples, observations from nature provided a clue, whereas with AIDS, there was no natural cure or prevention to be imitated.

Both empiricists and reductionists pursued promising leads, but by the 1990s none had progressed sufficiently to warrant FDA approval for a clinical trial in humans. When the presidential administration of Bill Clinton assumed control of the White House in January 1993, AIDS activists who had split from ACT UP to form the Treatment Action Group (TAG) issued a scathing report about the NIH's AIDS research program and demanded better organization. They persuaded Senator Edward Kennedy of Massachusetts to introduce a bill that reorganized the NIH's Office of AIDS Research (OAR). It transferred the entire AIDS budget at NIH to the OAR rather than dividing it among the various NIH institutes. In addition, the bill charged the OAR with developing each year a long-range strategic plan that balanced basic and applied research and required that the director of OAR not hold any other position at NIH. This effectively prohibited Anthony Fauci from serving simultaneously as director of NIAID and OAR, positions from which, since 1986, he had overseen all AIDS research.[71]

Even as this change in bureaucracy was in process, the United States was experiencing its own version of attempted political manipulation of a medical research project. In September 1992 the Senate subcommittee that oversaw the $253 billion budget of the Department of Defense included a recommendation that $20 million go to the Walter Reed Army Institute of Research to conduct studies of the candidate vaccine based on the surface protein gp160 of HIV, which was made by the company MicroGeneSys and called VaxSyn. It also stipulated that the trial could only be stopped if the secretary of defense, the NIH director, and the FDA commissioner all agreed that it should not go forward and submitted their reasons in writing. Former senator Russell Long of Louisiana led the lobbying effort through his law firm.[72]

FDA commissioner David Kessler and NIH director Bernadine Healy strongly and publicly objected to this attempt to circumvent the drug and vaccine approval process. In November 1992 they convened a blue-ribbon panel that included themselves, Assistant Secretary of Defense Enrique Mendez Jr., NIAID director Anthony Fauci, NCI director Sam Broder, Upjohn CEO Ted Cooper, Aaron Diamond researcher David Ho, and Nobel laureate Fred Robbins, as well as Frank Volvovitz, CEO of MicroGeneSys. Volvovitz argued passionately that the seriousness of the AIDS crisis demanded quick action to test a promising vaccine product. Fauci and others argued just as passionately that no large human trial should proceed until safety and efficacy trials had been completed and various candidate products compared with each other.

The debate over this single-candidate vaccine dragged on until 1996 with bizarre twists. In April 1993 the Department of Defense suggested that NIH take over the $20 million and conduct a phase II trial comparing candidate vaccines. MicroGeneSys, however, wanted payment for supplying the vaccine, a highly unusual situation. For most clinical trials, pharmaceutical firms provided the vaccine at no cost. This also raised suspicion that MicroGeneSys's underlying motive in pushing the single trial had been to receive a large share of the $20 million as payment for supplied vaccine. NIH refused to go forward with a trial for which one manufacturer insisted on payment while others agreed to supply the candidate vaccines at no cost, and the money reverted to the Army. AIDS activists, who initially had strongly supported the proposed test of VaxSyn, now staged a demonstration at MicroGeneSys headquarters wearing T-shirts proclaiming, "MicroGeneSys AIDS Extortionists." During 1994 the Army conducted its own review of VaxSyn. The major pharmaceutical firm Wyeth-Ayerst, which had previously been willing to fund large-scale production of the vaccine if approved, terminated its relationship with MicroGeneSys. Political leadership in Congress stepped away from support of the product. By the time the Army completed the phase II trial evaluating safety and efficacy in April 1996, its findings appeared anticlimactic. Analysis of the data showed "no clinical improvement that could be attributed to the vaccine used as an adjunct therapy for HIV infection."[73]

It is worth stating that this attempt to politicize AIDS vaccine research for the benefit of a single company never enjoyed the kind of blind government support that the South African government under Thabo Mbeki was able to provide for the drug Virodene. No U.S. official held sufficient power to ignore distinguished scientists' criticism of the proposal, and no U.S. official was persuaded to ignore scientific consensus about HIV and AIDS in order to promote a single product. The story of VaxSyn was, however, another example in which faith in a product exacerbated by a public health emergency and the opportunity to make money led to a situation in which political officials rather than scientists could have determined which candidate vaccine was worth an investment. The many critics of scientific peer review are correct in concluding that the process is not perfect, but, like democracy itself, it so far has been the best system devised to select, on the basis of merit, those research projects that will best utilize taxpayer funds.

In 1993 epidemiologist Donald Francis left the CDC and joined Genentech to work on another candidate subunit AIDS vaccine, this one based on gp120, which, with gp41, makes up gp160, the full envelope protein of HIV. The gp120 candidate vaccines developed by several companies, however, did not gain support within the federal scientific community for a large-scale human trial because phase II studies were inconclusive. Francis persuaded Robert Nowinski, the successful founder of multiple biotech companies, to join him in forming VaxGen, a spin-off company from Genentech, which had abandoned AIDS vaccine research. Francis planned for VaxGen to produce the gp120 vaccine, dubbed AIDSVAX, and to conduct human trials in the United States and Thailand, a country in which AIDS was ravaging injecting drug users, sex workers, their spouses, and their children. The Thai government was desperate to do something, anything that would slow the epidemic.

The actual trials of gp120 vaccines did not begin until 2003. Because AIDSVAX elicited only a humoral response to HIV, VaxGen combined AIDSVAX with a vaccine known as ALVAC-HIV, produced by the French pharmaceutical firm Aventis-Pasteur, which caused a cellular immune response and used genetic elements of several different HIV strains encapsulated in a harmless canarypox virus as the vaccine's vector. Ultimately, the trial cost $105 million and enrolled more than sixteen thousand subjects. As the results came in, once again they were uniformly disappointing. The vaccine provided no more protection than a placebo. To make matters worse, however, the vaccine also appeared to make some recipients even more susceptible to HIV infection than they would have been ordinarily.[74]

In July 2008 NIAID announced that it intended to return to a basic research approach to an AIDS vaccine, that too little was understood about how HIV functions to push forward with further human trials on existing candidate vaccines.[75] This announcement came two months before the U.S. stock market declined precipitately and the U.S. economy entered a prolonged recession that witnessed cutbacks in AIDS assistance programs across the country.[76] In a profile of NIAID director Anthony S. Fauci in 2009, he stated,

> We may not ever have an AIDS vaccine in the classical sense of being 95% protective. . . . We still don't know how, why, or if a body makes a robust neutralizing antibody and T-cell response that can both block acquisition and prevent disease progression. The reason we don't know this, is because the body doesn't do it in natural infection. With other viruses, nature tells us just follow me and I'll lead you to a vaccine. With HIV, nature is telling us if you follow me, you're going to be in trouble. We're going to have to push the envelope with HIV vaccinol-

ogy in ways that we never had to do before. I feel that as we probe the scientific secrets of HIV, we may get there.[77]

Two institutional entities created in the 1990s became the leaders of AIDS vaccine research in the third decade of the epidemic. At the NIH, a dedicated Vaccine Research Center (VRC) was authorized by President Clinton in 1997 and launched in 1999 as a joint effort of NIAID, NCI, and OAR. The VRC funded vaccine research in laboratories across the United States and also supported intramural NIH researchers in its Bethesda laboratories. In 1994 a number of scientists who supported the empiricist model of vaccine making organized a meeting at the Rockefeller Foundation's villa in Bellagio, Italy. From this meeting emerged the International AIDS Vaccine Initiative (IAVI), which focused its vaccine research on the strains of HIV most prevalent in the developing world. Both of these institutions have concentrated intensely on promoting vaccine development, but as the third decade of the epidemic closes, both are promoting more basic research into the molecular immunology of HIV rather than emphasizing empirical trials of vaccine candidates.[78]

Other Preventive Techniques
With hope fading that a conventional preventive vaccine for AIDS would be soon forthcoming, medical researchers turned their efforts to techniques targeted to specific populations. In 2009, after anecdotal evidence had suggested for several years that male circumcision seemed to reduce the incidence of HIV transmission to female partners of men, researchers produced persuasive data that male circumcision reduced HIV transmission by 50 to 60 percent. Although they could not explain exactly why circumcision helped, they could strongly recommend it as an effective way to reduce transmission.[79]

In July 2010, at the Eighteenth International AIDS Conference in Vienna, Austria, participants hailed the finding that a vaginal microbicide gel had been shown to be 50 percent effective if used once up to twelve hours before and once up to twelve hours after sexual intercourse. Women in sub-Saharan Africa suffered the most new HIV infections throughout the first decade of the twenty-first century, and this microbicide gave them the power of prevention. It was especially advantageous for those who might not be able to insist that their partners use a condom. Moreover, the trial from which these data were reported was the first of a topical antiretroviral product. By providing proof that the right microbicide could prevent HIV in women, it opened the door for intense work to refine and intensify the gel to attain more complete protection.[80]

A different approach to prevention was identified in May 2011, when emerging data from a large clinical trial scheduled to end in 2015 caused its data and safety monitoring board (DSMB) to terminate the trial early. Led by study chair Myron Cohen, director of the Institute for Global Health and Infectious Diseases at the University of North Carolina–Chapel Hill, the study, which began in 2005, enrolled 1,763 couples, 97 percent of whom were heterosexual, in nine countries around the world. One person in each couple was HIV positive; the other was HIV negative. The infected partners in one group in the study were given antiretroviral drugs while their immune systems were still at levels considered healthy (more than 500 CD4+ T cells per cubic millimeter of blood, according to guidelines in the United States; more than 350 cells per cubic millimeter, according to World Health Organization guidelines). The infected partners of the second group were given antiretroviral drugs only after their CD4+ T cells fell below 250 cells per cubic millimeter of blood or when they experienced an AIDS-related event such as *Pneumocystis* pneumonia. The DSMB found twenty-eight infections in the previously uninfected partners in study participants. Of those, twenty-seven occurred in the partners of infected study subjects who did not receive the antiretroviral drugs while their immune systems were still healthy. Only one infection occurred in the partners of infected study subjects who were treated early with antiretroviral drugs. Statistically, this represented a 96 percent reduction in HIV transmission to the HIV-uninfected partner if antiretroviral drugs were started immediately after diagnosis.[81]

Anthony Fauci, director of NIAID, which sponsored the trial, hailed the results. "Previous data about the potential value of antiretrovirals in making HIV-infected individuals less infectious to their sexual partners came largely from observational and epidemiological studies," he said. "This new finding convincingly demonstrates that treating the infected individual—and doing so sooner rather than later—can have a major impact on reducing HIV transmission." Similarly, Margaret Chan, director general of the World Health Organization, called this a "crucial development, because we know that sexual transmission accounts for about 80 percent of all new infections." Michel Sidibe, who succeeded Peter Piot as director of UNAIDS in January 2009, predicted that this finding would be "a serious game changer" that would "drive the prevention revolution forward. It makes HIV treatment a new priority prevention option."[82]

This study, however, does not answer a different question: does the early administration of antiretroviral drugs place an unacceptably heavy burden of negative side effects on those who take the drugs when their immune systems are still in the healthy range? Documented side effects, which vary by individual, include peripheral neuropathy (nerve damage), lipodystrophy (fat redistribution), elevated cholesterol and triglycerides (risk factors for heart attack and stroke), and liver damage.[83] A new study that seeks to answer this question will follow four thousand HIV-infected men and women in thirty countries, all of whom have CD4+ T cell counts above five hundred cells per cubic millimeter and who have never before taken antiretroviral therapy. Half will be assigned randomly to receive immediate therapy; the other half will not receive therapy until their CD4+ counts fall below 350 cells per cubic millimeter or an AIDS-related event occurs. Fauci observed, "Some epidemiological evidence suggests that HIV infected patients remain healthier when they begin treatment at higher CD4 counts. However, there are also concerns about the health complications and side effects associated with lifelong antiretroviral use and the possibility that the virus may become resistant to medication."[84] Depending on the results of this trial, public health officials and physicians will be able to make a more rational recommendation about when antiretroviral therapy should begin, balancing its promise to prevent the spread of HIV with its impact on the bodies of infected people.

Conclusion

During the third decade of the AIDS pandemic, after ART was developed and began being used to help HIV-infected people, the world started to respond robustly to the serious economic and national security threats posed by AIDS. Major funding by governments, nongovernmental organizations, and the private sector began to have an impact in the developing world, the areas in which the disease had caused the most misery and death. UNAIDS has repeatedly set goals, such as the "three-by-five" initiative, aimed at getting antiretroviral therapy to 3 million people by 2005.[85] Though this goal was not met, the effort highlighted the continuing need for more involvement.

Efforts to produce a vaccine have not been successful. They have illustrated the limitations of responding to a medical problem when the underlying
biological mechanisms are novel and thus do not provide natural models for
medicine to imitate. Political initiatives in South Africa and the United States to
promote one line of research on a therapy or vaccine to the exclusion of others,
however well intentioned, demonstrated that the political, cultural, and economic frameworks in which the response to HIV/AIDS has been constructed
are similar to those framing earlier epidemics.

The emergence of male circumcision and female microbicides as partially
effective prevention strategies also demonstrated the need to utilize many different interventions to address the epidemic. The finding that antiretroviral
therapy can serve to reduce transmission drastically holds the promise of controlling the pandemic if the side effects of early therapy are tolerable to those
infected. Bioethical issues for physicians treating infected individuals must be
weighed carefully alongside the desire to reduce transmission of the virus within
a worldwide population. There may never be a medical magic bullet to control
HIV/AIDS as antibiotics controlled bacterial infections and vaccines controlled
smallpox and polio. Nonetheless, the most recent medical information holds
considerable promise that the AIDS pandemic may be halted or severely cur-
tailed if human political, social, religious, and cultural entities have the will to
implement the tools that have been demonstrated effective in scientific trials.[86]

Epilogue: AIDS at 30

"Fulfilling the UNAIDS vision of zero new infections will require a hard look at the societal structures, beliefs and value systems that present obstacles to effective HIV prevention efforts."

—UNAIDS, *Global Report 2010*[1]

As the HIV/AIDS pandemic enters its fourth decade, where does it stand? UNAIDS reported in its 2010 *Global Report* that 33 million people in the world are living with HIV/AIDS. The figures on AIDS-related deaths by region between 1990 and 2009 provide a graphic picture of the epidemic around the world. Figure 9.1 shows the number of deaths as heavy lines, with the lighter lines on either side representing the statistical error probability. The graph for North America and Western and Central Europe—the industrialized Western democracies—shows deaths peaking in the early 1990s and dropping after 1996, when combination antiretroviral therapy was introduced. Deaths in Central and South America began to level off around 2005, as did deaths in Asia. Deaths in the Caribbean reached a peak around 2003 but began to decline rapidly after that date. Sub-Saharan Africa's graph shows a similar pattern, with one exception: the number of deaths in this region are measured in millions instead of the thousands that characterize the rest of the world. The dramatic drop in deaths in sub-Saharan Africa and the Caribbean track closely with increased funding of international donors for diagnosis, treatment, and prevention efforts. The moderating trends in Asia and Central and South America reflect not only increased international assistance but also a large investment by many of the wealthy countries in those regions. The only trend line for deaths that still climbs in 2009 is the one for Eastern Europe and Central Asia, the regions in which injecting drug use is fueling the epidemic and governments have no harm-reduction programs in place.

Looking back over the three decades of the HIV/AIDS epidemic, medical science can take pride in how quickly the syndrome was identified, the causative agent found, a diagnostic test prepared, and an effective therapy developed. The original diagnostic test has been refined many times so that in 2011 it is possible to learn one's HIV status in twenty minutes via a cheek swab test. The FDA posts a long list of antiretroviral drugs now available to treat HIV infection and its complications.[2] Although it seemed interminable for those living with HIV/AIDS or caring for a person with HIV/AIDS, in historical perspective, the period from first recognition of the disease in 1981 to the introduction of combination antiretroviral therapy in 1996—fifteen years—is stunningly

GLOBAL REPORT
Figure 2.3
Annual AIDS-related deaths by region, 1990-2009

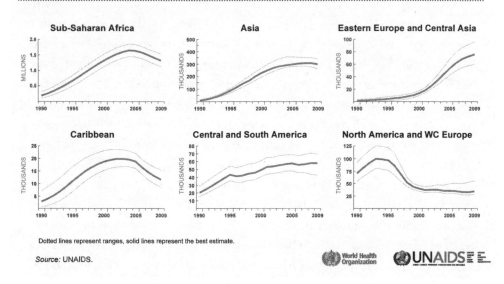

Dotted lines represent ranges, solid lines represent the best estimate.

Source: UNAIDS.

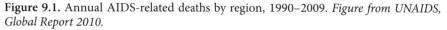

Figure 9.1. Annual AIDS-related deaths by region, 1990–2009. *Figure from UNAIDS, Global Report 2010.*

short. "There is probably not anything the equivalent in medicine, apart from maybe the development of penicillin, in terms of night-and-day difference," stated Paul Volberding, one of the earliest physicians involved in HIV/AIDS in San Francisco, in a film he made in 2009 to capture the history of HIV/AIDS, *Life Before the Lifeboat*.[3] In contrast, HIV/AIDS challenged everything known about making a preventive vaccine, and as the fourth decade of the epidemic begins, none is yet even strongly promising. Figure 9.2 shows the most detailed three-dimensional image of HIV yet produced. Winner of the 2010 Visualization Challenge sponsored by the American Association for the Advancement of Science and the U.S. National Science Foundation, this image was created by a group at the Visual Science Company in Moscow, Russia, in only two colors to emphasize how HIV wraps itself in proteins from the host cell it infects, thus making it harder for the immune system to recognize it as an invader.

One of the unique characteristics of the HIV/AIDS epidemic has been the vigorous and continuous involvement of people with HIV/AIDS and their supporters, together known colloquially as "AIDS activists." It is hard to recall another medical challenge in which those already infected or most at risk took political action to force governments to respond to their demands for assistance. Indeed, the success of the HIV/AIDS activists and their red ribbons, which were first introduced in 1991 by Visual AIDS in New York as a simple symbol declaring solidarity among those living with HIV/AIDS, inspired many later groups of health lobbyists, beginning with advocates for more breast cancer research, who adopted a pink ribbon symbol, and moving on to many other groups with ribbons of various colors.[4]

More time needs to pass before the effect of HIV/AIDS on societal attitudes toward stigmatized groups at high risk for HIV infection can be evaluated. Homosexual men initially feared that the advent of HIV/AIDS would set back irreparably their crusade for greater civil rights. For many people, however, the need to confront the disease meant confronting the fact that their sons or their relatives, or their friends' sons, were gay. John-Manuel Andriote, a writer in Norwich, Connecticut, argued in his book, *Victory Deferred: How AIDS Changed Gay Life in America*, that because of AIDS, "gay people and their families, friends, neighbors and co-workers realized compassion is the supreme traditional value."[5] In many cases, this led to a reconsideration of the nature of homosexuality as an inborn orientation, not as a perverse lifestyle choice.

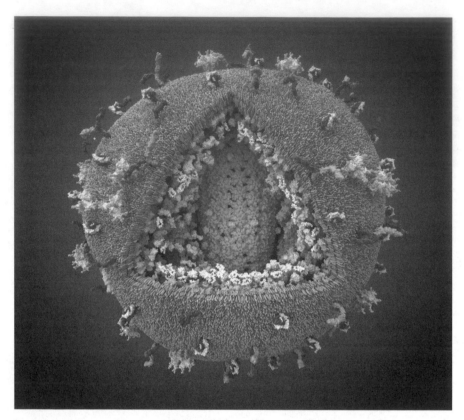

Figure 9.2. Human immunodeficiency virus in three dimensions. First place winner of the 2010 Visualization Challenge sponsored by the American Association for the Advancement of Science and the U.S. National Science Foundation. HIV was represented in two colors: orange, which represented viral proteins, and gray, which represented proteins from the infected host. The two-color scheme revealed how HIV "uses material from the host to sort of wrap itself in this membrane." *Courtesy of Ivan Konstantinov, Yury Stefanov, Aleksander Kovalevsky, and Yegor Voronin, Visual Science Company, Moscow, Russia.*

It may be argued that legislation approving same-sex marriage is one example of a positive outcome of this social phenomenon, but only time will provide the necessary perspective for this conclusion. Other people, of course, never budged from a belief that homosexuality was a free-will choice, that it was sinful, and that homosexuals had brought this terrible disease upon themselves. This attitude remains very strong in some countries, especially in central Africa, where homosexuals have recently been murdered and laws have been passed making homosexual acts capital offenses.[6]

Underdeveloped countries, however, are not the only places where stigma and bias have had negative consequences on the epidemic. In the District of Columbia, home of the U.S. Congress, Supreme Court, and president, the rate of HIV infection rose 22 percent between 2006 and 2009, to a rate of 3 percent of the total D.C. population. "Our [3 percent] rates are higher than West Africa," said Shannon L. Hader, director of the District's HIV/AIDS Administration, who once led the CDC's work in Zimbabwe. "They're on par with Uganda and some parts of Kenya."

To make matters worse, in February 2011, PreventionWorks, a program that made clean needles available to drug addicts, was cancelled because of lack of funds. *Washington Post* columnist Petula Devork commented on the shortsightedness of such a policy: "The average cost of lifetime care for someone with HIV/AIDS is about $385,200. . . . PreventionWorks was getting about $300,000 a year from the city budget. It collapsed while waiting for $130,000 in delayed funds."[7]

The other stigmatized group associated with HIV/AIDS is injecting drug users. Wary of authority, addicts have been the most difficult group to reach and the least sympathetic group for advocates to support. Epidemiologic data have clearly shown that harm-reduction strategies reduce the incidence of infection, yet punitive attitudes toward drug users have stymied treatment programs and needle exchanges in countries as varied as Russia and the United States. Western European countries and Australia, which adopted harm reduction early on, have kept the incidence of HIV infection low in this group and in their partners and children. Curiously, according to Peter Piot, not all authoritarian countries shun harm-reduction techniques. After he consulted with the Chinese government, which had in place harsh penalties for drug users, the leaders became convinced that harm reduction was the most effective strategy against AIDS and took action. Within one week, he stated,

the government issued decrees about how to deal with AIDS that were literally taken from UNAIDS publications. . . . They decided that they needed 300 methadone centers, that they would have needle exchange. They set a target, and in one year, there were 300 centers. . . . But it's still one country, two systems. On the one hand, the police still crack down on drug use, so if addicts have bad luck, they end up in a reeducation center for years or locked up and detoxed cold turkey. If they are lucky, they end up in a drop-in center for drug users, where they get methadone and clean needles. Both scenarios can happen in the same city.[8]

Whether more countries can be persuaded to adopt harm-reduction strategies will be the test for how the HIV/AIDS epidemic evolves in the future via this risk group.

Perhaps the most novel development during the first three decades of the epidemic was the consensus during the third decade that HIV/AIDS required a global response because it was a global threat. HIV/AIDS was clearly not a classic epidemic, such as a cholera outbreak, that would soon pass through the institution of public health measures, nor even a highly lethal epidemic like the 1918–1919 influenza epidemic or the medieval bubonic plague. Untreated, HIV killed 100 percent of people who developed full-blown AIDS, and the number of people who were either resistant to infection or never developed any illness from the infection was miniscule. The largest number of people who contracted HIV infection were young adults, and their deaths left a critical gap in hard-hit populations. AIDS orphans were left to mature with little adult guidance, and AIDS widows were forced into sex work to survive, a situation via which they often passed the virus to their patrons. In short, such a dismal situation was destabilizing to world security. Long-term illnesses caused by HIV/AIDS also led to employee absenteeism and a smaller market for goods, thus threatening world economy. Once these characteristics were grasped at the highest political levels, the global response became focused and has slowed deaths and new infections from HIV. To address the epidemic fully, however, UNAIDS has called for up to four times as much investment as has been made, but in a time of world economic slowdown, the commitment to HIV/AIDS programs is uncertain.

Finally, the HIV/AIDS epidemic will be viewed as all other epidemics, as a biological event occurring in historical time within human social, political, religious, and cultural institutions. Because HIV is transmitted sexually, religious and cultural beliefs about sex will always frame the willingness of individuals to support public health interventions. Conservative religious people in many faiths reject outright the need to discuss sexual activity that occurs outside their beliefs, let alone fund programs such as the distribution of condoms.

The medical community has created a new discipline called "implementation science," which is defined as "the scientific study of methods to promote the integration of research findings and evidence based interventions into health care policy and practice and hence to improve the quality and effectiveness of health services and care."[9] The task of this field is to demonstrate to funders of programs in HIV/AIDS diagnosis, therapy, and prevention the scientific data supporting one intervention as more effective than another so that the most efficacious and cost-effective programs may be identified. Those involved are hopeful that rigorous data will be convincing and will contribute to controlling the HIV/AIDS epidemic. Whether rational scientific data can overcome strong social, religious, and political beliefs that are in conflict with science remains to be seen.

Glossary

AIDS	acquired immune deficiency syndrome
antibody	protein used by the immune system to identify and neutralize foreign molecules or substances such as viruses and bacteria
antigen	substance or molecule that triggers the production of an antibody
ART	antiretroviral therapy (current usage for HAART)
ARV	AIDS-associated retrovirus, the name first given to the AIDS virus by the laboratory of Jay Levy at the University of California–San Francisco
ASFV	African swine fever virus
assay	test designed to reveal some property of a chemical, physical, or biological substance, such as the presence or absence of that substance
AZT	azidothymidine, first drug found partially effective against AIDS
B cells	white blood cells formed in the bone marrow that produce antibodies to foreign proteins
candidiasis	fungal infection (mycosis) of any of the *Candida* species of yeast; also known as thrush
capsid, viral	container in which a virus's genetic material is located
CCR-5	chemokine receptor type 5 (also known as CD195 [cluster of differentiation 195]), the second receptor used by HIV to enter macrophages

CD4	cluster of differentiation 4; a glycoprotein found on T cells that serves as a receptor for HIV
cellular immune system	body's response to infecting pathogens and cancers by activating various white blood cells to kill infected cells
chemokines	family of small proteins that is secreted by cells; one subgroup, known as β chemokines, suppresses HIV
clone	to produce an exact copy of an organism; in laboratory usage, to produce multiple exact copies of a fragment of DNA
codon, genetic	series of bases in DNA that directs the synthesis of one amino acid in a protein; a fragment of a gene
cryptosporidiosis	parasitic disease caused by the protozoan *Cryptosporidium*, which caused severe diarrhea in people with AIDS
CXCR-4	chemokine receptor type 4 (also known as CD184 [cluster of differentiation 184]), the second receptor used by HIV to enter T cells
cytokines	molecules that provide communication between cells; interleukins, interferons, and chemokines are subgroups of cytokines
cytomegalovirus	CMV, a widespread herpes virus that rarely causes disease unless the immune system is compromised
data and safety monitoring board	DSMB, committee with no direct connection to the drugs used in a drug trial but whose members monitor the data from the trial and have the authority to stop the trial if the candidate drug proves either harmful or especially effective
DNA	deoxyribonucleic acid; a double helix–shaped strand of genetic material that encodes genetic information for all known living organisms except for some viruses
efficacy	how well a candidate drug works in a drug trial
ELISA	enzyme-linked immunosorbent assay, a technique for detecting the presence of an antibody or antigen in a sample
epidemic	condition that exists in a population when the incidence of a disease during a given period substantially exceeds what past experience suggests is normal

etiology	study of disease causation
FACS machine	fluorescence-activated cell sorter, an instrument that sorts cells for study
gene	series of bases in DNA that directs the synthesis of a single protein
germ theory of infectious diseases	the theory that one microorganism is the cause of one disease
gp	glycoprotein, a viral protein with sugar chains attached; e.g., gp41 is glycoprotein 41
granulocyte	white blood cells characterized by their granular appearance that kill invading microbes
GRID	gay-related immune disorder, an early term used to describe AIDS
HAART	highly active anti-retroviral therapy
helper T cells	T cells that serve as the master cells of the immune system, directing both humoral and cellular immunity
herpes viruses	viruses in the herpesvirus family, members of which cause cold sores, genital lesions, chicken pox, and other diseases; herpes viruses persist in the body after the infection they cause subsides and may reactivate episodically
HIV	human immunodeficiency virus, the virus that causes AIDS, named by an international committee in 1986
HIV-1	first human immunodeficiency virus identified; most common throughout the world
HIV-2	second human immunodeficiency virus identified; less common, except in West Africa
HTLV-III	human T-cell lymphotropic virus number three, the name first given to the AIDS virus by the laboratory of Robert Gallo at the U.S. National Institutes of Health
humoral immune system	body's response to infecting pathogens by the production of antibodies to neutralize the foreign proteins
in vitro	literally "in glass"; study done in the laboratory but not in animals or humans
in vivo	literally "in life"; study done on living beings

IND	investigational new drug, a category assigned by the FDA to drugs undergoing review before marketing
IND, treatment	drug with IND status that may be used by physicians in advance of formal FDA approval because trial data have shown it to be effective
institutional review board	IRB, committee that oversees all human-subject research at a medical center
integrase	enzyme utilized by HIV to insert viral DNA into the host cell's DNA
interferon	protein released by a lymphocyte in the presence of a pathogen that helps trigger an immune response to eradicate the pathogen
interleukin-2	protein that recognizes the presence of infection in the body and signals the immune system to ramp up production of T cells that will kill the invading organism; also known as T-cell growth factor because it promotes the growth of T cells in laboratory culture.
Kaposi's sarcoma	KS, cancerous tumor caused by infection with human herpesvirus 8, which is normally held in check by the immune system but proves to be an opportunistic cancer in people with compromised immune systems
Koch's postulates	series of steps in the process of demonstrating that one microscopic pathogen causes one disease
LAV	lymphadenopathy associated virus, the name first given to the AIDS virus by the laboratory of Luc Montagnier at the Pasteur Institute
lentivirus	virus that has a long incubation period and the unique ability to replicate in nondividing cells
long-term nonprogressors	individuals who are infected with HIV but do not develop full-blown AIDS
lymphocyte	category of white blood cells, including T cells, B cells, and natural killer cells
lymphokines	proteins that direct the immune response by signaling between cells
macrophage	from the Greek "large eater," a white blood cell that engulfs and digests cellular debris and pathogens

memory B cells	B cells that have experienced exposure to a specific antigen and "remember" it, sometimes for the life of the infected person, in order to produce antibodies quickly if the antigen invades the body again
MIP 1-α	chemokine "macrophage inflammatory protein-1-α"
MIP 1-β	chemokine "macrophage inflammatory protein-1-β"
molecular biology	study of how the human body works at the level of molecules
monocyte	white blood cell that has several roles in the immune system; one of them is to replenish macrophages
MSM	men who have sex with men
murine animals	rodents that include mice and rats
NDA	new drug application (FDA classification)
NIH, extramural	program of grants awarded to medical researchers at universities across the United States and in some foreign countries
NIH, intramural	laboratories and clinics on NIH's campuses, primarily in Bethesda, Maryland, but also in Baltimore, North Carolina, and Montana
oncovirus	virus that causes cancer
p (e.g., p24, p25)	viral protein identified by its molecular weight—e.g., p24 is a protein with a molecular weight of 24,000 daltons
pandemic	worldwide epidemic
pathogen	a substance that causes disease
pathophysiology	disease process in the human body
PCP	*Pneumocystis carinii* pneumonia
PCR	polymerase chain reaction, a technique to amplify a piece of DNA so that a large quantity is easily available for study
peer review	evaluation of the merit of a grant proposal or publication by a panel of scientists in the same field as the person proposing
phase I drug trial	drug trial conducted to establish which dosage of a candidate drug works best; usually a very small number of people are involved
phase II drug trial	drug trial conducted to establish the effectiveness and

                       toxicity of a candidate drug; more people are treated in a phase II trial

phase III drug trial   drug trial conducted in a large population over a relatively long period to evaluate safety and effectiveness of a candidate drug before it is released to the public

placebo   drug with no effect, often called a sugar pill

placebo-controlled, double-blind drug trial   drug trial in which one group of participants receive a placebo while another receives the candidate drug; it is "double-blind" because neither patients nor physicians know which patients are receiving the placebo or the drug

plasma   liquid part of the blood from which whole cells have been removed

plasma B cells   B cells that produce large quantities of antibodies

Pneumocystis carinii   pathogen, now correctly recognized as *Pneumocystis jirovecii*, that is commonly found in the lungs of healthy people but causes a severe pneumonia in people whose immune systems are compromised

protease   enzyme utilized by HIV to cleave the components of new virions so that it may mature and infect new cells

protocol, medical research   detailed research plan designed to increase knowledge about a specific medical problem

PWA   people with AIDS

RANTES   chemokine "regulated-upon-activation, normal T expressed and secreted"

reagent, biological   substance that is used in the study of immunological and other processes in laboratories of molecular and cell biology

recombinant DNA technology   laboratory technique that permits manipulation, deletion, or addition of genes to an existing organism

retrovirus   RNA virus that utilizes the enzyme reverse transcriptase to convert itself into a form of DNA that can integrate into the genome of its host cell

reverse transcriptase   enzyme utilized by retroviruses to convert their RNA cores into a form of DNA that can be integrated into the host cell's genome

RNA	ribonucleic acid; a single helix–shaped strand of genetic material that contains genes that can direct the production of proteins; it serves as the sole genetic material for some viruses, including HIV
SARS	severe acute respiratory syndrome
sequence	to determine the order of bases—i.e., the genes—in a strand of DNA
serum	liquid part of the blood from which whole cells and clotting factors have been removed
SIDA	abbreviation for acquired immune deficiency syndrome in some other languages, e.g., *syndrome d'immunodéficience acquise* (French), *síndrome de inmunodeficiencia adquirida* (Spanish)
SIV	simian immunodeficiency virus
suppressor T cells	T cells that recognize when a microbial threat has been defeated and shut down the immune response
syndrome	collection of symptoms that characterize a disease
T cells	white blood cells that are processed in the thymus gland as they mature; they control or participate in the body's immune response.
T-cell growth factor	see interleukin-2
toxoplasmosis	parasitic disease caused by the protozoan *Toxoplasma gondi* that causes severe symptoms such as encephalitis in people with AIDS
vasculitis	inflammation of the blood vessels
VIH	abbreviation for human immunodeficiency virus in some other languages, e.g., *virus de l'immunodéficience humaine* (French); *virus de la inmunodeficiencia humana* (Spanish)
viral load	amount of HIV in a specific quantity of blood
virus	tiny infectious agent that can reproduce only inside the cells of a host organism; there are many types of viruses; all have genes made of DNA or RNA and a protein coat that surrounds and protects these genes; some also have a lipid, or fat, envelope surrounding them when they are outside the host cell

| Western blot | analytical technique that first sorts the proteins in a substance by the use of gel electrophoresis (which passes an electrical current through a gel matrix to sort the proteins), then transfers the sorted proteins to a membrane, and finally identifies individual proteins through the use of specific antibodies |
| zoonosis | disease caused by a microscopic pathogen transmitted from other animals to humans |

Notes

Prologue: Emergence in Silence

1. William H. McNeill, "Patterns of Disease Emergence in History," in *Emerging Viruses*, ed. Stephen S. Morse (New York: Oxford University Press, 1993), 29–36.

2. A month earlier, an article in the *New York Native*, the "most influential" newspaper in the gay community of the United States, had advised that rumors of a "gay cancer" had been denied by the U.S. Centers for Disease Control. See Lawrence Mass, "Disease Rumors Largely Unfounded," *New York Native*, May 18, 1981; Jack Begg, "Word for Word/Nameless Dread; 20 Years Ago, the First Clues to the Birth of a Plague," *New York Times*, June 3, 2001, Week in Review section, in *New York Times* Online AIDS Collection, http://topics.nytimes.com /topics/news/health/diseasesconditionsandhealthtopics/aids/index.html (*New York Times* Online AIDS Collection hereafter). Figures for 2010 incidence of HIV/AIDS are from Joint United Nations Programme on HIV/AIDS (UNAIDS), *Global Report: UNAIDS Report on the Global AIDS Epidemic, 2010* (Geneva, Switzerland: UNAIDS, 2010), 7.

3. Michael S. Gottlieb, Howard M. Schanker, Peng Thim Fan, Andrew Saxon, Joel D. Weisman, and Irving Pozalski, "*Pneumocystis* Pneumonia—Los Angeles," *Morbidity and Mortality Weekly Report* (*MMWR* hereafter) 30 (June 5, 1981): 250–52.

4. For good introductions and various points of view on the history of humans and disease organisms, see Rene Jules Dubos, *Mirage of Health: Utopias, Progress, and Biological Change* (New Brunswick, NJ: Rutgers University Press, 1959); Harry F. Dowling, *Fighting Infection: Conquests of the Twentieth Century* (Cambridge, MA: Harvard University Press, 1977); Harald Brüssow, "Europe, the Bull and the Minotaur: The Biological Legacy of a Neolithic Love Story," *Environmental Microbiology* 11 (November 2009): 2778–88.

5. In the years since 1981, much has been learned about *Pneumocystis* pneumonia and Kaposi's sarcoma. At the 2001 International Workshop on Opportunistic Protists, the name of *Pneumocystis carinii* was changed to *Pneumocystis jirovecii*,

although the taxonomical issue is not completely settled. In 1994 Yuan Chang and her colleagues at Columbia University discovered a new herpesvirus as the cause of Kaposi's sarcoma. For updated reviews of both AIDS-related illnesses, see Emilie Catherinot et al., "*Pneumocystis jirovecii* Pneumonia," *Infectious Disease Clinics of North America* (*Infect. Dis. Clin. North Am.* hereafter) 24 (March 2010): 107–38; Don Ganem, "KSHV and the Pathogenesis of Kaposi Sarcoma: Listening to Human Biology and Medicine," *Journal of Clinical Investigation* (*J. Clin. Invest.* hereafter) 120 (April 2010): 939–49.

6. Centers for Disease Control, "Current Trends Classification System for Human T-Lymphotropic Virus Type III/ Lymphadenopathy-Associated Virus Infections," *MMWR* 35 (May 23, 1986): 334–39; World Health Organization, "Acquired Immunodeficiency Syndrome (AIDS): WHO/CDC Case Definition for AIDS," *Weekly Epidemiological Record* (*Wkly. Epidemiol Rec.* hereafter) 61 (March 7, 1986): 69–73. Between 1984 and 2000 the term "AIDS-related complex" was also used to describe a "prodromal" phase of infection. Once the disease was defined solely as infection with HIV, this term fell out of use.

7. World Health Organization, "WHO Case Definitions for AIDS Surveillance in Adults and Adolescents," *Wkly. Epidemiol. Rec.* 69 (September 16, 1994): 273–75; Kenneth G. Castro et al., "1993 Revised Classification System for HIV Infection and Expanded Surveillance Case Definition for AIDS among Adolescents and Adults," *MMWR* 41 (December 18, 1992).

8. Richard M. Selik et al., "Increase in Deaths Caused by HIV Infection due to Changes in Rules for Selecting Underlying Cause of Death," *Journal of Acquired Immune Deficiency Syndrome* (*J. Acquir. Immune Defic. Syndr.* hereafter) 32 (January 1, 2003): 62–69.

9. Beatrice H. Hahn et al., "AIDS as a Zoonosis: Scientific and Public Health Implications," *Science* 287 (January 28, 2000): 607–14.

10. David Quammen, "Deadly Contact: How Animals and Humans Exchange Disease," *National Geographic*, October 2007, 79–105.

11. Victoria A. Harden, *Rocky Mountain Spotted Fever* (Baltimore: Johns Hopkins University Press, 1990).

12. Colin R. Parrish et al., "Cross-Species Virus Transmission and the Emergence of New Epidemic Diseases," *Microbiology and Molecular Biology Reviews* 72 (2008): 457–70; Quammen, "Deadly Contact"; Jon Cohen, "Searching for the Epidemic's Origins," *Science* 288 (June 23, 2000): 2164–65; Jared Diamond, "The Mysterious Origin of AIDS," *Natural History* 101, no. 9 (1992): 24–29; Jon Cohen, "Virology: AIDS Virus Traced to Chimp Subspecies," *Science* 283 (February 5, 1999): 772–73; Edward C. Holmes, "When HIV Spread Afar," *Proceedings of the National Academy of Sciences of the United States of America* (*Proc. Natl. Acad. Sci.* hereafter) 104 (November 20, 2007): 18351–52; Jon Cohen, "AIDS Research: Reconstructing the Origins of the AIDS Epidemic from Archived HIV Isolates," *Science* 318 (November 2, 2007): 731a.

13. Jonathan L. Heeney, Angus G. Dalgleish, and Robin A. Weiss, "Origins of HIV and the Evolution of Resistance to AIDS," *Science* 313 (July 28, 2006): 462–66.

14. Louise V. Wain et al., "Adaptation of HIV-1 to Its Human Host," *Molecular Biology and Evolution* 24 (August 2007): 1853–60; Paul M. Sharp and Beatrice H. Hahn, "AIDS: Prehistory of HIV-1," *Nature* 455 (October 2, 2008): 605–6;

Paul M. Sharp and Beatrice H. Hahn, "The Evolution of HIV-1 and the Origin of AIDS," Philosophical Transactions of the Royal Society of London, Series B, Biological Sciences 365 (August 27, 2010): 2487–94.

15. According to the U.S. Red Cross, in 2009, "the estimated risk that an HIV-infected donation would be available for transfusion is 1 in 1.5 million." See http://www.redcross.org/www-files/Documents/pdf/HIVAIDS/GivingBlood_lh_cr.pdf, (accessed July 24, 2011).

16. "Colonial Clue to the Rise of HIV," BBC News, October 1, 2008, http://news .bbc.co.uk/2/hi/health/7646255.stm; Heidi Ledford, "Tissue Sample Suggests HIV Has Been Infecting Humans for a Century," Nature News, October 1, 2008, http://www.nature.com/news/2008/081001/full/news.2008.1143.html; Laurence Dudley Stamp and William Thomas Wilson Morgan, Africa: A Study in Tropical Development (New York: Wiley, 1972), 302.

17. M. Thomas P. Gilbert et al., "The Emergence of HIV/AIDS in the Americas and Beyond," Proc. Natl. Acad. Sci. 104 (October 31, 2007): 18566–70; Jean-Francois Molez, "The Historical Question of Acquired Immunodeficiency Syndrome in the 1960s in the Congo River Basin Area in Relation to Cryptococcal Meningitis," American Journal of Tropical Medicine and Hygiene 58 (1998): 273–76. The country was renamed Zaire in 1971.

18. Michael Worobey et al., "Direct Evidence of Extensive Diversity of HIV-1 in Kinshasa by 1960," Nature 455 (October 2, 2008): 661–64; Paul M. Sharp and Beatrice H. Hahn, "AIDS: Prehistory of HIV-1," Nature 455 (October 2, 2008): 605–6; Gilbert et al., "Emergence of HIV/AIDS in the Americas and Beyond"; Jean William Pape et al., "The Epidemiology of AIDS in Haiti Refutes the Claims of Gilbert et al.," Proc. Natl. Acad. Sci. 105 (March 6, 2008): 1073; Jon Cohen, "HIV/AIDS: Latin America and Caribbean. The Caribbean," Science 313 (July 28, 2006): 470; Paul Farmer, AIDS and Accusation: Haiti and the Geography of Blame (Berkeley: University of California Press, 1992).

19. Peter Piot, interview, in "The Age of AIDS," Frontline, PBS, February 25, 2005, http://www.pbs.org/wgbh/pages/frontline/aids/interviews (accessed August 28, 2009).

20. Judith Williams, interview by Victoria A. Harden and Caroline Hannaway, February 20, 1997, Oral History Archive, Office of NIH History, National Institutes of Health, Bethesda, MD (NIH AIDS Oral Histories hereafter).

Chapter 1. What Is This New Disease?

1. Selma K. Dritz, "Charting the Epidemiological Course of AIDS, 1981 1984," interview by Sally Smith Hughes, 1992, in The AIDS Epidemic in San Francisco: The Medical Response, 1981–1984, vol. 1, Regional Oral History Office, Bancroft Library, University of California–Berkeley, 1995. All the interviews in The AIDS Epidemic in San Francisco are available on the Internet at http://bancroft.berkeley.edu/ROHO/collections/subjectarea/sci_tech/aids.html (San Francisco AIDS Oral Histories hereafter.)

2. Oxford English Dictionary, 2nd ed., s.v. "disease" (2004), Oxford University Press.

3. K. Codell Carter, "Koch's Postulates in Relation to the Work of Jacob Henle and Edwin Klebs," Medical History (Med. Hist. hereafter) 29 (1985): 353–74;

K. Codell Carter, "The Development of Pasteur's Concept of Disease Causation and the Emergence of Specific Causes in Nineteenth-Century Medicine," *Bulletin of the History of Medicine* (*Bull. Hist. Med.* hereafter) 65 (1991): 528–48; K. Codell Carter, *The Rise of Causal Concepts of Disease: Case Histories* (Burlington, VT: Ashgate, 2003).

4. Phyllis Allen Richmond, "American Attitudes toward the Germ Theory of Disease (1860–1880)," *Journal of the History of Medicine and Allied Sciences* 9 (1954): 428–54; "Rethinking the Reception of the Germ Theory of Disease: Comparative Perspectives," ibid., 52 (1997): 7–157; Nancy Tomes, *The Gospel of Germs: Men, Women, and the Microbe in American Life* (Cambridge, MA: Harvard University Press, 1999).

5. Robert A. Buerki, "Reception of the Germ Theory of Disease," *Pharmacy in History* 13 (1971): 158–68; John Farley, "Parasites and the Germ Theory of Disease," in *Framing Disease: Studies in Cultural History* (New Brunswick, NJ: Rutgers University Press, 1992), 33–49; Dowling, *Fighting Infection*; K. Codell Carter, "Ignaz Semmelweis, Carl Mayrhofer, and the Rise of Germ Theory," *Med. Hist.* 29 (1985): 33–53.

6. "The Nobel Prize in Physiology or Medicine 1901: Emil von Behring," Nobel prize.org, 2011, http://nobelprize.org/nobel_prizes/medicine/laureates/1901/index.html; "Emil von Behring: The Founder of Serum Therapy," Nobelprize .org, n.d., http://nobelprize.org/nobel_prizes/medicine/laureates/1901/behring -article.html.

7. Steven Wayne Collins, *The Race to Commercialize Biotechnology* (London: Routledge, 2004), 127.

8. There is a large literature describing or documenting the retrospective studies on stored sera and remembered experiences of patients with clinical features of the disease. Summaries may be found in general histories of AIDS, especially Jonathan Engel, *The Epidemic* (New York: Smithsonian Books/Collins, 2006); Mirko D. Grmek, *History of AIDS* (Princeton, NJ: Princeton University Press, 1990); Randy Shilts, *And the Band Played On: Politics, People and the AIDS Epidemic* (New York: St. Martin's Press, 1987); Thomas C. Quinn, interview by Victoria A. Harden and Caroline Hannaway, December 5, 1996; Peter Piot, interviews by Victoria A. Harden, January 4, 2008, April 8, 2009, June 16, 2010; Williams interview, all interviews in NIH AIDS Oral Histories.

9. Op. cit., Prologue, n. 2.

10. Shilts, *And the Band Played On*, passim. Randy Shilts died of AIDS in 1994.

11. Martin Duberman, *Stonewall* (New York: Penguin Books, 1994); David Carter, *Stonewall: The Riots That Sparked the Gay Revolution* (New York: St. Martin's Griffin, 2005); Barry D. Adam, *The Rise of a Gay and Lesbian Movement* (Boston: Twayne Publishers, 1987); David B. Feinberg, *Eighty-Sixed* (New York: Viking, 1989).

12. See, for example, comments on so-called gay bowel syndrome by a leader in the study of the sexually transmitted diseases before AIDS, King K. Holmes, professor of medicine at the University of Washington, in King K. Holmes, interview by Gerald Oppenheimer, July 1996, Oral History Research Office, Columbia University Libraries, Columbia University, New York (Columbia University AIDS Oral Histories hereafter); Sevgi O. Aral and King K. Holmes,

"Sexually Transmitted Diseases in the AIDS Era," *Scientific American* (*Sci. Am.* hereafter) 264 (February 1991): 62–69.

13. Larry Kramer, *Reports from the Holocaust: The Story of an AIDS Activist*, updated and expanded ed. (New York: St. Martin's Press, 1994), 14.

14. On the history of advances in molecular immunology, see Peter Keating and Alberto Cambrosio, *Biomedical Platforms: Realigning the Normal and the Pathological in Late-Twentieth-Century Medicine* (Cambridge, MA: MIT Press, 2003); National Institute of Allergy and Infectious Diseases, *New Initiatives in Immunology: NIAID Study Group Report*, NIH Publication No. 81-2215 (Bethesda, MD: National Institutes of Health, 1981); Debra Jan Bibel, *Milestones in Immunology: A Historical Exploration* (Madison, WI: Science Tech, 1981); Arthur M. Silverstein, *A History of Immunology* (San Diego: Academic Press, 1989).

15. Elizabeth Fee and Theodore M. Brown, "Michael S. Gottlieb and the Identification of AIDS," *American Journal of Public Health* (*Am. J. Public Health* hereafter) 96 (2006): 982–83.

16. Michael S. Gottlieb, "AIDS—Past and Future," *New England Journal of Medicine* (*N. Engl. J. Med.* hereafter) 344 (2001): 1788–91; Michael Gottlieb, interview by Gerald Oppenheimer, October 26, 1995, Columbia University AIDS Oral Histories.

17. M. S. Gottlieb et al., "*Pneumocystis* Pneumonia—Los Angeles," *MMWR* 30 (1981): 250–52.

18. A. Friedman-Kien et al., "Kaposi's Sarcoma and *Pneumocystis* Pneumonia in Homosexual Men—New York City and California," ibid., 30 (1981): 306–8; S. M. Friedman et al., "Follow Up on Kaposi's Sarcoma and *Pneumocystis* Pneumonia," ibid., 30 (1981): 409–10.

19. M. S. Gottlieb et al., "*Pneumocystis Carinii* Pneumonia and Mucosal Candidiasis in Previously Healthy Homosexual Men: Evidence of a New Acquired Cellular Immunodeficiency," *N. Engl. J. Med.* 305 (1981): 1425–31; F. P. Siegal et al., "Severe Acquired Immunodeficiency in Male Homosexuals, Manifested by Chronic Perianal Ulcerative Herpes Simplex Lesions," ibid., 305 (1981): 1439–44; H. Masur et al., "An Outbreak of Community-Acquired *Pneumocystis Carinii* Pneumonia: Initial Manifestation of Cellular Immune Dysfunction," ibid., 305 (1981): 1431–38.

20. Alvin Friedman-Kien, interview by Gerald Oppenheimer, March 24, 1995, Columbia University AIDS Oral Histories.

21. Friedman Kien et al., "Kaposi's Sarcoma and *Pneumocystis* Pneumonia among Homosexual Men," 306–8.

22. Henrik Klem Thomsen, Marianne Jacobsen, and Axel Malchow-Moller, "Kaposi Sarcoma among Homosexual Men in Europe," *Lancet* 318 (1981): 688.

23. Jean Baptiste Brunet et al., "Acquired Immunodeficiency Syndrome in France," *Lancet* 321 (1983): 700–701; Grmek, *History of AIDS*, 24–27; Rosa Haritos, "The Forging of a Collective Truth: A Sociological Analysis of the Discovery of the Human Immunodeficiency Virus" (Ph.D. dissertation, Columbia University, New York, 1993), 32–37; Shilts, *And the Band Played On*, 102–3.

24. L. Weinstein et al., "Intestinal Cryptosporidiosis Complicated by Disseminated Cytomegalovirus Infections," *Gastroenterology* 81 (1981): 584–91.

25. Gottlieb interview.
26. Marcus A. Conant, "Founding the KS Clinic, and Continued AIDS Activism," interview conducted by Sally Smith Hughes, 1992, San Francisco AIDS Oral Histories; Sally Smith Hughes, "The Kaposi's Sarcoma Clinic at the University of California, San Francisco: An Early Response to the AIDS Epidemic," *Bull. Hist. Med.* 71 (1997): 651–88.
27. Conant interview.
28. Subcommittee on Health and Environment, Committee on Energy and Commerce, *Kaposi's Sarcoma and Related Opportunistic Infections*, H. R. Doc. No. 97-125, at 49–50 (April 14, 1982).
29. Gottlieb interview; Dritz interview, San Francisco AIDS Oral Histories.
30. Herman E. Hilleboe, "Preventing Future Shock: Health Developments in the 1960's and Imperatives for the 1970's," *Am. J. Public Health* 62 (1972): 136–45.
31. Laurie Garrett, *The Coming Plague: Newly Emerging Diseases in a World Out of Balance* (New York: Penguin Books, 1995); Richard Preston, *The Hot Zone* (New York: Anchor Books, 1995).
32. Holmes interview.
33. A few examples of Holmes's fellows who became leaders in the response to AIDS include Thomas Quinn, Peter Piot, Lawrence Corey, and Joan Kreiss.
34. Elizabeth Etheridge, *Sentinel for Health: A History of the Centers for Disease Control* (Berkeley: University of California Press, 1992), 257–67, 305–7. On Legionnaires' disease, see also Gary L. Lattimer and Richard A. Ormsbee, *Legionnaires' Disease* (New York: Marcel Dekker, 1981), 1–8, quotation from 1; Gordon Thomas and Max Morgan-Witts, *Trauma: The Search for the Cause of Legionnaires' Disease* (London: H. Hamilton, 1981); Gordon Thomas and Max Morgan-Witts, *Anatomy of an Epidemic* (Garden City, NY: Doubleday, 1982).
35. "Toxic-Shock Syndrome—United States," *MMWR* 29 (1980): 229–30; "Follow-Up on Toxic-Shock Syndrome," *MMWR* 29 (1980): 441–45; Division of Health Sciences Policy, Division of Health Promotion and Disease Prevention, Institute of Medicine, *Toxic Shock Syndrome: Assessment of Current Information and Future Research Needs: Report of a Study* (Washington, DC: National Academy Press, 1982).
36. "Centers for Disease Control: Organization, Mission, and Functions" (Centers for Disease Control, March 1983), CDC library, Atlanta, GA; Etheridge, Sentinel for Health.
37. James W. Curran, interview by Victoria A. Harden and Caroline Hannaway, May 19, 1998, NIH AIDS Oral Histories. In this interview, Curran states that the task force was formed immediately after publication of the first *MMWR* article on June 5, 1981. In later testimony at the first congressional hearing on AIDS, Curran stated that the task force had been formed in mid-June, after reports of Kaposi's sarcoma from New York City. This mid-June date is no doubt the correct date because no reports of Kaposi's sarcoma had come to the CDC by June 5, 1981. See House Committee on Energy and Commerce, Subcommittee on Health and Environment, Kaposi's Sarcoma and Related Opportunistic Infections, 97th Cong. (1982) (Waxman AIDS hearing hereafter), 7.
38. Waxman AIDS hearing.
39. Ibid., 8.

40. Ibid. In a personal communication to the author, James Curran corrected this statement, stating that there had been one request between 1967 and 1980.

41. Waxman AIDS hearing, 8.

42. When the definition used by the task force became the criterion for deciding which sick people received free medical care, however, people with other manifestations cried foul and demanded a change in the definition. This problem continued for more than a decade. See "Supplemental Security Income for the Aged, Blind and Disabled; Presumptive Disability and Presumptive Blindness; Categories of Impairments—AIDS—Social Security Administration, HHS. Final rule," *Federal Register* 53, no. 26 (February 9, 1988): 3739–42; "AIDS Patients Eligible for Benefits under New Social Security Regulation," *Public Health Reports* (*Public Health Rep.* hereafter) 103 (1988): 327.

43. "Current Trends Update on Acquired Immune Deficiency Syndrome (AIDS)—United States," *MMWR* 31 (1982): 507–8, 513–14.

44. "Draft Oral History of Activities of the Department of Health, New York, New York, Relating to AIDS" (unpublished document, n.d.). I thank Dr. David Sencer for making this document available to me.

45. Dritz interview.

46. Ibid. New York City also had such a liaison group and held monthly meetings to coordinate efforts. See Federal Response to AIDS: Hearings before a Subcommittee of the Committee on Government Operations, House of Representatives, 98th Cong., (1983), 258.

47. "A Cluster of Kaposi's Sarcoma and *Pneumocystis Carinii* Pneumonia among Homosexual Male Residents of Los Angeles and Orange Counties, California," *MMWR* 31 (1982): 305–7.

48. H. W. Jaffe et al., "National Case-Control Study of Kaposi's Sarcoma and *Pneumocystis Carinii* Pneumonia in Homosexual Men: Part 1. Epidemiologic Results," *Annals of Internal Medicine* (*Ann. Intern. Med.* hereafter) 99 (1983): 145–51. I thank Dr. Harold Jaffe for making a copy of the epidemiological questionnaire on which this study was based available to me.

49. "Epidemiologic Aspects of the Current Outbreak of Kaposi's Sarcoma and Opportunistic Infections," *N. Engl. J. Med.* 306 (1982): 248–52; Etheridge, *Sentinel for Health*, 327.

50. Ibid., 331; Curran interview.

51. "Opportunistic Infections and Kaposi's Sarcoma among Haitians in the United States," *MMWR* 31 (1982): 353–54, 360–61.

52. Dritz interview.

53. Etheridge, *Sentinel for Health*, 331.

54. Arthur S. Levine, MD, special assistant for scientific coordination, Division of Cancer Treatment, NCI, "RE: Update on the Epidemic of Acquired Immunodeficiency—Kaposi [*sic*] Sarcoma—Opportunistic Infection," confidential memorandum to director, NCI, through acting director, NCI, July 2, 1982, "Kaposi's Sarcoma 1981–1982," Intramural Research 5-15, Office of the Director files, Office of NIH History, National Institutes of Health, Bethesda, MD (OD files, NIH hereafter). The descriptor "4-H" groups had no relationship with the 4-H clubs that promoted a fourfold development of young people: "head, heart, hands, and health."

55. See prologue for a discussion of why Haiti has the oldest AIDS epidemic in the Western Hemisphere. On July 28, 1983, New York City no longer listed Haitians as a high-risk group, by order of New York City health commissioner David Sencer.

56. Levine, memorandum to director, NCI, July 2, 1982.

57. James B. Wyngaarden, director, NIH, "RE: Working Group on Epidemic of Acquired Immunosuppression, Opportunistic Infections, and Kaposi's Sarcoma," memorandum, to BID directors, July 13, 1982; and "Summary Minutes of NIH Kaposi Sarcoma Working Group (KSWG)," July 20, 1982, both in "Kaposi's Sarcoma, 1981–1982," Intramural Research 5-15, OD files, NIH. This group became known colloquially as the "Gordon committee," after its chairman, Robert S. Gordon Jr.

58. Special assistant to the director, NIH, "RE: First Meeting of the PHS AIDS Executive Task Force," May 25, 1984, Robert S. Gordon Jr. Notebook, "PHS Executive Task Force on AIDS, 1984," Office of NIH History, National Institutes of Health, Bethesda, MD.

59. J. Vilaseca et al., "Kaposi's Sarcoma and Toxoplasma Gondii Brain Abscess in a Spanish Homosexual," *Lancet* 319 (1982): 572; K. Shibusawa, "Medical Episodes: Kaposi's Sarcoma among Homosexual Men," *Kango: Japanese Journal of Nursing* 34 (February 1982): 74; K. A. Jørgensen and S. O. Lawesson, "Nitrosation Reagents (e.g. Amyl Nitrite) as Possible Cause of Kaposi's Sarcoma in Homosexual Men," *Ugeskrift for Laeger* 144 (1982): 3727–28; J. Geerling, "Acquired Immunodeficiency and Kaposi's Sarcoma in Homosexual Men," *Nederlands Tijdschrift Voor Geneeskunde* 126 (1982): 631–33.

60. These generalizations about different subgroups of physicians are distilled from the author's numerous interviews with practitioners in each group.

61. Friedman-Kien interview.

62. William H. Foege, "RE: Kaposi's Sarcoma and Opportunistic Infections," memorandum to Vincent T. DeVita Jr., July 30, 1981, "Kaposi's Sarcoma, 1981–1982," Division of Cancer Treatment files, Office of NIH History, National Institutes of Health, Bethesda, MD (DCT files, NCI, NIH hereafter).

63. Bruce Chabner, acting director, DCT, NCI, "RE: Kaposi's Sarcoma Conference," memorandum to director, Center for Disease Control, through director, NCI, and acting director, NIH, August 6, 1981, "Kaposi's Sarcoma, 1981–1982," DCT files, NCI, NIH.

64. Ibid.

65. Summary of the Workshop on Kaposi's Sarcoma, sponsored by the Division of Cancer Treatment and Division of Cancer Cause and Prevention, National Cancer Institute and Centers for Disease Control, National Institutes of Health, September 15, 1981, copy in "Kaposi's Sarcoma 1981–1982," Intramural Research 5–15, OD files, NIH; W. D. DeWys et al., "Workshop on Kaposi's Sarcoma: Meeting Report," *Cancer Treatment Reports* 66 (1982): 1387–90.

66. William A. Blattner, memorandum to acting director, Division of Cancer Treatment, NCI, October 13, 1981, "Kaposi's Sarcoma, 1981–1982," DCT files, NCI, NIH.

67. Etheridge, *Sentinel for Health*, 333.

68. Richard M. Titmuss, *The Gift Relationship: From Human Blood to Social Policy* (New York: Pantheon Books, 1971); Susan E. Lederer, *Flesh and Blood: Organ*

Transplantation and Blood Transfusion in Twentieth-Century America (Oxford: Oxford University Press, 2008).

69. Harvey G. Klein, interviews by Victoria A. Harden and Dennis Rodrigues, January 29, and February 8, 1993, NIH AIDS Oral Histories.

70. Etheridge, *Sentinel for Health*, 333, 335.

71. Rudolf Virchow, *Collected Essays on Public Health and Epidemiology*, ed. L. J. Rather (Canton, MA: Science History Publications, 1985), 33–36.

72. Charles L. Heatherly, ed., *Mandate for Leadership: Policy Management in a Conservative Administration* (Washington, DC: Heritage Foundation, 1981), 270–91, as quoted in Fitzhugh Mullan, *Plagues and Politics: The Story of the United States Public Health Service* (New York: Basic Books, 1989), 194; Karen Davis, "Reagan Administration Health Policy," *Journal of Public Health Policy* (*J. Public Health Policy* hereafter) 2 (1981): 312–32, quotation from 318; Etheridge, *Sentinel for Health*, 325.

73. C. Everett Koop, "The Early Days of AIDS as I Remember Them," in *AIDS and the Public Debate: Historical and Contemporary Perspectives*, ed. Caroline Hannaway, Victoria A. Harden, and John Parascandola (Washington, DC: IOS Press, 1995), 9–18.

74. H. R. Doc. 97-125, at 1, 46.

75. Ibid., 10.

76. "Current Trends Prevention of Acquired Immune Deficiency Syndrome (AIDS): Report of Inter-Agency Recommendations," *MMWR* 32 (1983): 101–3; Curran interview.

77. *MMWR* 32 (1983): 101–3.

78. Kramer, *Reports from the Holocaust*, 8–23.

79. H. R. Doc. 97–125, at 44–45.

80. Michael Callen and Dan Turner, "A History of the People with AIDS Self-Empowerment Movement," *The Body: The Complete HIV/AIDS Resource*, December 1997, http://www.thebody.com/content/art31074.html.

81. Peter L. Allen, *The Wages of Sin: Sex and Disease, Past and Present* (Chicago: University of Chicago Press, 2000), 120.

Chapter 2. Searching for the Cause of AIDS

1. Karl R. Popper, *Conjectures and Refutations* (London: Routledge & Kegan Paul, 1963), 216.

2. M. A. Conant, "Speculations on the Viral Etiology of Acquired Immune Deficiency Syndrome and Kaposi's Sarcoma," *Journal of Investigative Dermatology* 83 (July 1984): 57s–62s.

3. K. W. Sell et al., "Cyclosporin Immunosuppression as the Possible Cause of AIDS," *N. Engl. J. Med.* 309 (1983): 1065; also published in the *AIDS Memorandum* 1 (October 1983): 6–8.

4. William A. Blattner, interview by Victoria A. Harden and Dennis Rodrigues, March 2, 1990; James J. Goedert, interview by Victoria A. Harden and Dennis Rodrigues, March 10, 1993, both in NIH AIDS Oral Histories.

5. Blattner interview.

6. J. E. Osborn, "Co-factors and HIV: What Determines the Pathogenesis of AIDS?" *BioEssays: News and Reviews in Molecular, Cellular and Developmen-*

tal Biology 5, no. 6 (December 1986): 287–89; I. L. Livingston, "Co-factors, Host Susceptibility, and AIDS: An Argument for Stress," *Journal of the National Medical Association* 80 (January 1988): 49–59; S. D. Holmberg et al., "Herpes-viruses as Co-factors in AIDS," *Lancet* 332 (1988): 746–47; I. H. Chowdhury et al., "Mycoplasma Can Enhance HIV Replication In Vitro: A Possible Cofactor Responsible for the Progression of AIDS," *Biochemical and Biophysical Research Communications* 170 (1990): 1365–70; M. B. Vasudevachari, T. C. Mast, and N. P. Salzman, "Suppression of HIV-1 Reverse Transcriptase Activity by Mycoplasma Contamination of Cell Cultures," *AIDS Research and Human Retroviruses* (*AIDS Res. Hum. Retroviruses* hereafter) 6 (1990): 411–16.

7.   See, for example, U.S. President's NIH Study Committee, *Biomedical Science and Its Administration: A Study of the National Institutes of Health* (Washington, DC: Government Printing Office, February 1965); National Institute of Mental Health, *Finding the Balance: Report of the NIMH Intramural Research Program (IRP) Planning Committee* (Bethesda, MD: National Institutes of Health, February 1997); U.S. President's Biomedical Research Panel, *Report of the President's Biomedical Research Panel, DHEW Publication Nos. (OS) 76-500–76-509* (Washington, DC: Government Printing Office, 1976); National Academy of Sciences, *Responding to Health Needs and Scientific Opportunity: The Organizational Structure at the National Institutes of Health* (Washington, DC: National Academy Press, October 1984).

8.   Victoria A. Harden and Dennis Rodrigues, "Context for a New Disease: Aspects of Biomedical Research Policy in the United States before AIDS," in *AIDS and Contemporary History*, ed. Virginia Berridge and Philip Strong (Cambridge: Cambridge University Press, 1993), 182–202.

9.   National Institute of Allergy and Infectious Diseases, *AIDS Memorandum*, 9 issues, August 1983–December 1984, http://www.history.nih.gov/NIHInOwn Words/docs/page_36.html.

10.   Hughes, "Kaposi's Sarcoma Clinic at the University of California, San Francisco: An Early Response to the AIDS Epidemic," *Bull. Hist. Med.* 71 (1997): 651–88.

11.   National Cancer Act of 1971, Pub. L. No. 92-216 (1971), http://www.history .nih.gov/research/downloads/PL92-218.pdf.

12.   Robert Gallo and Jay Levy were clinical associates at NIH; Françoise Barré-Sinoussi was a visiting fellow under the John E. Fogarty International Center program. Jean-Claude Chermann worked in the NCI Viral Leukemia and Lymphoma Branch with Peter Fischinger. Luc Montagnier was not trained as a retrovirologist, but he had studied with many of the earliest virus-cancer leaders in the United States and Europe, and he established a collaboration with Robert Gallo soon after he set up his viral oncology laboratory at the Pasteur Institute. See Luc Montagnier, *Virus: The Codiscoverer of HIV Tracks Its Rampage and Charts the Future*, trans. Stephen Sartarelli (New York: W. W. Norton, 2008), 53–54; Rosa Haritos, "The Forging of a Collective Truth: A Sociological Analysis of the Discovery of the Human Immunodeficiency Virus" (PhD dissertation, Columbia University, New York, 1993), 150–53. No scholarly study of the Special Virus Cancer Program has been written, and the lack of such work has led to a conspiracy theory widely publicized on the Internet that AIDS was

developed in the supposedly "secret" SVCP. The late Carl Baker, director of NCI from 1970 to 1972, conducted interviews with key surviving scientists and administrators involved in the program and wrote an administrative history. Edward Beeman, a physician who held a postdoctoral fellowship at NIH in the late 1940s, wrote a biography of Robert Huebner, one of the key leaders of the SVCP. Both manuscripts are available on the website of the Office of NIH History: http://www.history.nih.gov/research/publications.html.

13. National Cancer Advisory Board (NCAB), *National Cancer Program: 1974 Report of the National Cancer Advisory Board* (Washington, DC: U.S. Department of Health, Education, and Welfare, 1974), http://tobaccodocuments.org /ti/TIMN0097121-7135.pdf. See also Barbara J. Culliton, "Cancer Select Committee Calls Virus Program a Closed Shop," *Science* 182 (1973): 1110–12; Barbara J. Culliton, "Virus Cancer Program: Review Panel Stands by Its Criticism," *Science* 184 (1974): 143–45; R.A. Rettig, *Cancer Crusade: The Story of the National Cancer Act of 1971* (Princeton, NJ: Princeton University Press, 1977).

14. Robert C. Gallo, *Virus Hunting: AIDS, Cancer and the Human Retrovirus: A Story of Scientific Discovery* (New York: Basic Books, 1991), 59–124; R. E. Gallagher and R. C. Gallo, "Type C RNA Tumor Virus Isolated from Cultured Human Acute Myelogenous Leukemia Cells," *Science* 187 (1975): 350–53.

15. Doris A. Morgan, Francis W. Ruscetti, and Robert Gallo, "Selective In Vitro Growth of T Lymphocytes from Normal Human Bone Marrows," *Science* 193 (1976): 1007–8.

16. B. J. Poiesz, F. W. Ruscetti, A. F. Gazdar, P. A. Bunn, J. D. Minna, and R. C. Gallo, "Detection and Isolation of Type C Retrovirus Particles from Fresh and Cultured Lymphocytes of a Patient with Cutaneous T-cell Lymphoma," *Proc. Natl. Acad. Sci.* 77 (1980): 7415–19; Robert C. Gallo, "History of the Discoveries of the First Human Retroviruses: HTLV-1 and HTLV-2," *Oncogene* 24 (2005): 5926–30.

17. Bernard J. Poiesz et al., "Isolation of a New Type C Retrovirus (HTLV) in Primary Uncultured Cells of a Patient with Sezary T-Cell Leukemia," *Nature* 294 (1981): 268–71. The "L" in the name "HTLV" was later changed to "lymphotropic" to indicate the virus's tendency to infect T cells rather than just to cause the disease lymphoma.

18. Jay A. Levy, "Animal Virology and the Discovery of the AIDS Virus," interview by Sally Smith Hughes, 1993, San Francisco AIDS Oral Histories.

19. Ibid.

20. Montagnier, *Virus*, 16–27; "Luc Montagnier—Autobiography," Nobelprize.org, 2008, http://nobelprize.org/nobel_prizes/medicine/laureates/2008/montagnier -autobio.html; "Luc Montagnier Biography (1932–)," faqs.org, 2011, http:// www.faqs.org/health/bios/61/Luc-Montagnier.html.

21. Montagnier, *Virus*, 27–32.

22. Pasteur had been granted a section of this Paris suburb to house the rabbits and dogs used in his research when their presence became a nuisance for the neighborhood around his institute on Rue d'Ulm in Paris.

23. For biographical information on Chermann, see Jean-Claude Chermann and Olivier Galzi, *Tout le monde doitconnaitrecette histoire* (Paris: Stock, 2009); for biographical information on Barré-Sinoussi, see "Françoise Barré-Sinoussi

Autobiography," Nobelprize.org, 2008, http://nobelprize.org/nobel_prizes/medicine/laureates/2008/barre-sinoussi-autobio.html.

24. Montagnier, *Virus*, 53–54; Haritos, "Forging of a Collective Truth," 150–53.
25. Lily E. Kay, *The Molecular Vision of Life: Caltech, the Rockefeller Foundation, and the Rise of the New Biology* (New York: Oxford University Press, 1993); Rudolf Hausmann, *To Grasp the Essence of Life: A History of Molecular Biology* (New York: Springer, 2002).
26. Hepatitis viruses provide the best example of the older system. All hepatitis viruses cause inflammation of the liver with certain common symptoms, especially jaundice. The viruses themselves, however, differ markedly in their morphology and genetics. The virus that causes hepatitis A is an RNA virus in an icosahedral-shaped capsid with no envelope proteins. It is transmitted by contaminated food and drinking water. Hepatitis B, however, is caused by a virus transmitted by blood-to-blood contact and through sex. It is a DNA virus with a circular core surrounded by an icosahedral capsid but also with envelope proteins that bind the virus to susceptible cells and enable entry into the cell. Such differences between hepatitis viruses became known only as techniques permitted analysis at the molecular level, and some scientists might argue that these two viruses (and there are actually five hepatitis viruses known) should be called by different names because of the great difference between the causative viruses. The issue of naming viruses had not been resolved by the time an AIDS virus was discovered, and discussions about evolving standards of nomenclature became a part of determining what the AIDS virus would be called officially.
27. P. H. Bartels and G. B. Olsen, "Computer Analysis of Lymphocyte Images," in *Methods of Cell Separation*, vol. 3, ed. Nicholas Catsimpoolas (New York: Plenum Press, 1980), 9.
28. According to a search of the National Library of Medicine's database MEDLINE.
29. *Medical World News*, August 16, 1982, 7–10, as cited in Haritos, "Forging of a Collective Truth," 54–56.
30. Ibid., 47.
31. Montagnier, *Virus*, 48.
32. The other discovery was the understanding that microscopic germs caused infection when the body was opened and the development of antiseptic and aseptic practices to prevent infection during surgery.
33. Lois N. Magner, *A History of Medicine* (New York: Marcel Dekker, 1992), 285.
34. Hal Hellman, *Great Feuds in Medicine* (New York: John Wiley and Sons, 2001); Hal Hellman, *Great Feuds in Science* (New York: John Wiley and Sons, 1999); Hal Hellman, *Great Feuds in Technology* (New York: John Wiley and Sons, 2004).
35. Victoria A. Harden, "Koch's Postulates and the Etiology of AIDS: An Historical Perspective," *History and Philosophy of the Life Sciences* 14 (1992): 245–65; K. Codell Carter, "Koch's Postulates in Relation to the Work of Jacob Henle and Edwin Klebs," *Med. Hist.* 29 (1985): 353–74.
36. E. P. Gelmann et al., "Proviral DNA of a Retrovirus, Human T-cell Leukemia Virus, in Two Patients with AIDS," *Science* 220 (1983): 862–65; R. C. Gallo

et al., "Isolation of Human T-cell Leukemia Virus in Acquired Immune Deficiency Syndrome (AIDS)," ibid., 865–67.

37. M. Essex et al., "Antibodies to Cell Membrane Antigens Associated with Human T-cell Leukemia Virus in Patients with AIDS," *Science* 220 (1983): 859–62.

38. F. Barré-Sinoussi et al., "Isolation of a T-Lymphotropic Retrovirus from a Patient at Risk for Acquired Immune Deficiency Syndrome (AIDS)," *Science* 220 (1983): 868–71.

39. Jean-Claude Chermann, F. Barré-Sinoussi, and Luc Montagnier, "Retrovirus et Syndrome Immunodeficience Acquise (SIDA)," *Bulletin de l'Académie Nationale de Médecine* 168 (1984): 288–95; Chermann et al., "Isolation of a New Retrovirus in a Patient at Risk for Acquired Immunodeficiency Syndrome," *Antibiotics and Chemotherapy* (*Antibiot. Chemother.* thereafter) 32 (1984): 48–53.

40. M. Popovic et al., "Detection, Isolation, and Continuous Production of Cytopathic Retroviruses (HTLV-III) from Patients with AIDS and Pre-AIDS," *Science* 224 (1984): 497–500.

41. R.C. Gallo et al., "Frequent Detection and Isolation of Cytopathic Retroviruses (HTLV-III) from Patients with AIDS and at Risk for AIDS," *Science* 224 (1984): 500–503.

42. J. Schupbach et al., "Serological Analysis of a Subgroup of Human T-Lymphotropic Retroviruses (HTLV-III) Associated with AIDS," *Science* 224 (1984): 503 5.

43. M. G. Sarngadharan et al., "Antibodies Reactive with Human T-Lymphotropic Retroviruses (HTLV-III) in the Serum of Patients with AIDS," *Science* 224 (1984): 506–8.

44. Bijan Safai et al., "Seroepidemiological Studies of Human T-Lymphotropic Retrovirus Type III in Acquired Immunodeficiency Syndrome," *Lancet* 323 (1984): 1438–40.

45. Jean L. Marx, "Strong New Candidate for AIDS Agent," *Science* 224 (1984): 474–77.

46. J. A. Levy et al., "Isolation of Lymphocytopathic Retroviruses from San Francisco Patients with AIDS," *Science* 225 (1984): 840–42.

47. Paul A. Luciw et al., "Molecular Cloning of AIDS-Associated Retrovirus," *Nature* 312 (1984): 760–63; M. Ollero et al., "Antibodies to the AIDS-Associated Retrovirus in Hemophiliacs and Other Individuals from Southern Spain: Lack of Correlation with Lymphocytes Sub-populations," *AIDS Research* 1 (1984): 439.

48. R. Cheingsong-Popov et al., "Prevalence of Antibody to Human T-Lymphotropic Virus Type III in AIDS and AIDS-Risk Patients in Britain," *Lancet* 324 (1984): 477–80; B. G. Gazzard et al., "Clinical Findings and Serological Evidence of HTLV-III Infection in Homosexual Contacts of Patients with AIDS and Persistent Generalised Lymphadenopathy in London," *Lancet* 324 (1984): 480–83; Giovanni B. Rossi et al., "Recovery of HIV-Related Retroviruses from Italian Patients with AIDS or AIDS-Related Complex and from Asymptomatic At-Risk Individuals," *Annals of the New York Academy of Sciences* 511 (1987): 390; "Antibodies to a Retrovirus Etiologically Associated with Acquired Immunodeficiency Syndrome (AIDS) in Populations with Increased Incidences of the Syndrome," *MMWR* 33 (1984): 377–79.

49. Animal models were searched for and even created with mice whose genes had been manipulated to make them susceptible. By 1986 it was clear that studying animal infections similar to AIDS or nonpathological infections of animals with HIV would be the mechanisms available. See Lois Ann Salzman, ed., *Animal Models of Retrovirus Infection and Their Relationship to AIDS* (Orlando: Academic Press, 1986); N.W. King, "Simian Models of Acquired Immunodeficiency Syndrome (AIDS): A Review," *Veterinary Pathology* 23 (1986): 345–53; D. E. Mosier, "Animal Models for Retrovirus-Induced Immunodeficiency Disease," *Immunological Investigations* 15 (1986): 233–61.

50. Montagnier, *Virus*, 41.

51. Bernadine Healy, M.D., speech given to the Science Diplomats Club, Cosmos Club, Washington, DC, October 7, 1992, quoted in Walter A. Brown, "What about the Mozarts of Science?" *The Scientist*, May 14, 2001.

52. Gallo, *Virus Hunting*, 191–95. The full text of the press conference is reproduced in Nikolas Kontaratos, *Dissecting a Discovery: The Real Story of How the Race to Uncover the Cause of AIDS Turned Scientists against Disease, Politics against Science, Nation against Nation* (Philadelphia: Xlibris, 2007), 395–401, quotation from 398.

53. Donald P. Francis, "Defining AIDS and Isolating the Human Immunodeficiency Virus (HIV)," interview by Sally Smith Hughes, 1993, 1994, San Franscisco AIDS Oral Histories.

54. Ibid.; Gallo, *Virus Hunting*, 191–93.

55. Francis interview.

56. The full text of the press conference is reproduced in Kontaratos, *Dissecting a Discovery*, 395–401.

57. Montagnier, *Virus*, 69.

58. Robert C. Gallo, Mikulas Popovic, and Mangalasseril G. Sarngadharan, "Serological Detection of Antibodies to HTLV-III in Sera of Patients with AIDS and Pre-AIDS Conditions," U.S. patent 4,520,113, filed April 23, 1984, issued May 28, 1985.

59. Luc Montagnier et al., "Human Immunodeficiency Viruses Associated with Acquired Immune Deficiency Syndrome (AIDS), a Diagnostic Method for AIDS and Pre-AIDS, and a Kit Therefor," U.S. patent 4,708,818, filed October 8, 1985, issued November 24, 1987.

60. The Bayh-Dole Act was signed on December 12, 1980, as Pub. L. 96–517. The text of the Federal Technology Transfer Act, Pub. L. 99-502, signed October 20, 1986, is available at http://history.nih.gov/research/downloads/PL99-502.pdf.

61. Gallo, *Virus Hunting*, 205–11; Montagnier, *Virus*, 69–74; Kontaratos, *Dissecting a Discovery*, 135–50.

62. John Roberts, "Dispute over HIV Ownership Ends," *British Medical Journal* 309 (1994): 219–20.

63. Kontaratos, *Dissecting a Discovery*, 147–48; "Settling the AIDS Virus Dispute," *Nature* 326 (1987): 425–26.

64. R. C. Gallo and L. Montagnier, "The Chronology of AIDS Research," *Nature* 326 (1987): 435–36.

65. A similarly confusing naming dispute that played out in the scientific literature occurred between 1913 and 1917 over the name of the tick that transmitted Rocky Mountain spotted fever in Montana. Two U.S. federal agencies each

claimed the right to name the tick. See Victoria A. Harden, *Rocky Mountain Spotted Fever* (Baltimore: Johns Hopkins University Press, 1990), 91.

66. John Coffin et al., "Human Immunodeficiency Viruses," *Science* 232 (1986): 697; Coffin et al., "What to Call the AIDS Virus?" *Nature* 321 (1986): 10. For a detailed discussion of the issues in resolving the name of the AIDS virus, see Haritos, "Forging of a Collective Truth," 265–82.

67. The original papers were Luciw et al., "Molecular Cloning of AIDS-Associated Retrovirus," *Nature* 312 (1984): 760–63; Lee Ratner et al., "Complete Nucleotide Sequence of the AIDS Virus, HTLV-III," ibid. 313 (1985): 277–84; L. Ratner, R. C. Gallo, and F. Wong-Staal, "HTLV-III, LAV, ARV Are Variants of Same AIDS Virus," ibid. 313 (1985): 636–37.

68. H. G. Guo et al., "Sequence Analysis of Original HIV-1," *Nature* 349 (1991): 745–46; S. Wain-Hobson et al., "LAV Revisited: Origins of the Early HIV-1 Isolates from Institut Pasteur," *Science* 252 (1991): 961–65; Kontaratos, *Dissecting a Discovery*, 206–21. The AIDS virus isolated in Robin Weiss's laboratory had also been contaminated with LAI.

69. The citation, introduction, video, and text of the Nobel lectures are available at "The Nobel Prize in Physiology or Medicine 2008," Nobelprize.org, 2011, http://nobelprize.org/nobel_prizes/medicine/laureates/2008/index.html.

70. Abraham Verghese, "A Prize Tarnished: Euro-bias Robs Gallo of a Nobel Prize," Forbes.com, October 6, 2008, http://www.forbes.com/2008/10/06/nobel -medicine-gallo-oped-cx_av_1006verghese.html. See chapter 1 for a discussion of the controversy over the first Nobel prize awarded in Physiology or Medicine in 1901.

71. "Nobel Prize in Medicine for Jean-Claude Chermann," http://www.nobel chermann.com/index_eng.html; Anne Jeanblanc, "Sida: 'l'oublié du Nobel' n'a pas dit son dernier mot," *Le Point*, November 16, 2009. Chermann's own history of his contributions to the search for the AIDS virus are in Chermann and Galzi, *Tout le monde doitconnaitrecette histoire*.

72. "1986 Winners, Albert Lasker Clinical Medical Research Award," Lasker Foundation, 2011, http://www.laskerfoundation.org/awards/1986_c_description.htm.

73. "Nobel Prize in Medicine for Jean-Claude Chermann."

74. Anders Vahlne, "A Historical Reflection on the Discovery of Human Retroviruses," *Retrovirology* 6, no. 1 (2009): 40.

Chapter 3. Clinical Research, Epidemic of Fear, and AIDS in the Worldwide Blood Supply

1. Anthony S. Fauci, interviews by Victoria A. Harden and Dennis Rodrigues, July 3, 1986; March 7, 1989; and June 29, 1993, NIH AIDS Oral Histories.

2. See, for example, descriptions of work by university and community physicians and nurses in San Francisco, California, in *The AIDS Epidemic in San Francisco: The Medical Response, 1981–1984*, Regional Oral History Office, Bancroft Library, University of California, Berkeley, CA, 1995–2000; the efforts of physicians in New York in Ronald Bayer and Gerald M. Oppenheimer, *AIDS Doctors: Voices from the Epidemic* (Oxford, UK: Oxford University Press, 2000); the initial response of physicians in France in Grmek, *History of AIDS*, and in Montagnier, *Virus*.

3. Thomas Waldmann, interview by Victoria A. Harden and Dennis Rodrigues, March 14, 1990, NIH AIDS Oral Histories.

4. Ibid.

5. Ibid.

6. Fauci, interviews. The date of admission is in Richard M. Krause, letter to Edward N. Brandt Jr., January 15, 1982, "Kaposi's Sarcoma 1981–1982," Intramural Research 5–15, OD Files, NIH.

7. Sandeep Khot, Buhm Soon Park, and W. T. Longstreth Jr., "The Vietnam War and Medical Research: Untold Legacy of the U.S. Doctor Draft and the NIH 'Yellow Berets,'" *Academic Medicine* 86 (2011): 502–8.

8. John E. Fogarty International Center for Advanced Study in the Health Sciences, "Fogarty International Center Establishes Sheldon M. Wolff, M.D. Fellowship on International Health," press release, March 28, 2001, http://www.nih.gov/news/pr/mar2001/fic-28.htm.

9. Fauci, interviews, NIH AIDS Oral Histories.

10. Ibid.

11. Donald C. Drake, "Life, Death and Hope: How Science Tussles with AIDS," *Philadelphia Inquirer*, June 9, 1983; Donald C. Drake, "Testing a Drug on AIDS, From Beginning to an End," *Philadelphia Inquirer*, August 21, 1983; Donald Resio, personal communication to the author via telephone, April 12, 2010. I am grateful to Dr. Resio for providing a personal perspective on the efforts to treat his twin brother at the NIH.

12. The study also demonstrated the adoptive transfer of delayed-type hypersensitivity and an increase in the total number of peripheral blood helper T lymphocytes in the AIDS patient. See Fauci interviews; H. Clifford Lane, interview by Victoria A. Harden and Dennis Rodrigues, March 12, 1990, NIH AIDS Oral Histories; Moyer material, Public Health Service Supplementary Budget Data, Justification of Appropriation Estimates for Committee on Appropriations, manuscript, Office of NIH History, National Institutes of Health, Bethesda, MD, FY 1986, 18–19; A. H. Rook et al., "Interleukin-2 Enhances the Depressed Natural Killer and Cytomegalovirus-Specific Cytotoxic Activities of Lymphocytes from Patients with the Acquired Immune Deficiency Syndrome," *J. Clin. Invest.* 72 (1983): 398–403; H. C. Lane et al., "Abnormalities of B Cell Activation and Immunoregulation in Patients with the Acquired Immunodeficiency Syndrome," *N. Engl. J. Med.* 309 (1983): 453–58.

13. Lane et al., "Abnormalities of B Cell Activation," 453–58; Lane et al., "Partial Immune Reconstitution in a Patient with the Acquired Immunodeficiency Syndrome," *N. Engl. J. Med.* 311 (1984): 1099–1103; J. Laurence, "The Immune System in AIDS," *Sci. Am.* 253 (December 1985): 84–93; K. M. Zunich and H. C. Lane, "The Immunology of HIV Infection," *Journal of the American Academy of Dermatology* 22 (1990): 1202–5.

14. Lane interview.

15. Robert B. Nussenblatt, interview by Victoria A. Harden and Dennis Rodrigues, April 25, 1990, NIH AIDS Oral Histories; Moyer material, FY 1986, 19, 22; FY 1987, 21–22; FY 1988, 9. See also the more general discussion of NEI contributions in Moyer material, FY 1985, 17.

16. Nussenblatt interview; Moyer material, FY 1990, 66; M. R. Rodrigues et al.,

"Unilateral Cytomegalovirus Retinochorioditis and Bilateral Cystoid Bodies in a Bisexual Male with the Acquired Immunodeficiency Syndrome," *Ophthalmology* 90 (1983): 1577–82; A. G. Palestine et al., "Treatment of Cytomegalovirus Retinitis with Dihydroxy Propoxymethyl Guanine," *American Journal of Ophthalmology* 101 (1986): 95–101; Henry Masur et al., "Effect of 9-(1,3-Dihydroxy-2-Propoxymethyl) Guanine on Serious Cytomegalovirus Disease in Eight Immunosuppressed Homosexual Men," *Ann. Intern. Med* 104 (1986): 41–44; M. A. Polis et al., "Increased Survival of a Cohort of Patients with Acquired Immunodeficiency Syndrome and Cytomegalovirus Retinitis Who Received Sodium Phosphonoformate (Foscarnet)," *American Journal of Medicine* 94 (1993): 175–80.

17. Resio, personal communication.
18. Moyer material, FY 1985, 11; FY 1986, 16; G. M. Shaw et al., "HTLV-III Infection in Brains of Children and Adults with AIDS Encephalopathy," *Science* 227 (1985): 177–82.
19. NIDR investigators also studied the gastrointestinal manifestations of cytomegalovirus infection. See Moyer material, FY 1985, 10; FY 1986, 14; FY 1987, 17.
20. Moyer material, FY 1985, 10; FY 1986, 14; FY 1987, 17; P. D. Smith et al., "Monocyte Function in the Acquired Immune Deficiency Syndrome: Defective Chemotaxis," *J. Clin. Invest.* 74 (1984): 2121–28.
21. Barbara Fabian Baird, interview by Victoria A. Harden and Dennis Rodrigues, March 17, 1993, NIH AIDS Oral Histories.
22. David Henderson, interview by Victoria A. Harden, Dennis Rodrigues, and Caroline Hannaway, June 13, 1996, NIH AIDS Oral Histories.
23. Baird interview.
24. Federal Response to AIDS: Hearings before a Subcommittee of the Committee on Government Operations, 98th Cong., 82–83 (1983).
25. Drake, "Life, Death and Hope."
26. Baird interview.
27. Christine Grady, interview by Victoria A. Harden and Caroline Hannaway, January 30, 1997, NIH AIDS Oral Histories.
28. Lois Salzman, interview by Victoria A. Harden and Ruth Harris, June 29, 1998, NIH AIDS Oral Histories.
29. Ryan White and Ann Marie Cunningham White, *Ryan White: My Own Story* (New York: Dial Books, 1991); "Chronology of Ryan White's Fight to Attend School," United Press International, November 25, 1985; Lisa Perlman, "Health Officer Says AIDS Victim Ryan White Can Return to School," Associated Press, February 13, 1986; Dirk Johnson, "Ryan White Dies of AIDS at 18; His Struggle Helped Pierce Myths," *New York Times*, April 9, 1990, *New York Times* Online AIDS Collection; "Ricky Ray Program Office Set to Close," National Hemophilia Foundation, 2006, http://www.hemophilia.org/NHFWeb/MainPgs/MainNHF.aspx?menuid=117&contentid=360; "President Clinton Signs Ricky Ray Hemophilia Relief Fund into Law; Community Rejoices," PR Newswire, November 13, 1998, http://www.encyclopedia.com/doc/1G1-53218176.html; Hemophilia Federation of America, http://hemophiliafed.org/.
30. Darden Asbury Pyron, *Liberace: An American Boy* (Chicago: University of Chicago Press, 2000), 369, 392–409.

31. Greg Louganis, *Breaking the Surface*, with Eric Marcus (New York: Random House, 1995); Alan Hines, *Breaking the Surface: The Greg Louganis Story*, directed by Stephen Hilliard Stern (Studio City, CA: Ariztical Entertainment, 2003), DVD.

32. Arthur Ashe, *Days of Grace: A Memoir*, with Arnold Rampersad (New York: Ballantine, 1993). Information about the Arthur Ashe Institute for Urban Health is at http://www.arthurasheinstitute.org/arthurashe/home/.

33. Rick Weinberg, "Magic Johnson Announces He's HIV Positive," ESPN 25: ESPN Counts Down the 100 Most Memorable Moments of the Past 25 Years, 2009, http://sports.espn.go.com/espn/espn25/story?page=moments/7; Richard W. Stevenson, "Magic Johnson Ends His Career, Saying He Has AIDS Infection," *New York Times*, November 8, 1991; Michael Specter, "When AIDS Taps Hero, His 'Children' Feel Pain," *New York Times*, November 9, 1991; Karen De Witt, "On Capitol Hill, the Battle for AIDS Funds Heats Up," *New York Times*, November 9, 1991, all in *New York Times* Online AIDS Collection.

34. Elizabeth Glaser and Laura Palmer, *In the Absence of Angels: A Hollywood Family's Courageous Story* (New York: Putnam, 1991); Allison Spensley et al., "Preventing Mother-to-Child Transmission of HIV in Resource-Limited Settings: The Elizabeth Glaser Pediatric AIDS Foundation Experience," *Am. J. Public Health* 99 (2009): 631–37; Christian Pitter et al., "Cost-Effectiveness of Cotrimoxazole Prophylaxis among Persons with HIV in Uganda," *J. Acquir. Immune Defic. Syndr.* 44 (2007): 336–43; Jeffrey T. Safrit et al., "Immunoprophylaxis to Prevent Mother-to-Child Transmission of HIV-1," *J. Acquir. Immune Defic. Syndr 35.* (2004): 169–77; Paul M. Glaser, "A Parent's Perspective on the Need for Pediatric Clinical Research," *Seminars in Pediatric Surgery* 11, no. 3 (August 2002): 147–50; C. M. Wilfert, "Prevention of Mother-to-Child Transmission of HIV-1," *Antiviral Therapy* 6 (2001): 161–77.

35. Bruce Lambert, "Kimberly Bergalis Is Dead at 23; Symbol of Debate over AIDS Tests," *New York Times*, December 9, 1991, *New York Times* Online AIDS Collection.

36. Stephen Barr, "The 1990 Florida Dental Investigation: Is the Case Really Closed?" *Ann. Intern. Med.* 124 (1996): 250–54; "Possible Transmission of Human Immunodeficiency Virus to a Patient during an Invasive Dental Procedure," *MMWR* 39 (1990): 489–93; "Epidemiologic Notes and Reports Update: Transmission of HIV Infection during an Invasive Dental Procedure—Florida," *MMWR* 40 (1991): 21–27, 33; "Epidemiologic Notes and Reports Update: Transmission of HIV Infection during Invasive Dental Procedures—Florida," *MMWR* 40 (1991): 377–81. I also thank Dr. Harold Jaffe of the CDC for his perspective on this case.

37. Eric A. Feldman and Ronald Bayer, eds., *Blood Feuds: AIDS, Blood, and the Politics of Medical Disaster* (New York: Oxford University Press, 1999). See also Harvey M. Sapolsky and Stephen L. Boswell, "The History of Transfusion AIDS: Practice and Policy Alternatives," in *AIDS: The Making of a Chronic Disease*, ed. Elizabeth Fee and Daniel M. Fox (Berkeley: University of California Press, 1992), 170–93; Anne Marie Moulin, "Reversible History: Blood Transfusion and the Spread of AIDS in France," in *AIDS and the Public Debate*, 170–86.

38. Priscilla Hitchcock, letter to the Hon. Don Ritter, n.d., copy in Congressional Correspondence, 1981–82, OD files, NIH.

39. Ibid.

40. Richard M. Titmuss, *The Gift Relationship: From Human Blood to Social Policy* (New York: Pantheon Books, 1971).

41. "Judith Graham Pool," in *The Biographical Dictionary of Women in Science: L-Z*, ed. Marilyn Bailey Ogilvie and Joy Dorothy Harvey (London: Taylor & Francis, 2000), 1039–40.

42. R. Palmer Beasley et al., "Hepatocellular Carcinoma and Hepatitis B Virus: A Prospective Study of 22,707 Men in Taiwan," *Lancet* 318 (1981): 1129–33.

43. Immunization Practices Advisory Committee, CDC, "The Safety of Hepatitis B Virus Vaccine," *MMWR* 32 (1983): 134–36.

44. Ronald Bayer, "Blood and AIDS in America: Science, Politics, and the Making of an Iatrogenic Catastrophe," in *Blood Feuds*, 30–31.

45. Arthur Ammann et al., "Epidemiologic Notes and Reports: Possible Transfusion-Associated Acquired Immune Deficiency Syndrome (AIDS)—California," *MMWR* 31 (1982): 652 54.

46. Donald C. Drake, "The Disease Detectives Puzzle over Methods of Control," *Philadelphia Inquirer*, January 9, 1983.

47. Cited in Robin Marantz Henig, "AIDS: A New Disease's Deadly Odyssey," *New York Times*, February 6, 1983, *New York Times* Online AIDS Collection.

48. Drake, "Disease Detectives Puzzle over Methods of Control."

49. There are multiple accounts of this meeting. Some of the most complete include Marantz Henig, "AIDS: A New Disease's Deadly Odyssey"; Bayer, "Blood and AIDS in America," 22–25; Curran interview; Drake, "Disease Detectives Puzzle over Methods of Control."

50. Drake, "Disease Detectives Puzzle over Methods of Control."

51. "Current Trends Prevention of Acquired Immune Deficiency Syndrome (AIDS): Report of Inter-Agency Recommendations," *MMWR* 32 (1983): 101–3.

52. Bayer, "Blood and AIDS in America."

53. CDC, NIH, FDA in collaboration with many professional associations, "Recommendations for Preventing Transmission of Infection with Human T-Lymphotropic Virus Type III/ Lymphadenopathy-Associated Virus in the Workplace," *MMWR* 34 (1985): 691–95.

54. The name "Western blot" came about as a bit of scientific humor. Another test, which detected DNA, was developed by Edwin Southern and called the "Southern blot." Since the Western blot had been developed at Stanford University in California, one scientist decided to play off the earlier-named test and dubbed it the "Western blot." While the Western blot remains in wide use, the Southern blot and another test known as the Northern blot are no longer used because other methods have been developed that replaced them.

55. Moulin, "Reversible History," 178; Monika Steffen, "The Nation's Blood: Medicine, Justice, and the State in France," in *Blood Feuds*, 106–7.

56. Sherry Glied, "The Circulation of the Blood: AIDS, Blood, and the Economics of Information," in *Blood Feuds*, table 11-2, 341. Germany did not mandate heat treatment, but its state health service would not reimburse for the use of untreated products.

57. David L. Kirp, "The Politics of Blood: Hemophilia Activism in the AIDS Crisis," in *Blood Feuds*, 293–321; William Felstiner, Richard Abel, and Austin Sarat, "The Emergence and Transformation of Disputes: Naming, Blaming, Claiming . . . ," *Law and Society Review* 15 (1980): 3–4; R. D. Eckert, "The AIDS Blood-Transfusion Cases: A Legal and Economic Analysis of Liability," *San Diego Law Review* 29 (1992): 203–98.

58. Glied, "Circulation of the Blood," 335–36.

59. Steffen, "Nation's Blood," 95–126; Moulin, "Reversible History," 170–86; Rone Tempest, "Transfusions AIDS-Tainted; Doctors on Trial," *Los Angeles Times*, July 21, 1992, available online at http://articles.latimes.com/1992-07-21/news/mn-4337_1_blood-products.

60. Alex Lefebvre, "France: Court Dismisses Charges in Tainted Blood Scandal," *World Socialist*, June 28, 2003, http://www.wsws.org/articles/2003/jun2003/fran-j28.shtml.

61. Steffen, "Nation's Blood," 121.

62. "State Admits HIV Guilt," *Japan Times*, February 17, 1996, 1, as cited in Eric A. Feldman, "HIV and Blood in Japan: Private Conflict into Public Scandal," in *Blood Feuds*, 78.

63. Ibid., 81.

64. Theodore R. Marmor, Patricia A. Dillon, and Stephen Scher, "The Comparative Politics of Contaminated Blood: From Hesitancy to Scandal," in *Blood Feuds*, 351–66.

65. Lauren B. Leveton, Harold C. Sox Jr., and Michael A. Stoto, eds., *HIV and the Blood Supply: An Analysis of Crisis Decisionmaking* (Washington, DC: National Academies Press, 1995).

66. Ronald Bayer, "Blood and AIDS in America: Science, Politics, and the Making of an Iatrogenic Catastrophe," in *Blood Feuds*, 42.

67. Ricky Ray Hemophilia Relief Fund Act of 1998, Pub. L. 105-369; "Ricky Ray Trust Fund Will Terminate in November 2003," HRSA Archive, September 24, 2002, http://archive.hrsa.gov/newsroom/NewsBriefs/2002/rickyray.htm.

68. Jessica Martucci, "Negotiating Exclusion: MSM, Identity, and Blood Policy in the Age of AIDS," *Social Studies of Science* 40 (2010): 215–41; "Constitutionality of Gay Blood Donor Ban Challenged in Court," *HIV/AIDS Policy & Law Review/Canadian HIV/AIDS Legal Network* 14 (December 2009): 19–20; Charlene Galarneau, "Blood Donation, Deferral, and Discrimination: FDA Donor Deferral Policy for Men Who Have Sex with Men," *American Journal of Bioethics* 10 (February 2010): 29–39.

69. Center for Biologics Evaluation and Research, "Procleix Ultrio Assay," February 24, 2011, http://www.fda.gov/BiologicsBloodVaccines/BloodBloodProducts/ApprovedProducts/LicensedProductsBLAs/BloodDonorScreening/InfectiousDisease/ucm092027.htm. The window period was taken from data presented on the website of its distributor, Novartis Diagnostics Global, http://www.novartisdiagnostics.com/products/procleix-assays/index.shtml.

70. For example, see the webpage of an Australian campaign, "Gay Blood Donation," 2008, http://www.gayblooddonation.org/index.html.

71. Hospital Infections Program, Division of Viral Diseases, Division of Host Factors, Division of Hepatitis and Viral Enteritis, AIDS Activity, Center for In-

fectious Diseases, Office of Biosafety, CDC, and Division of Safety, NIH, "Current Trends: Acquired Immune Deficiency Syndrome (AIDS): Precautions for Clinical and Laboratory Staffs," *MMWR* 31 (1982): 577–80; AIDS Activity, Division of Host Factors, Division of Viral Diseases, Hospital Infections Program, Center for Infectious Diseases, Office of Biosafety, CDC, "Acquired Immunodeficiency Syndrome (AIDS): Precautions for Health-Care Workers and Allied Professionals," ibid. 32 (1983): 450–51.

Chapter 4. AIDS as a Cultural Phenomenon

1. Stephen J. Gould, *An Urchin in the Storm: Essays about Books and Ideas* (New York: W. W. Norton, 1988), 153.
2. Charles E. Rosenberg, *Explaining Epidemics and Other Studies in the History of Medicine* (Cambridge, UK: Cambridge University Press, 1992), 285.
3. Milton Friedman and Rose Friedman, "The Tide Is Turning," in *The United States in the 1980s*, Peter Duignan and Alvin Rabushka, eds., Hoover Institution Publication 228 (Stanford, CA: Hoover Institute, Stanford University, 1980), 3.
4. Daniel Defert, "AIDS as a Challenge to Religion," in *AIDS in the World II: Global Dimensions, Social Roots, and Responses*, eds. Jonathan M. Mann and D. J. M. Tarantola (New York: Oxford University Press, 1996), 447–48.
5. Ibid.
6. Karen Davis, "Reagan Administration Health Policy," *J. Public Health Policy* 2 (December 1981): 313.
7. Peg McGlinch and Peter Barton Hutt, "Hollow Government: Resource Constraints and Workload Expansion at the Food and Drug Administration [redacted version]," April 30, 2001, http://leda.law.harvard.edu/leda/data/742/McGlinch01_redacted.html; Lynn Etheridge, "Reagan, Congress, and Health Spending," *Health Affairs* 2, no. 1 (1983): 14–24; Davis, "Reagan Administration Health Policy."
8. Elizabeth W. Etheridge, *Sentinel for Health: A History of the Centers for Disease Control* (Berkeley: University of California Press, 1992), 324.
9. Charles Everett Koop, *Koop: The Memoirs of America's Family Doctor* (New York: Random House, 1991), 248. Edward Brandt died on August 25, 2007. See Lawrence K. Altman, "Edward N. Brandt Jr., a Leader on AIDS, Dies at 74," *New York Times*, September 1, 2007, *New York Times* Online AIDS Collection.
10. Mullan, *Plagues and Politics*, 154–62.
11. Koop, *Koop*, 256–57.
12. Robert Gordon, files of the NIH AIDS representative to the PHS Executive Committee on AIDS, copy in the Office of NIH History, National Institutes of Health, Bethesda, MD; "PHS Executive Task Force on AIDS," "AIDS Meeting 9-9-85," Office of AIDS Research files, Office of NIH History, National Institutes of Health, Bethesda, MD.
13. Koop, *Koop*, 250.
14. Associated Press, "Report of AIDS Jokes Roils San Franciscans," *New York Times*, October 3, 1986, *New York Times* Online AIDS Collection.
15. Koop, *Koop*, 251.

16. C. Everett Koop, "The Early Days of AIDS as I Remember Them," in *AIDS and the Public Debate*, 11.

17. Ibid., 13.

18. Koop, *Koop*, 273; Koop, "Early Days of AIDS," 14; Philip M. Boffey, "Surgeon General Urges Frank Talk to Young on AIDS," *New York Times*, October 23, 1986, *New York Times* Online AIDS Collection; C. Everett Koop, "Statement by C. Everett Koop, M.D., Surgeon General," October 22, 1986, Folder 3, Box 54a, C. Everett Koop Papers, Profiles in Science, National Library of Medicine, Bethesda, MD, http://profiles.nlm.nih.gov/QQ/; Office of the Surgeon General, *Surgeon General's Report on Acquired Immune Deficiency Syndrome* (Washington, DC: U.S. Public Health Service, 1986).

19. Dr. Mason believed that Congress's instruction that he, an executive branch employee, bypass the normal clearance process was "probably unconstitutional," but no one challenged him at the time and so he moved forward. James O. Mason, "Understanding AIDS—An Information Brochure Mailed to All U.S. Households," unpublished document, n.d. I am grateful to Dr. Mason for making this document available to me.

20. Ibid.; Office of the Surgeon General and Centers for Disease Control, *Understanding AIDS* (Washington, DC: U.S. Public Health Service, 1988). In 1992, under Surgeon General Antonia C. Novello, a third report was also mailed. See Office of the Surgeon General, *Surgeon General's Report on Acquired Immune Deficiency Syndrome*; Office of the Surgeon General and Centers for Disease Control, "Understanding AIDS," 1988, C. Everett Koop Papers; Office of the Surgeon General, *Surgeon General's Report to the American Public on HIV Infection and AIDS* (Washington, DC: U.S. Public Health Service, 1992).

21. Ryan White Care Act, Pub. L. No. 101-381 (1990); Ryan White HIV/AIDS Treatment Extension Act of 2009, Pub. L. No. 111-87 (2009).

22. Public Health Service, *AIDS Operational Plan* (Washington, DC: Department of Health and Human Services, 1983), copy in OAR files, NIH.

23. James C. Hill, interview by Victoria A. Harden, October 4, 1988, NIH AIDS Oral Histories.

24. Title XVIII: Research with Respect to Acquired Immune Deficiency Syndrome, Subtitle A: Office of AIDS Research, in National Institutes of Health Revitalization Act of 1993, Pub. L. No. 103–43 (1993).

25. Allan M. Brandt, "AIDS: From Public History to Public Policy," in *AIDS and the Public Debate*, 128; John Donnelly, "Hemophilia, Ricky, AIDS: 'It Didn't Need to Happen,'" *Miami Herald*, December 15, 1992.

26. Lawrence K. Altman, "Many Questions Cloud Start of AIDS Testing," *New York Times*, June 10, 1987; "Victim of AIDS Gains Waiver," *New York Times*, April 7, 1989; Philip J. Hilts, "Agency Says AIDS Should Not Bar Entry to U.S.," *New York Times*, February 27, 1990; Warren E. Leary, "Visa Rules Eased for Foreigners with AIDS," *New York Times*, April 14, 1990; "Gay Men's Crisis Unit to Shun AIDS Session," *New York Times*, May 8, 1990; Philip J. Hilts, "Bar on H.I.V.-Infected Immigrants Is Retained in Final Capitol Test," *New York Times*, May 25, 1993, all from *New York Times* Online AIDS Collection; Reuters, "Obama Lifts Ban on U.S. Entry of Those with HIV/AIDS," October 30, 2009.

27. David L. Kirp and Ronald Bayer, "The Second Decade of AIDS: The End of Exceptionalism?" in *AIDS in the Industrialized Democracies: Passions, Politics and Policies*, David L. Kirp and Ronald Bayer, eds. (New Brunswick, NJ: Rutgers University Press, 1992), 361.

28. Virginia Berridge, *AIDS in the UK: The Making of Policy, 1981–1994* (Oxford, UK: Oxford University Press, 1996), 56–59, quotations from 59.

29. Ibid., 66–78, quotation from 78.

30. Ibid., 157–59, 182–208.

31. Ibid., 182–208; Virginia Berridge, "'Unambiguous Voluntarism'? AIDS and the Voluntary Sector in the United Kingdom, 1981–1992," in *AIDS and the Public Debate*, 153–69. See also Ewin Ferlie, "The NHS Responds to HIV/AIDS," and John Street, "A Fall in Interest? British AIDS Policy, 1986–1990," in *AIDS and Contemporary History*, eds. Virginia Berridge and Philip Strong (Cambridge, UK: Cambridge University Press, 1993), 203–23, 224–39.

32. Michael Fumento, *The Myth of Heterosexual AIDS* (New York: Basic Books, 1990).

33. Berridge, *AIDS in the UK*, 238 44.

34. See Jesús M. de Miguel and David L. Kirp, "Spain: An Epidemic of Denial," and Eric A. Feldman and Shohei Yonemoto, "Japan: AIDS as a 'Non issue,'" in *AIDS in the Industrialized Democracies*, 168–84, 339–60.

35. Ronald Bayer and David L. Kirp, "Introduction: An Epidemic in Political and Policy Perspective," in *AIDS in the Industrialized Democracies*, 4.

36. "Response to AIDS by the New York City Department of Health during the Early Days of the Epidemic," unpublished manuscript, personal collection of David Sencer, Atlanta, GA. I am grateful to Dr. Sencer for making this document available to me.

37. Mervyn F. Silverman, "Public Health Director, The Bathhouse Crisis: 1983–1984," interview by Sally Smith Hughes, 1993, in San Francisco AIDS Oral Histories. Frank Lynn, "McGrath Proposes Closing Homosexuals' Bathhouses," *New York Times*, October 2, 1985; Robert D. McFadden, "Cuomo and Koch Reconsidering Their Opposition to Closing of Bathhouses," *New York Times*, October 5, 1985, both in *New York Times* Online AIDS Collection.

38. Institute of Medicine of the National Academy of Sciences, *Confronting AIDS: Directions for Public Health, Health Care and Research* (Washington, DC: National Academies Press, 1986); June E. Osborn, "The National Commission on AIDS," in *AIDS and the Public Debate*, 77–78.

39. Presidential Commission on the Human Immunodeficiency Virus Epidemic, *The Presidential Commission on the Human Immunodeficiency Virus Epidemic Report* (Washington, DC: 1988), http://www.eric.ed.gov/PDFS/ED299531.pdf.

40. Osborn, "National Commission on AIDS," 79.

41. National Commission on AIDS, *The Twin Epidemics of Substance Abuse and HIV: A Report* (Washington, DC: 1991).

42. National Commission on AIDS, *HIV Disease in Correctional Facilities: Report of the National Commission on AIDS* (Washington, DC: 1991).

43. National Commission on AIDS, *The Challenge of HIV/AIDS in Communities of Color* (Washington, DC: 1992); Osborn, "National Commission on AIDS," 82–83.

44. National Commission on AIDS, *AIDS: An Expanding Tragedy: The Final Report of the National Commission on AIDS* (Washington, DC: 1993); Osborn, "National Commission on AIDS," 84.

45. For an overview history of the Gay Men's Health Crisis, see Philip M. Kayal, *Bearing Witness: Gay Men's Health Crisis and the Politics of AIDS* (Boulder, CO: Westview Press, 1993); Susan Maizel Chambré, *Fighting for Our Lives: New York's AIDS Community and the Politics of Disease* (New Brunswick, NJ: Rutgers University Press, 2006).

46. P. A. Kawata and J. M. Andriote, "NAN—a National Voice for Community-Based Services to Persons with AIDS," *Public Health Rep.* 103 (1988): 300–301.

47. Paul A. Kawata, "Community-Based Response to AIDS," in *AIDS and the Historian*, eds. Victoria A. Harden and Guenter B. Risse, NIH Publication No. 91-1584 (Bethesda, MD: National Institutes of Health, 1991), 118–19.

48. Chambré, *Fighting for Our Lives*, 120.

49. Larry Kramer, *The Normal Heart and The Destiny of Me: Two Plays* (New York: Grove Press, 2000), 40.

50. Ibid., 15.

51. Chambré, *Fighting for Our Lives*, 120–23; Kramer, *Reports from the Holocaust*, 137–39; "ACT UP Capsule History 1987," ACT UP/New York, http://www.actupny.org/documents/cron-87.html.

52. Lindsay Knight, *UNAIDS: The First 10 Years: 1996–2007* (Geneva, Switzerland: Joint United Nations Programme on HIV/AIDS [UNAIDS], 2008), 10.

53. Sandra D. Lane, "Needle Exchange: A Brief History," publications from the Kaiser Forums, sponsored by the Henry J. Kaiser Family Foundation, Aegis Law Library, 1993, http://www.aegis.com/law/journals/1993/HKFNE009.html.

54. Ibid.; "Syringe Access," San Francisco AIDS Foundation, 2010, http://www.sfaf.org/hpp.

55. Warwick Anderson, "The New York Needle Trial: The Politics of Public Health in the Age of AIDS," *Am. J. Public Health* 81 (1991): 1506–17.

56. *Federal Response to AIDS*, 258.

57. Anderson, "New York Needle Trial," 1507.

58. Ibid., 1509, 1512.

59. Ibid., 1512.

60. Roy Porter, "Epidemic of Fear," *New Society*, March 4, 1988, 24–25, as cited in Anderson, "New York Needle Trial," 1515.

61. D. Paone et al., "New York City Syringe Exchange: Expansion, Risk Reduction, and Seroincidence," *International Conference on AIDS* 10 (1994): 274.

62. S. B. Thomas and S. C. Quinn, "The Tuskegee Syphilis Study, 1932 to 1972: Implications for HIV Education and AIDS Risk Education Programs in the Black Community," *Am. J. Public Health* 81 (1991): 1498–1505; James Howard Jones, *Bad Blood: The Tuskegee Syphilis Experiment* (New York: Simon & Schuster, 1981); Susan M. Reverby, *Examining Tuskegee: The Infamous Syphilis Study and Its Legacy* (Chapel Hill: University of North Carolina Press, 2009).

63. Mark D. Smith, "AIDS and Minority Health," in *AIDS and the Public Debate*, 103–5.

64. Cleve Jones, *Stitching a Revolution: The Making of an Activist*, with Jeff Dawson (San Francisco: Harper, 2001); "History," The AIDS Memorial Quilt, The NAMES Project Foundation, http://www.aidsquilt.org/history.htm.

65. Information from the website for amfAR, http://www.amfar.org. In 2005 the name of the organization was shortened to the Foundation for AIDS Research.
66. Information from the website for the Elizabeth Taylor AIDS Foundation, http://www.elizabethtayloraidsfoundation.org/.
67. "Programs: HIV/AIDS," Magic Johnson Foundation, http://www.magic johnson.com/foundation/hiv-overview.php; Elton John AIDS Foundation, http://www.ejaf.org/; Deidre Woollard, "Maison Martin Margiela Shirt Goes Japanese for World AIDS Day," *Luxist*, October 13, 2010, http://www.luxist .com/2010/10/13/maison-martin-margiela-shirt-goes-japanese-for-world -aids-day/; AIDES, http://www.aides.org/en; Coalition PLUS, coalition inter- nationale sida, http://www.coalitionplus.org/.
68. Sue Cross, "Falwell Wants Attack on 'Gay Plague,'" Associated Press, July 5, 1983, as cited in "Jerry Falwell and AIDS: A Brief History of a Judgmental Response," *One More Dying Quail* (blog), February 21, 2007, http://onemore dyingquail.blogspot.com/2007/02/jerry-falwell-and-aids-brief-history-of .html; Bill Press, "The Sad Legacy of Jerry Falwell," *Milford (MA) Daily News*, May 18, 2007, http://www.milforddailynews.com/opinion/x1987843539.
69. Susan Sontag, *AIDS and Its Metaphors* (New York: Farrar, Straus and Giroux, 1989), 93.

Chapter 5. AIDS Therapy

1. Quoted in Martin Delaney, "The Development of Combination Therapies for HIV Infection," *AIDS Res. Hum. Retroviruses* 26 (2010): 9.
2. Kramer, *Normal Heart and the Destiny of Me*, 85.
3. One overview history is Rudolf Hausmann, *To Grasp the Essence of Life: A His- tory of Molecular Biology* (New York: Springer, 2002).
4. Donald S. Fredrickson, *The Recombinant DNA Controversy: A Memoir: Science, Politics, and the Public Interest 1974–1981* (Washington, DC: ASM Press, 2001).
5. Some of the best public information on molecular biology and genetics is on- line; see, for example, Wellcome Trust Sanger Institute's "Yourgenome.org," http://www.yourgenome.org/.
6. W. Fiers et al., "Complete Nucleotide Sequence of Bacteriophage MS2 RNA: Primary and Secondary Structure of the Replicase Gene," *Nature* 260 (1976): 500–507.
7. J. L. Marx, "AIDS Virus Genomes," *Science* 227 (1985): 503; B. H. Hahn et al., "Molecular Cloning and Characterization of the HTLV-III Virus Associated with AIDS," *Nature* 312 (1984): 166–69; M. Alizon et al., "Molecular Cloning of Lymphadenopathy-Associated Virus," *Nature* 312 (1984): 757–60; Lee Ratner et al., "Complete Nucleotide Sequence of the AIDS Virus, HTLV-III," *Nature* 313 (1985): 277–84; M. A. Muesing et al., "Nucleic Acid Structure and Expres- sion of the Human AIDS/Lymphadenopathy Retrovirus," *Nature* 313 (1985): 450–58; L. Ratner, R. C. Gallo, and F. Wong-Staal, "HTLV-III, LAV, ARV Are Variants of Same AIDS Virus," *Nature* 313 (1985): 636–37; R. Sanchez-Pescador et al., "Nucleotide Sequence and Expression of an AIDS-Associated Retrovirus (ARV-2)," *Science* 227 (1985): 484–92.
8. For the most recent detailed information about the structure and function of HIV genes, see the website maintained by the Los Alamos Laboratory, U.S.

Department of Energy, and the National Institutes of Health, U.S. Department of Health and Human Services, "Landmarks of the HIV Genome," http://www .hiv.lanl.gov/content/sequence/HIV/MAP/landmark.html.

9. D. J. Bauer, "A History of the Discovery and Clinical Application of Antiviral Drugs," *British Medical Bulletin* 41 (1985): 310.

10. Ibid., 311–12.

11. Samuel Broder, interview by Victoria A. Harden and Caroline Hannaway, February 2, 1997, NIH AIDS Oral Histories.

12. Ibid.

13. Ibid.

14. Robert Yarchoan, interview by Victoria A. Harden and Caroline Hannaway, April 30, 1998, NIH AIDS Oral Histories.

15. Ibid.

16. Ibid.

17. Ibid.

18. Broder interview; Yarchoan interview; H. Mitsuya et al., "Functional Properties of Antigen-Specific T Cells Infected by Human T-Cell Leukemia-Lymphoma Virus (HTLV-I)," *Science* 225 (1984): 1484–86.

19. Broder interview.

20. Linda J. Wastila and Louis Lasagna, "The History of Zidovudine (AZT)," *Journal of Clinical Research and Pharmacoepidemiology* 4 (1990): 25–37, quotation from 26–27; H. Mitsuya et al., "3'-Azido-3'-deoxythymidine (BW A509U): An Antiviral Agent That Inhibits the Infectivity and Cytopathic Effect of Human T-Lymphotropic Virus Type III/Lymphadenopathy-Associated Virus in Vitro," *Proc. Natl. Acad. Sci.* 82 (1985): 7096–7100.

21. For an overview of FDA involvement with AIDS drugs through 1993, see James Harvey Young, "AIDS and the FDA," in *AIDS and the Public Debate*, 47–66; and the timeline on the FDA website, http://www.fda.gov/ForConsumers/ByAudience/ForPatientAdvocates/HIVandAIDSActivities/ucm117935.htm.

22. Wastilla and Lasagna, "History of Zidovudine (AZT)," 31.

23. Ibid., 27; R. Yarchoan et al., "Administration of 3'-azido-3'-deoxythymidine, an Inhibitor of HTLV-III/LAV Replication, to Patients with AIDS or AIDS-Related Complex," *Lancet* 327 (1986): 575–80.

24. Wastilla and Lasagna, "History of Zidovudine (AZT)," 28–29.

25. Ibid., 29–30.

26. See also Emily H. Thomas and Daniel M. Fox, "The Cost of AZT," *AIDS & Public Policy Journal* 2 (1987): 17–21.

27. Arno and Feiden, *Against the Odds*, 57, 58.

28. Ibid., 126–30.

29. Ibid., 135–37.

30. Ibid., 138–39, quotation from 138.

31. Robert Yarchoan, personal communication to the author, October 16, 2010.

32. Arno and Feiden, *Against the Odds*, 137–41, 267–72; Teresa Riordan, "Patents; A Court Ruling Extends Burroughs-Wellcome's Monopoly on the AIDS Drug AZT," *New York Times*, November 28, 1994; "AIDS Drug Patent Challenged in Suit," *New York Times*, March 20, 1991, both in *New York Times* Online AIDS

Collection; *Burroughs Wellcome Co. v. Barr Labs, Depositions of Dr. Samuel Broder, Dr. Robert Yarchoan, and Dr. Hiroaki Mitsuya*, 1992–93, copies in Office of the General Counsel, Department of Health and Human Services, Public Health Division, Bethesda, MD; Broder interview.

33. Andrea L. Ciaranello et al., "Access to Medications and Medical Care after Participation in HIV Clinical Trials: A Systematic Review of Trial Protocols and Informed Consent Documents," *HIV Clinical Trials* 10 (2009): 13–24; L. H. Glantz, "Research with Children," *American Journal of Law and Medicine* 24 (1998): 213–44.

34. A. Rubinstein, "Pediatric AIDS," *Current Problems in Pediatrics* 16 (1986): 361–409; M. L. Belfer, P. K. Krener, and F. B. Miller, "AIDS in Children and Adolescents," *Journal of the American Academy of Child and Adolescent Psychiatry* 27 (1988): 147–51.

35. P. A. Pizzo et al., "Effect of Continuous Intravenous Infusion of Zidovudine (AZT) in Children with Symptomatic HIV Infection," *N. Engl. J. Med* 319 (1988): 889–96; P. A. Pizzo, "Emerging Concepts in the Treatment of HIV Infection in Children," *Journal of the American Medical Association* (JAMA hereafter) 262 (1989): 1989–92; P. A. Pizzo, "Practical Issues and Considerations in the Design of Clinical Trials for HIV-Infected Infants and Children," *J. Acquir. Immune. Defic. Syndr.* 3, Suppl. 2 (1990): S61–63; K. Hein, "Lessons from New York City on HIV/AIDS in Adolescents," *New York State Journal of Medicine* 90 (1990): 143–45; T. A. DiLorenzo et al., "The Evaluation of Targeted Outreach in an Adolescent HIV/AIDS Program," *Journal of Adolescent Health* (*J. Adolesc. Health* hereafter) 14 (1993): 301–6; H. Kunins et al., "Guide to Adolescent HIV/AIDS Program Development," *J. Adolesc. Health* 14, Suppl. 5 (1993): 1S–140S; J. F. Blair and K. K. Hein, "Public Policy Implications of HIV/AIDS in Adolescents," *Future of Children* 4, no. 3 (1994): 73–93.

36. M. E. Horowitz and P. A. Pizzo, "Pediatric AIDS: A Perspective for the Oncologist," *Oncology* (Williston Park, NY) 4 (December 1990): 21–27, discussion, 27–28, 30.

37. Blair and Hein, "Public Policy Implications of HIV/AIDS in Adolescents."

38. Yarchoan interview. Complete lists of currently available AIDS drugs of all classes are available on numerous websites concerned with AIDS therapy.

39. Ramunas Kondratas, "Biologics Control Act of 1902," in *The Early Years of Federal Food and Drug Control*, ed. James Harvey Young (Madison, WI: American Institute of the History of Pharmacy, 1982), 8–27.

40. James Harvey Young, "The 'Elixir Sulfanilamide' Disaster," *Emory University Quarterly* 14 (1958): 230–37.

41. Morton Mintz, "'Heroine' of FDA Keeps Bad Drug off of Market," *Washington Post*, July 15, 1962; L. Bren, "Frances Oldham Kelsey. FDA Medical Reviewer Leaves Her Mark on History," *FDA Consumer* 35 (April 2001): 24–29.

42. Suzanne White Junod, "FDA and Clinical Drug Trials: A Short History," in *A Quick Guide to Clinical Trials: For People Who May Not Know It All* (Rockville, MD: Bioplan Assn., 2008), 21–51; Harry M. Marks, *The Progress of Experiment: Science and Therapeutic Reform in the United States, 1900–1990* (Cambridge, UK: Cambridge University Press, 2000); A. M. Lilienfeld, "Ceteris Paribus: The Evolution of the Clinical Trial," *Bull. Hist. Med.* 56 (1982): 1–18.

43. My discussion follows Arno and Feiden, *Against the Odds*, 60–68.

44. "AIDS Treatment News Mission and History," http://www.aidsnews.org/about .html.

45. The two best overview books on the history of patent medicines and health quackery remain James Harvey Young, *Toadstool Millionaires: A Social History of Patent Medicines in America before Federal Regulation* (Princeton, NJ: Princeton University Press, 1961); James Harvey Young, *The Medical Messiahs: A Social History of Health Quackery in Twentieth-Century America* (Princeton, NJ: Princeton University Press, 1967).

46. James Harvey Young, "AIDS and Deceptive Therapies," in *American Health Quackery*, 259.

47. Ibid., 256–85.

48. See, for example, Stephen Barrett, "AIDS-Related Quackery and Fraud," *Quackwatch*, December 13, 2001, http://www.quackwatch.com/01Quackery RelatedTopics/aids.html; "Where's the Harm in Fake AIDS Cures?" *AVERT*, September 10, 2010, http://www.avert.org/cure-for-aids.htm.

49. A. G. Palestine et al., "Ophthalmic Involvement in Acquired Immunodeficiency Syndrome," *Ophthalmology* 91 (1984): 1092–99; M. M. Rodrigues et al., "Unilateral Cytomegalovirus Retinochoroiditis and Bilateral Cytoid Bodies in a Bisexual Man with the Acquired Immunodeficiency Syndrome," ibid., 1577–82.

50. Arno and Feiden, *Against the Odds*, 158–68, quotation from 158.

51. Ibid., 161.

52. Online images of this demonstration are included in the "Action on AIDS" segment of a National Library of Medicine Web exhibit "Against the Odds," http:// apps.nlm.nih.gov/againsttheodds/exhibit/action_on_aids/action_on_aids .cfm, and on ACT UP's website, "ACTUP Capsule History 1988," http://www .actupny.org/documents/cron-88.html. Another account of the demonstration and its aftermath is in Susan Maizel Chambré, *Fighting for Our Lives: New York's AIDS Community and the Politics of Disease* (New Brunswick, NJ: Rutgers University Press, 2006), 150–51.

53. Arno and Feiden, *Against the Odds*, 164–67, quotation from 164.

54. Loyola University Health System, "Expensive New Blood Pressure Meds No Better than Generics, According to Long-Term Data," *ScienceDaily*, August 14, 2010, http://www.sciencedaily.com/releases/2010/08/100813082715.htm.

55. Arno and Feiden, *Against the Odds*, 168–71.

56. Ibid.

57. Gina Kolata, "Ideas and Trends; The Philosophy of the 'New F.D.A.' Is Mostly a Matter of Packaging," *New York Times*, May 19, 1991, *New York Times* Online AIDS Collection. For a summary of mechanisms developed to increase the speed with which the FDA reviewed and approved drugs, see U.S. Food and Drug Administration, "Speeding Access to Important New Therapies: HIV Specific Resources," September 10, 2009, http://www.fda.gov/ForConsumers/ ByAudience/ForPatientAdvocates/SpeedingAccesstoImportantNewTherapies/ ucm181838.htm.

58. My discussion is adapted from Harden, "Koch's Postulates and the Etiology of AIDS," 245–65.

59. P. H. Duesberg et al., "Sequences and Functions of Rous Sarcoma Virus RNA," *Hämatologie Und Bluttransfusion* 19 (1976): 327–40; L. H. Wang et al., "Distribution of Envelope-Specific and Sarcoma-Specific Nucleotide Sequences from Different Parents in the RNAs of Avian Tumor Virus Recombinants," *Proc. Natl. Acad. Sci.* 73 (1976): 1073–77; L. Wang et al., "Mapping Oligonucleotides of Rous Sarcoma Virus RNA That Segregate with Polymerase and Group-Specific Antigen Markers in Recombinants," *Proc. Natl. Acad. Sci* 73 (1976): 3952–56.

60. Peter H. Duesberg, "Retroviruses as Carcinogens and Pathogens: Expectations and Reality," *Cancer Research* 47 (1987): 1199–1220, quotation from 1200.

61. Peter H. Duesberg, "Human Immunodeficiency Virus and Acquired Immunodeficiency Syndrome: Correlation but Not Causation," *Proc. Natl. Acad. Sci.* 86 (1989): 755–64; Peter Duesberg, "HIV Is Not the Cause of AIDS," Policy Forum, *Science* 421 (1988): 514–17; "Blattner and Colleagues Respond to Duesberg," Policy Forum, *Science* 421 (1988): 514–17; W. Blattner, R. C. Gallo, and H. M. Temin, "HIV Causes AIDS," Policy Forum, *Science* 421 (1988): 514–17; "Duesberg's Response to Blattner and Colleagues," Policy Forum, *Science* 421 (1988): 514–17.

62. Peter H. Duesberg, *Inventing the AIDS Virus* (Washington, DC: Regnery Publishing, 1997).

63. Duesberg adopted an older theory of chromosomal aberrations as the cause of cancer. See P. Duesberg et al., "Aneuploidy and Cancer: From Correlation to Causation," *Contributions to Microbiology* 13 (2006): 16–44; Peter H. Duesberg, "Chromosomal Chaos and Cancer," *Sci. Am.* 296 (May 2007): 52–59.

64. My discussion of all the arguments on both sides is taken from the policy forum papers in *Science.*

65. Seth C. Kalichman, *Denying AIDS: Conspiracy Theories, Pseudoscience, and Human Tragedy* (New York: Springer, 2009).

66. Kary Mullis, *Dancing Naked in the Mind Field* (New York: Vintage Books, 2000), 171–86.

67. Robert S. Root-Bernstein, *Rethinking AIDS: The Tragic Cost of Premature Consensus* (New York: Free Press, 1993).

68. J. Sonnabend, S. S. Witkin, and D. T. Purtilo, "Acquired Immunodeficiency Syndrome, Opportunistic Infections, and Malignancies in Male Homosexuals: A Hypothesis of Etiologic Factors in Pathogenesis," *JAMA* 249 (1983): 2370–74.

69. My discussion of the development of HAART follows that of Delaney, "Development of Combination Therapies for HIV Infection," 1–9. See also Viviana Simon and David D. Ho, "HIV-1 Dynamics in Vivo: Implications for Therapy," Nature Reviews, *Microbiology* 1 (2003): 181–90.

70. I thank Dr. Robert Yarchoan for the detailed information about how HIV resistance to AZT-class drugs developed. Yarchoan, personal communication to the author, October 16, 2010.

71. T. D. Copeland and S. Oroszlan, "Genetic Locus, Primary Structure, and Chemical Synthesis of Human Immunodeficiency Virus Protease," *Gene Analysis Techniques* 5 (1988): 109–15; Manuel A. Navia et al., "Three-Dimensional Structure of Aspartyl Protease from Human Immunodeficiency Virus HIV-1," *Nature* 337 (1989): 615–20.

72. For a detailed discussion of one pharmaceutical company's internal collaboration on HIV protease inhibitors, see R. Gordon Douglas Jr., "AIDS Therapies and Vaccines: A Pharmaceutical Industry Perspective," in *AIDS and the Public Debate*, 86–97.

73. R. M. Gulick et al., "Treatment with Indinavir, Zidovudine, and Lamivudine in Adults with Human Immunodeficiency Virus Infection and Prior Antiretroviral Therapy," *N. Engl. J. Med.* 337 (1997): 734–39; Delaney, "Development of Combination Therapies for HIV Infection," 5; Gina Kolata, "Researchers Find Early Battlers of H.I.V.," *New York Times*, January 29, 1995, *New York Times* Online AIDS Collection.

74. John W. Mellors et al., "Prognosis in HIV-1 Infection Predicted by the Quantity of Virus in Plasma," *Science* 272 (1996): 1167–70; Delaney, "Development of Combination Therapies for HIV Infection," 5.

75. Delaney, "Development of Combination Therapies for HIV Infection," 5. Dates of approval of each drug are given on "HIV-AIDS Historical Timeline," U.S. Food and Drug Administration, May 13, 2009, http://www.fda.gov/ForConsumers/ByAudience/ForPatientAdvocates/HIVandAIDSActivities/ucm151079.htm.

76. X. Wei et al., "Viral Dynamics in Human Immunodeficiency Virus Type 1 Infection," *Nature* 373 (1995): 117–22; A. S. Perelson et al., "HIV-1 Dynamics in Vivo: Virion Clearance Rate, Infected Cell Life-Span, and Viral Generation Time," *Science* 271 (1996): 1582–86.

77. D. D. Ho, "Time to Hit HIV, Early and Hard," *N. Engl. J. Med.* 333 (1995): 450–51.

78. Lawrence K. Altman "The Doctor's World: Discussing Possible AIDS Cure Raises Hope, Anger and Question: What Exactly Is Meant by 'Cure'?" *New York Times*, July 16, 1996, *New York Times* Online AIDS Collection.

79. T. W. Chun et al., "Presence of an Inducible HIV-1 Latent Reservoir During Highly Active Antiretroviral Therapy," *Proc. Natl. Acad. Sci.* 94 (1997): 13193–97; T. W. Chun and A. S. Fauci, "Latent Reservoirs of HIV: Obstacles to the Eradication of Virus," *Proc. Natl. Acad. Sci.* 96 (1999): 10958–61; D. Fins et al., "Latent Infection of CD4+ T Cells Provides a Mechanism for Lifelong Persistence of HIV-1, Even in Patients on Effective Combination Therapy," *Nature Medicine* (*Nat. Med.* hereafter) 5 (1999): 512–17.

80. David W. Dunlap, "Surviving AIDS: Now What?" *New York Times*, August 1, 1996, *New York Times* Online AIDS Collection.

81. A. G. Dalgliesh et al., "The CD4 (T4) Antigen Is an Essential Component of the Receptor of the AIDS Retrovirus," *Nature* 312 (1984): 763–67; D. Classman et al., "T-Lymphocyte T4 Molecule Behaves as the Receptor for Human Retrovirus LAV," *Nature* 312 (1984): 20–27. My discussion of these two discoveries is adapted from M. Patricia D'Souza and Victoria A. Harden, "Chemokines and HIV-1 Second Receptors. Confluence of Two Fields Generates Optimism in AIDS Research," *Nat. Med.* 2 (1996): 1293–1300.

82. P. J. Maddon et al., "The T4 Gene Encodes the AIDS Virus Receptor and Is Expressed in the Immune System and the Brain," *Cell* 47 (1986): 333–48.

83. Y. Feng et al., "HIV-1 Entry Cofactor: Functional cDNA Cloning of a Seven-Transmembrane, G Protein-Coupled Receptor," *Science* 272 (1996): 872–77.

84. C. M. Walker et al., "CD8+ Lymphocytes Can Control HIV Infection in Vitro by Suppressing Virus Replication," *Science* 234 (1986): 1563–66; C. Mackewicz and J. A. Levy, "CD8+ Cell Anti-HIV Activity: Nonlytic Suppression of Virus Replication," *AIDS Res. Hum. Retroviruses* 8 (1992): 1039–50; C. E. Mackewicz, H. Ortega, and J. A. Levy, "Effect of Cytokines on HIV Replication in CD4+ Lymphocytes: Lack of Identity with the CD8+ Cell Antiviral Factor," *Cellular Immunology* 153 (1994): 329–43.

85. F. Cocchi et al., "Identification of RANTES, MIP1-alpha, and MIP1-beta as the Major HIV-Suppressive Factors Produced by CD8+ T Cells," *Science* 270 (1995): 1811–15.

86. M. Samson et al., "Molecular Cloning and Functional Expression of a New Human CC-Chemokine Receptor Gene," *Biochemistry* 35 (1996): 3362–67.

87. T. Dragic et al., "HIV-1 Entry into CD4+ Cells Is Mediated by the Chemokine Receptor CD-CKR-5," *Nature* 381 (1996): 667–73; H. Deng et al., "Identification of a Major Co-Receptor for Primary Isolates of HIV-1," *Nature* 381 (1996): 661–67; G. Alkhatib et al., "CC CKR5: A Rantes., MIP-1á, MIP-1β Receptor as a Fusion Cofactor for Macrophage-Tropic HIV-1," *Science* 272 (1996): 1955–58; B. J. Doranz et al., "A Dual-Tropic Primary HIV-1 Isolate That Uses Fusin and the Chemokine Receptors CKR-5, CKR-3, and CKR-2b as Fusion Cofactors," Cell 85 (1996): 1149–58; C. Hyeryun et al., "The β-Chemokine Receptors CCR3 and CCR5 Facilitate Infection by Primary HIV-1 Isolates," *Cell* 85 (1996): 1135–48.

88. Olivier Lambotte et al., "HIV Controllers: A Homogeneous Group of HIV-1-Infected Patients with Spontaneous Control of Viral Replication," *Clinical Infectious Diseases* 41 (2005): 1053–56. The variation consists of a thirty-two base pair deletion in the gene encoding CCR-5. Robert Yarchoan, personal communication to the author, October 16, 2010.

89. Paul and Fauci quotations from Lawrence K. Altman, "A Discovery Energizes AIDS Researchers," *New York Times*, August 10, 1996, *New York Times* Online AIDS Collection.

90. The full list of anti-HIV drugs approved by the FDA is at "HIV and AIDS Activities: Antiretroviral Drugs Used in the Treatment of HIV Infection," May 20, 2011, http://www.fda.gov/ForConsumers/ByAudience/ForPatientAdvocates/HIVandAIDSActivities/ucm118915.htm.

91. Tina Rosenberg, "The Man Who Was Cured of HIV and What It Means for a Cure for AIDS," *New York Magazine*, June 6, 2011, 26–31.

92. Laura Douglas-Brown, "Reflections on AIDS," *Emory Magazine* 86 (Autumn 2010): 58–59; Timothy Rodrigues, "No Obits," *Bay Area Reporter*, August 13, 1998, 1.

Chapter 6. Communicating AIDS

1. See, for example, the articles in Workshop 4, "Documenting AIDS History: Preserving the Records of the Scientific, Institutional, and Popular Response to a New Disease," in *AIDS and the Historian*, 128–61. The American Association for the History of Medicine organized an AIDS History Group to help forestall the loss of documentation.

2. Baron William Thomson Kelvin, *Popular Lectures and Addresses* (London: Macmillan, 1891), 1: 80.

3. Stephen Jay Gould, *Leonardo's Mountain of Clams and the Diet of Worms: Essays on Natural History* (New York: Harmony Books, 1998), 155.

4. Ruth M. Kulstad, "Publishing AIDS Papers in the Early 1980s," in *AIDS and the Public Debate*, 107–23.

5. Ibid., quotation from 108.

6. Ibid., 120.

7. Ibid., 114–15.

8. A. S. Relman, "Introduction to AIDS: The Emerging Ethical Dilemmas," *Hastings Center Report, Special Supplement* (1985).

9. Ruth M. Kulstad, ed., *AIDS: Papers from Science, 1982–1985* (Washington, DC: American Association for the Advancement of Science, 1986); Helene M. Cole and George D. Lundberg, eds., *AIDS, from the Beginning* (Chicago: American Medical Association, 1986).

10. J. Oleske et al., "Immune Deficiency Syndrome in Children," *JAMA* 249 (1983): 2345–49.

11. James Kinsella, *Covering the Plague: AIDS and the American Media* (New Brunswick, NJ: Rutgers University Press, 1989), 56–58.

12. "SPJ Code of Ethics," Society of Professional Journalists, 1996, http://www.spj .org/ethicscode.asp.

13. "American Society of Newspaper Editors Statement of Principles," American Society of Newspaper Editors, 1996, http://www.asne.org/kiosk/archive/ principl.htm. See also "NASW Code of Ethics," National Association of Science Writers, 2011, http://www.nasw.org/nasw-code-ethics.

14. Norman Fairclough, *Media Discourse* (London: Edward Arnold, 1995); Thomas S. McCoy, *Voices of Difference: Studies in Critical Philosophy and Mass Communication* (Cresskill, NJ: Hampton Press, 1993), as cited in Nilanjana Bardhan, "Transnational AIDS-HIV News Narratives: A Critical Exploration of Overarching Frames," *Mass Communication and Society* 4 (2001): 283–309, quotation from 284.

15. M. E. McCombs, "The Evolution of Agenda-Setting Research: Twenty-Five Years in the Marketplace of Ideas," *Journal of Communications* 43 (1993): 58–67, as cited in Bardhan, "Transnational AIDS-HIV News Narratives," 288.

16. Ibid.

17. Kinsella, *Covering the Plague*, 29.

18. Ibid., 59–71, quotation from 71.

19. Ibid., 75.

20. Ibid., 126–36.

21. Ibid., 145.

22. Lawrence Mass, "Disease Rumors Largely Unfounded," *New York Native*, May 18, 1981.

23. Kinsella, *Covering the Plague*, 25.

24. Ibid., 31–33.

25. Ibid., 36–47; David M. Halbfinger, "A Mini-War of Gay Newspapers: A New Weekly Draws Fire Even before Its First Issue," *New York Times*, October 22, 1997, *New York Times* Online AIDS Collection.

26. Kinsella, *Covering the Plague*, 164.

27. Shilts, *And the Band Played On*, xi.

28. The number of books about AIDS is large and growing. The following is merely a sampling of some of the types of literature dealing with the epidemic. Literary works: Emmanuel Sampath Nelson, *AIDS—The Literary Response* (New York: Twayne Publishers, 1992); Timothy F. Murphy and Suzanne Poirier, *Writing AIDS: Gay Literature, Language, and Analysis* (New York: Columbia University Press, 1993); John Preston, ed., *Personal Dispatches: Writers Confront AIDS* (New York: St. Martin's Press, 1990). Specialized audiences: David McBride, *From TB to AIDS: Epidemics among Urban Blacks since 1900* (Albany: State University of New York Press, 1991); Kathryn Whetten-Goldstein and Trang Quyen Nguyen, *"You're the First One I've Told": New Faces of HIV in the South* (New Brunswick, NJ: Rutgers University Press, 2002). Sociological, cultural, and linguistic analysis: Steven Epstein, *Impure Science: AIDS, Activism, and the Politics of Knowledge* (Berkeley: University of California Press, 1996); Paula A. Treichler, *How to Have Theory in an Epidemic: Cultural Chronicles of AIDS* (Durham, NC: Duke University Press, 1999).

29. Randy Shilts and Arnold Schulman, *And the Band Played On*, directed by Roger Spottiswoode (New York: Home Box Office, 1993).

30. Kontaratos, *Dissecting a Discovery*, 169–77.

31. The text of the Freedom of Information Act with 1996 amendments relating to electronic records is available online at http://www.justice.gov/oip/foia_updates/Vol_XVII_4/page2.htm.

32. Bruce Nussbaum, *Good Intentions: How Big Business and the Medical Establishment Are Corrupting the Fight against AIDS* (New York: Atlantic Monthly Press, 1990), xiii–xvi, 14–16, 18.

33. Roger Lewin, "The Scientists Wear Black Hats," review of *Good Intentions*, by Bruce Nussbaum, *New York Times*, November 4, 1990, 20.

34. Jon Cohen, "John Crewdson: Science Journalist as Investigator," *Science* 254 (1991): 946–49.

35. Kontaratos, *Dissecting a Discovery*, 190; Robert C. Gallo, personal communication to author, May 20, 2010.

36. John Crewdson, "The Great AIDS Quest," *Chicago Tribune*, November 19, 1989.

37. Kontaratos, *Dissecting a Discovery*, 180.

38. Both sides of the investigations into Gallo's laboratory are examined exhaustively in John Crewdson, *Science Fictions*, http://www.sciencefictions.net/; Bernadine Healy, "The Dangers of Trial by Dingell," *New York Times*, July 3, 1996, Books section, http://www.nytimes.com/books/98/09/20/specials/baltimore-trial.html; Kontaratos, *Dissecting a Discovery*.

39. U.S. Department of Health and Human Services, Department Appeal Board, Research Integrity Adjudications Panel, Docket No. A-93-100, Decision No. 1446, November 3, 1993.

40. Christopher Martyn, review of *Science Fictions: A Scientific Mystery, a Massive Cover-up, and the Dark Legacy of Robert Gallo*, by John Crewdson, *Br. Med. J.* 324 (2002): 1341.

41. Daniel S. Greenberg, review of *Science Fictions* by John Crewdson, *New Scientist*, April 6, 2002, 48.

42. Tony Kushner, "Foreword," in Kramer, *Normal Heart and The Destiny of Me*, xxv.

43. Frank Rich, "Marching Out of the Closet, Into History," review of *Angels in America*, by Tony Kushner, *New York Times*, November 10, 1992, *New York Times* Online AIDS Collection.

44. John Leonard, "Winged Victory," review of *Angels in America* by Tony Kushner, *New York Magazine*, December 8, 2003, http://nymag.com/nymetro/arts/tv/reviews/n_9578/.

45. David Bianculli, review of *Angels in America* by Tony Kushner, *Fresh Air*, NPR, December 5, 2003, http://www.npr.org/templates/story/story.php?storyId=1534243.

46. John Hartl, "How Hollywood Portrays AIDS: From 'An Early Frost' to 'Yesterday': Filmmakers, Pioneers and Cowards," *Today*, NBC, June 5, 2006, http://www.msnbc.msn.com/id/12856549/.

47. Stewart Kampel, "L.I. Actor Stars in AIDS Film," *New York Times*, May 26, 1986, *New York Times* Online AIDS Collection.

48. Hartl, "How Hollywood Portrays AIDS."

49. Janet Maslin, "Tom Hanks as an AIDS Victim Who Fights the Establishment," review of *Philadelphia*, directed by Jonathan Demme, *New York Times*, December 22, 1993, *New York Times* Online AIDS Collection.

50. "6000 A Day: An Account of Catastrophe Foretold," Icarus Films, October 11, 2010, http://icarusfilms.com/new2002/six000.html; "Dominant 7: Philip Brooks and Laurent Bocahut," Anne Aghion Films, 2008, http://www.anneaghionfilms.com/bio_dominant7.html.

51. "It's My Life," Icarus Films, October 11, 2010, http://icarusfilms.com/new2002/mlife.html; Ginger Thompson, "In Grip of AIDS, South African Cries for Equity," *New York Times*, May 10, 2003, *New York Times* Online AIDS Collection.

52. "Pandemic: Facing Aids," Netflix, 2003, http://www.netflix.com/Movie/Pandemic_Facing_Aids/60032875?trkid=1767; Bill and Melinda Gates Foundation, "Rory Kennedy Film Focuses on Global HIV/AIDS Epidemic," press release, July 8, 2002, http://www.gatesfoundation.org/press-releases/Pages/new-film-global-aids-pandemic-020708.aspx.

53. *AIDS Jaago*, directed by Mira Nair, Farhan Akhtar, Santosh Sivan, and Vishal Bhardwaj (Film Karavan, 2009).

54. Louise Hogarth, "Does Anyone Die of AIDS Anymore?" Fanlight Productions, 2002, http://www.fanlight.com/catalog/films/362_dadoa.php; *The Gift*, directed by Louise Hogarth (Brighton, MA: Dream Out Loud Productions, 2003) DVD.

55. Matt James et al., "Leveraging the Power of the Media to Combat HIV/AIDS," *Health Affairs* 24 (2005): 854–57, quotation from 854.

56. Ibid.

57. I am following the analysis in William H. Helfand, "Images of AIDS: The Poster Record," in *AIDS and the Historian*, 66–93.

58. Ibid., 89.

59. Ibid., 74–75.

60. Online sources of AIDS posters and images include "Historical HIV/AIDS Posters," AVERT Organization, 2011, http://www.avert.org/aids-posters.htm;

"AIDS Posters," UCLA Louise M. Darling Biomedical Library, History and Special Collections Division, http://digital.library.ucla.edu/aidsposters/; "Visual Culture and Health Posters: HIV/AIDS: Visuals," Profiles in Science, National Library of Medicine, http://profiles.nlm.nih.gov/VC/Views/Exhibit/visuals/hiv.html.

61. Alive & Well AIDS Alternatives, 2007, http://www.aliveandwell.org/; Christine Maggiore, *What If Everything You Thought You Knew About AIDS Was Wrong?* (Studio City, CA: American Foundation for AIDS Alternatives, 1999).

62. Jonny Steinberg, "AIDS Denial: A Lethal Delusion," *New Scientist*, July 2009, 32–36.

63. Nathan Geffen, *Encouraging Deadly Choices: AIDS Pseudo-Science in the Media*, Center for Social Science Working Paper No. 182 (Rondebosch: University of Cape Town, 2007), 6–7. See also Nathan Geffen, *Debunking Delusions: The Inside Story of the Treatment Action Campaign* (Auckland Park: Jacana Media, 2010).

64. Celia Farber, "Out of Control: AIDS and the Corruption of Medical Science," *Harper's Magazine*, March 2006; John Moore and Nicoli Nattrass, "Deadly Quackery," *New York Times*, June 4, 2006, Opinion Section, http://www.nytimes.com/2006/06/04/opinion/04moore.html?ref=aids; Gal Beckerman, "*Harper's* Races Right Over the Edge of a Cliff," *Columbia Journalism Review*, March 8, 2006, http://www.cjr.org/behind_the_news/harpers_races_right_over_the_e.php; Richard Kim, "Harper's Publishes AIDS Denialist," *The Notion: The Nation's Group Blog*, March 2, 2006, http://www.thenation.com/blog/harpers-publishes-aids-denialist; Steinberg, "AIDS Denial: A Lethal Delusion," 12.

65. "The Origin of AIDS," Snopes.com: Rumor Has It, August 1, 2007, http://www.snopes.com/medical/disease/aids.asp.

66. "Talk:AIDS Denialism," Wikipedia, January 5, 2011, http://en.wikipedia.org/wiki/Talk:AIDS_denialism.

67. *House of Numbers*, produced and directed by Brent W. Leung, 2009; Warner Brothers release, 2011, http://www.houseofnumbers.com; Jeannette Catsoulis, "AIDS Seen from a Different Angle," review of *House of Numbers*, produced and directed by Brent W. Leung, *New York Times*, September 4, 2009, *New York Times* Online AIDS Collection.

Chapter 7. The Global Epidemic

1. Lindsay Knight, *UNAIDS, The First 10 Years: 1996–2007* (Geneva, Switzerland: UNAIDS, 2008), 7.

2. Richard Krause, interview by Victoria A. Harden, November 17, 1988, NIH AIDS Oral Histories.

3. Ibid. Since there was active TB in the ward and the cause of AIDS was not known, the Americans used masks, gowns, and gloves. According to Jean William Pape, their Haitian host, that created a real problem for the Haitians because after the Americans left, the Haitian nurses and physicians were unwilling to work again until they were provided with similar precautions. J. W. Pape, personal communication to Thomas Quinn and the author, February 4, 2007.

4. Thomas C. Quinn, interviews by Victoria A. Harden and Caroline Hannaway, December 5 and 16, 1996, NIH AIDS Oral Histories.

5.   M. Boncy et al., "Acquired Immunodeficiency in Haitians," *N. Engl. J. Med.* 308 (1983): 1419–20; J. W. Pape et al., "Characteristics of the Acquired Immunodeficiency Syndrome (AIDS) in Haiti," *N. Engl. J. Med.* 309 (1983): 945–50; "GHESKIO: The Haitian Group for the Study of Kaposi's Sarcoma and Opportunistic Infections," 2007, http://www.gheskio.org/about%20main.html.

6.   Quinn interviews.

7.   N. Clumeck et al., "Acquired Immune Deficiency Syndrome in Black Africans," *Lancet* 321 (1983): 642; M Cavaille-Coll et al., "Immunological Evaluation of Acquired Immune Deficiency Syndrome Patients in France: Preliminary Results," *Antibiot. Chemother.* 32 (1983): 105–11; H. Taelman et al., "Acquired Immune Deficiency Syndrome in 3 Patients from Zaire," *Annales De La Société Belge De Médecine Tropicale* 63 (1983): 73–74.

8.   For information about Haitians in Zaire in the 1960s, see the prologue.

9.   Jon Cohen, "The Rise and Fall of Projet SIDA," *Science* 278 (1997): 1565–68. I am largely following Cohen's account, along with oral histories from Quinn and Piot, personal communication from James Curran, and the publications resulting from the program.

10.   Cohen, "The Rise and Fall of Projet SIDA."

11.   Peter Piot et al., "Acquired Immunodeficiency Syndrome in a Heterosexual Population in Zaire," *Lancet* 324 (1984): 65–69. Piot enjoys noting that this highly quoted publication was originally turned down by a *Lancet* editor as being "only of local interest" and not suitable for *Lancet*'s worldwide audience. See Piot interview, January 4, 2008; April 8, 2009; and June 16, 2010, NIH AIDS Oral Histories.

12.   Piot interviews.

13.   J. M. Mann et al., "Surveillance for AIDS in a Central African City: Kinshasa, Zaire," *JAMA* 255 (1986): 3255–59; J. M. Mann et al., "Natural History of Human Immunodeficiency Virus Infection in Zaire," *Lancet* 328 (1986): 707–9; J. Mann et al., "Condom Use and HIV Infection among Prostitutes in Zaire," *N. Engl. J. Med.* 316 (1987): 345; A. E. Greenberg et al., "The Association between Malaria, Blood Transfusions, and HIV Seropositivity in a Pediatric Population in Kinshasa, Zaire," *JAMA* 259 (1988): 545–49; R. Colebunders et al., "Herpes Zoster in African Patients: A Clinical Predictor of Human Immunodeficiency Virus Infection," *Journal of Infectious Diseases* 157 (1988): 314–18; B. Tandaert et al., "The Association of Tuberculosis and HIV Infection in Burundi," *AIDS Res. Hum. Retroviruses* 5 (1989): 247–51; P. Nguyen-Dinh et al., "Absence of Association between Plasmodium Falciparum Malaria and Human Immunodeficiency Virus Infection in Children in Kinshasa, Zaire," *Bulletin of the World Health Organization* 65 (1987): 607–13; J. M. Mann et al., "ELISA Readers and HIV Antibody Testing in Developing Countries," *Lancet* 327 (1986): 1504; V. Batter et al., "High HIV-1 Incidence in Young Women Masked by Stable Overall Seroprevalence among Childbearing Women in Kinshasa, Zaïre: Estimating Incidence from Serial Seroprevalence Data," *AIDS (London)* 8 (1994): 811–17; John Iliffe, *The African AIDS Epidemic: A History* (Athens: Ohio University Press, 2006), 13–14.

14.   Iliffe, *African AIDS Epidemic*, 13.

15. Cohen, "Rise and Fall of Projet SIDA."
16. Ibid.; interviews with Peter Piot, Thomas Quinn, James Curran, Anthony Fauci, Richard Krause, NIH AIDS Oral Histories.
17. Cohen, "Rise and Fall of Projet SIDA."
18. Ibid.
19. A. M. T. Lwegaba, "Preliminary Report of 'An Unusual Wasting Disease' Complex Nicknamed 'Slim' A Slow Epidemic of Rakai District, Uganda," November 1984, photocopy of typescript, Uganda Ministry of Health Library, Kampala, Uganda, as cited in Iliffe, *African AIDS Epidemic*, 23; D. Serwadda et al., "Slim Disease: A New Disease in Uganda and Its Association with HTLV-III Infection," *Lancet* 2 (October 19, 1985): 849–52.
20. Iliffe, *African AIDS Epidemic*, 16–17.
21. Ibid., 15–16.
22. Ibid., 19.
23. Ibid., 21–22.
24. Maryinez Lyons, "Women's Destiny and AIDS in Uganda," in *AIDS and the Public Debate*, 192.
25. Iliffe, *African AIDS Epidemic*, 25.
26. Figures are from national documents published by each country as cited in ibid., 38–39.
27. Ibid., 43.
28. Figures from the United Nations Development Program and UNAIDS as cited in ibid., 43–47.
29. F. Barin et al., "Serological Evidence for Virus Related to Simian T-Lymphotropic Retrovirus III in Residents of West Africa," *Lancet* 326 (1985): 1387–89; Iliffe, *African AIDS Epidemic*, 48–49.
30. Iliffe, *The African AIDS Epidemic*, 53–56.
31. Ibid., 56–57.
32. Lawrence K. Altman, "Global Program Aims to Combat AIDS 'Disaster,'" *New York Times*, November 21, 1986, *New York Times* Online AIDS Collection.
33. Philip J. Hilts, "Leader in U.N.'s Battle on AIDS Resigns in Dispute over Strategy," *New York Times*, March 17, 1990, *New York Times* Online AIDS Collection.
34. Quotation from "The Power of Leadership," chapter 6 in "The Age of AIDS," Part 1, *Frontline*, PBS, 2006, http://www.pbs.org/wgbh/pages/frontline/aids/view/6.html; David Miller, "A New Strain of HIV? The Impact of HIV Infection on Formal Caregivers and Options for Management," in *Psychosocial and Biomedical Interactions in HIV Infection*, eds. Kenneth H. Nott and Kav Vedhara (London: Taylor & Francis, 2000), 297–332.
35. "World AIDS Day," World AIDS Campaign, 2009, http://www.worldaids campaign.org/en/World-AIDS-Day.
36. Quotations from "At the Brink," chapter 8 in "The Age of AIDS," Part 1, *Frontline*, PBS, 2006, http://www.pbs.org/wgbh/pages/frontline/aids/view/8.html.
37. Ibid.
38. Jonathan Mann, ed., *Global AIDS Policy Coalition, AIDS in the World* (Cambridge, MA: Harvard University Press, 1992); Jonathan Mann, ed., *Global AIDS*

Policy Coalition, AIDS in the World II: Global Dimensions, Social Roots, and Responses (New York: Oxford University Press, 1996).

39. For biographical information on Merson, see Duke Medicine News and Communications, "Michael Merson Named Leader of Duke Global Health Institute," DukeHealth.org, July 26, 2006, http://dukemednews.org/news/article .php?id=9810; "Horizon International Scientific Review Board: Michael H. Merson, M.D.," Horizon Solutions Site, April 29, 2003, http://www.solutions -site.org/artman/publish/article_84.shtml.

40. Philip J. Hilts, "Upheaval in the East; W.H.O. Emergency Team Is Sent to Romania to Assess AIDS Cases," *New York Times*, February 8, 1990; Youssef M. Ibrahim, "Culture and Stigma Slow AIDS Reports in Mideast," *New York Times*, February 18, 1990; Philip J. Hilts, "Poorer Countries Are Hit Hardest by Spread of AIDS, U.N. Reports," *New York Times*, June 13, 1990, *New York Times* Online AIDS Collection.

41. Peter B. Gray, "HIV and Islam: Is HIV Prevalence Lower Among Muslims?" *Social Science and Medicine* 58 (2004): 1751–56.

42. Laura M. Kelley and Nicholas N. Eberstadt, *Behind the Veil of a Public Health Crisis: HIV/AIDS in the Muslim World* (Seattle, WA: National Bureau of Asian Research, 2005).

43. P. Kandela, "Arab Nations: Attitudes to AIDS," *Lancet* 341 (1993): 884, as cited in ibid., 4.

44. Ibid.

45. R. M. Khanani et al., "Human Immunodeficiency Virus-Associated Disorders in Pakistan," *AIDS Res. Hum. Retroviruses* 4 (1988): 149–54.

46. Ministry of Health, Government of Pakistan, "National AIDS Control Programme," http://www.nacp.gov.pk.

47. "Five Million HIV/AIDS Cases in Indonesia by 2010," Antara News, November 16, 2009, http://www.antaranews.com/en/news/1258315607/five-million -hiv-aids-cases-in-indonesia-by-2010.

48. Ibid.

49. "Indonesia: Anti-AIDS Condom Campaign Splits Muslims," Adnkronos International, November 29, 2009, http://www.adnkronos.com/AKI/English/ Security/?id=1.0.1612628060.

50. Quinn interviews.

51. E. A. Simoes et al., "Evidence for HTLV-III Infection in Prostitutes in Tamil Nadu (India)," *Indian Journal of Medical Research* 85 (1987): 335–38.

52. "Indian Council of Medical Research," http://www.icmr.nic.in/; A. Pradesh, "Overview of HIV and AIDS in India," AVERT, 2011, http://www.avert.org/ aidsindia.htm; D. N. Kakar and S. N. Kakar, *Combating AIDS in the 21st Century: Issues and Challenges* (New Delhi: Sterling, 2001), 32; "National AIDS Control Organisation," http://www.nacoonline.org/NACO.

53. Pradesh, "HIV and AIDS in India."

54. Ibid.

55. Reuters, "Drug Users Raise Risk of HIV in India," UNODC, June 12, 2007, http://www.unodc.org/india/drug_users_risk.html.

56. Department of AIDS Control, *Annual Report 2008–2009* (New Delhi: Ministry

of Health and Family Welfare, Government of India, 2009), 6, http://nacoon
line.org/upload/Publication/Annual_Report_NACO_2008-09.pdf.

57. Quinn interviews; R. C. Bollinger, S. P. Tripathy, and T. C. Quinn, "The Human
Immunodeficiency Virus Epidemic in India. Current Magnitude and Future
Projections," *Medicine* 74 (1995): 97–106; Harjot Kaur Singh et al., "The Indian
Pediatric HIV Epidemic: A Systematic Review," *Current HIV Research* 6 (2008):
419–32; Gita Sinha, David H. Peters, and Robert C. Bollinger, "Strategies for
Gender-Equitable HIV Services in Rural India," *Health Policy and Planning* 24
(2009): 197–208.

58. Renée Sabatier et al., *AIDS and the Third World* (London: Panos Institute,
1989), 173.

59. Christine Gorman, "Sex, AIDS and Thailand," *Time*, July 12, 2004, http://www
.time.com/time/magazine/article/0,9171,662826,00.html.

60. Ellen Nakashima, "Cracks Start to Show in Thailand's Model Anti-AIDS Program," *Washington Post*, July 10, 2004.

61. Sabatier et al., *AIDS and the Third World*, 169–75.

62. Ofelia T. Monzon, "Mann, Jonathan, 1947–98," UNESCO Profiles of Famous
Educators, http://www.ibe.unesco.org/publications/ThinkersPdf/manne.pdf.

63. "Acquired Immunodeficiency Syndrome (AIDS): Testing for LAV/HTLV-III
Antibody," *Wkly. Epidemiol. Rec.* 61 (1986): 226.

64. Kong-lai Zhang and Shao-Jun Ma, "Epidemiology of HIV in China," *Br. Med. J.*
324 (2002): 803–4.

65. Joanne Csete and Siddharth Dube, "An Inappropriate Tool: Criminal Law and
HIV in Asia," *AIDS (London)* 24, Suppl. 3 (2010): S80–S85.

66. Leslie Chang, "China May Apply Lessons from SARS to Fight AIDS," *Wall
Street Journal*, August 4, 2001.

67. Jon Cohen, "The Overlooked Epidemic," *Science* 313 (2006): 468–69.

68. UNAIDS, *Report on the Global AIDS Epidemic* (Geneva, 2010), 40–44.

69. Cohen, "Overlooked Epidemic."

70. Shawn C. Smallman, *The AIDS Pandemic in Latin America* (Chapel Hill: University of North Carolina Press, 2007), 5.

71. Ibid., 7; "Pope: Condom Use Can Be Justified to Halt AIDS," *CBS News*,
November 20, 2010, http://www.cbsnews.com/stories/2010/11/20/world/
main7073896.shtml.

72. "Vatican Maintains Stance on Condoms at HIV/AIDS Summit," *PBS News
Hour*, PBS, May 30, 2011, http://www.pbs.org/newshour/bb/health/jan-june
11/vatican_05-30.html.

73. Jon Cohen, "Peru: A New Nexus for HIV/AIDS Research," *Science* 313 (2006):
488–90. The NIAID grant number is 5U01AI069438-05.

74. Jon Cohen, "Late for the Epidemic: HIV/AIDS in Eastern Europe," *Science*
329 (2010): 160–64. On the epidemic in this region, see also Judyth L. Twigg,
ed., *HIV/AIDS in Russia and Eurasia*, 2 vols. (New York: Palgrave Macmillan,
2007).

75. Cohen, "Late for the Epidemic," quotation from 161.

76. The full text of the Vienna Declaration and lists of signatories are available at
http://www.viennadeclaration.com/.

77. Lindsay Knight, *UNAIDS: The First Ten Years, 1996–2006* (Geneva: UNAIDS, 2008), 18.
78. GPA Management Committee, *Report of the Ad Hoc Working Group of the GPA Management Committee* (Geneva: World Health Organization, 1992), 4, as cited in ibid., 19–22.
79. Piot interviews, NIH AIDS Oral Histories.
80. Ibid.
81. Ibid.

Chapter 8. The Third Decade

1. William J. Clinton and William Gates, "Priorities in Ending the Epidemic," Sixteenth International AIDS Conference, August 14, 2006, http://dawn.thot .net/aids2006_clinton_gates_speeches.html.
2. Knight, *UNAIDS: The First Ten Years*, 110; Piot interviews, NIH AIDS Oral Histories.
3. Barton Gellman, "Death Watch: The Global Response to AIDS in Africa," *Washington Post*, July 5, 2000. The author experienced such a response first-hand in the 1990s when she questioned military personnel at a professional meeting about the threat of AIDS to world stability. In their minds at that time, there was no issue with AIDS.
4. Ibid.
5. Ibid.
6. Ibid.
7. Knight, *UNAIDS*, 58–61.
8. Ibid., 61.
9. Piot interviews, NIH AIDS Oral Histories.
10. Knight, *UNAIDS*, 92-93.
11. Ibid., 92–94, quotations from 93, 94.
12. Ibid., 106.
13. Ibid.
14. Piot interviews, NIH AIDS Oral Histories.
15. Knight, *UNAIDS*, 112.
16. UN General Assembly, "United Nations Millennium Declaration," September 8, 2000, http://www.un.org/millennium/declaration/ares552e.pdf.
17. Knight, *UNAIDS*, 132–34.
18. UN General Assembly, "Declaration of Commitment on HIV/AIDS," August 2, 2001, http://www.un.org/ga/aids/coverage/FinalDeclarationHIVAIDS.html; "UN General Assembly Special Session on HIV/AIDS," June 25–27, 2001, http://www.un.org/ga/aids/coverage/.
19. Knight, *UNAIDS*, 134.
20. Ibid., 68.
21. Bernhard Schwartländer, Ian Grubb, and Jos Perriëns, "The 10-Year Struggle to Provide Antiretroviral Treatment to People with HIV in the Developing World," *Lancet* 368, no. 9534 (August 5, 2006): 541–46.
22. Knight, *UNAIDS*, 69.
23. Ibid., 75–76.
24. James Myburgh, "The Virodene Affair (I)," Politicsweb.co.za, September 17,

2007, http://www.politicsweb.co.za/politicsweb/view/politicsweb/en/page 71619?oid=83156&sn=Detail&pid=71619; James Myburgh, "The Virodene Affair (II)," Politicsweb.co.za, September 18, 2007, http://www.politicsweb .co.za/politicsweb/view/politicsweb/en/page71619?oid=83179&sn=Detail; James Myburgh, "The Virodene Affair (III)," Politicsweb.co.za, September 18, 2007, http://www.politicsweb.co.za/politicsweb/view/politicsweb/en/ page71619?oid=83213&sn=Detail; James Myburgh, "The Virodene Affair (IV)," Politicsweb.co.za, September 20, 2007, http://www.politicsweb.co.za/ politicsweb/view/politicsweb/en/page71619?oid=83231&sn=Detail&p id=71619; James Myburgh, "The Virodene Affair (V)," Politicsweb.co.za, September 21, 2007, http://www.politicsweb.co.za/politicsweb/view/politicsweb/ en/page71619?oid=83253&sn=Detail&pid=71619, quotation from part IV. The story is also told in Lesley Lawson, *Side Effects: The Story of AIDS in South Africa* (Cape Town: Double Storey, 2008).

25. K. Morris, "Short Course of AZT Halves HIV-1 Perinatal Transmission," *Lancet* 351, no. 9103 (February 28, 1998): 651; P. Vuthipongse et al., "Administration of Zidovudine during Late Pregnancy and Delivery to Prevent Perinatal HIV Transmission—Thailand, 1996–1998," *MMWR* 47, no. 8 (March 6, 1998): 151–54; R. S. Sperling et al., "Maternal Viral Load, Zidovudine Treatment, and the Risk of Transmission of Human Immunodeficiency Virus Type 1 from Mother to Infant," *N. Engl. J. Med.* 335, no. 22 (November 28, 1996): 1621–29. The debates over the ethics of the lower-dose trials in developing countries are in M. Angell, "The Ethics of Clinical Research in the Third World," *N. Engl. J. Med.* 337, no. 12 (September 18, 1997): 847–49; Marcia Angell et al., "AIDS Studies Violate Helsinki Rights Accord," *New York Times*, September 24, 1997; Danstan Bagenda et al., "A Look at Ethics and AIDS—We're Trying to Help Our Sickest People, Not Exploit Them in the Researcher's Code of Conduct, Contradictions Abound," *Washington Post*, September 28, 1997; M. Angell, "Investigators' Responsibilities for Human Subjects in Developing Countries," *N. Engl. J. Med.* 342, no. 13 (2000): 967–69; J. Cohen, "Ethics of AZT Studies in Poorer Countries Attacked," *Science* 276, no. 5315 (May 16, 1997): 1022.

26. Myburgh, "Virodene Affair (IV)."

27. Samantha Power, "The AIDS Rebel," *New Yorker*, May 19, 2003; Anne-Marie O'Connor, "S. African AIDS Activist Makes a Striking Impact; Zackie Achmat Inspires L.A. Audiences and Celebrates a Triumph Won at Home," *Los Angeles Times*, November 24, 2003.

28. I am following the discussion of Mark Heywood, "South Africa's Treatment Action Campaign: Combining Law and Social Mobilization to Realize the Right to Health," *Journal of Human Rights Practice* 1, no. 1 (March 1, 2009): 15–16. See also the South African Constitution, http://www.info.gov.za/documents/ constitution/index.htm. The right to health care is in Section 27.

29. Heywood, "South Africa's Treatment Action Campaign," 18.

30. Ibid., 32.

31. African National Congress, *Annual Report*, 1999, as cited in ibid.

32. Myburgh, "Virodene Affair (V)."

33. Anthony Brink, "AZT: A Medicine from Hell," *Citizen*, October 1988, 6, http:// www.virusmyth.com/aids/hiv/abazt.htm; E Papadopulos-Eleopulos et al., "A

Critical Analysis of the Pharmacology of AZT and Its Use in AIDS," *Current Medical Research and Opinion* 15, Suppl. 1 (1999): S1–45.

34. Presidential AIDS Advisory Panel Report, Pretoria and Johannesburg, South Africa, July 6, 2000, 10, http://www.info.gov.za/otherdocs/2001/aidspanel pdf.pdf; Lawson, *Side Effects*; Myburgh, "Virodene Affair (V)."

35. Myburgh, "Virodene Affair (V)."

36. Ibid.; Lawson, *Side Effects*, 249–52.

37. Mark Gevisser, *Thabo Mbeki: The Dream Deferred* (Johannesburg: Jonathan Ball, 2007); Chris McGreal, "Mbeki Admits He Is Still AIDS Dissident Six Years On," *Guardian*, November 6, 2007, http://www.guardian.co.uk/world/2007/nov/06/southafrica.aids.

38. South African Press Association, "DA Calls for Release of AIDS Report," July 14, 2003, http://www.aegis.com/news/sapa/2003/sa030702.html.

39. Reuters, "Factbox: South Africa's new HIV/AIDS Plan," March 14, 2007, http://www.reuters.com/article/2007/03/14/us-aids-safrica-factbox-idUSL 1426358120070314.

40. Pride Chigwedere et al., "Estimating the Lost Benefits of Antiretroviral Drug Use in South Africa," *J. Acquir. Immune Defic. Syndr.* 49 (2008): 410–15; Celia W. Dugger, "Study Cites Toll of AIDS Policy in South Africa," *New York Times*, November 26, 2008, International/Africa section.

41. Schwartländer, Grubb, and Perriëns, "10-Year Struggle to Provide Antiretroviral Treatment"; Knight, *UNAIDS*, 121.

42. Piot interviews, NIH AIDS Oral Histories.

43. Schwartländer, Grubb, and Perriëns, "10-Year Struggle to Provide Antiretroviral Treatment," 541.

44. Piot interviews, NIH AIDS Oral Histories; Schwartländer, Grubb, and Perriëns, "10-Year Struggle to Provide Antiretroviral Treatment."

45. Schwartländer, Grubb, and Perriëns, "10-Year Struggle to Provide Antiretroviral Treatment."

46. Government of Japan, "G8 Communiqué Okinawa 2000," G8 Information Centre, University of Toronto Library, July 23, 2000, http://www.g8.utoronto .ca/summit/2000okinawa/finalcom.htm.

47. "'Three Ones' Key Principles" (presented by UNAIDS staff at the Consultation on Harmonization of International AIDS Funding, April 25, 2004, Washington, DC; Knight, *UNAIDS*, 188.

48. Piot interviews, NIH AIDS Oral Histories

49. Knight, *UNAIDS*, 128–29.

50. B. Schwartländer et al., "AIDS: Resource Needs for HIV/AIDS," *Science* 292, no. 5526 (June 29, 2001): 2434–36.

51. Knight, *UNAIDS*, 129.

52. For biographical information on Feachem, see "Professor Sir Richard Feachem—Bio," *UCSF Global Health Sciences*, September 2, 2010, http://global healthsciences.ucsf.edu/about/bios/feachem_richard.aspx.

53. "Governance and Core Documents," http://www.theglobalfund.org/en/ library/documents/; see also within http://www.theglobalfund.org/en/—there is a link to a spreadsheet detailing pledges and contributions, 2001–2011.

54. Africa Region, *Intensifying Action Against HIV/AIDS in Africa: Responding to*

a Development Crisis (Washington, DC: World Bank, 1999); World Bank, *The World Bank's Global HIV/AIDS Program of Action* (Washington, DC, 2005); Marelize Gorgens-Albino et al., *The Africa Multi-Country AIDS Program, 2000–2006: Results of the World Bank's Response to a Development Crisis* (Washington, DC: World Bank, 2007); World Bank, "HIV/AIDS—Multi-Country HIV/AIDS Program (MAP)," 2011, http://go.worldbank.org/l3A0B15ZN0; World Bank, "AIDS—Data, Global HIV/AIDS Program of Action," 2008, http://go.worldbank.org/319J9LLS90.

55. United States Leadership against HIV/AIDS, Tuberculosis, and Malaria Act of 2003, Pub. L. No. 108-25 (2003); Tom Lantos and Henry J. Hyde, United States Global Leadership Against HIV/ AIDS, Tuberculosis, and Malaria Reauthorization Act of 2008, Pub. L. No. 110-293 (2008).

56. HIV Policy Program, "U.S. Federal Funding for HIV/AIDS: The President's FY 2012 Budget Request," Kaiser Family Foundation, March 24, 2011, http://www .kff.org/hivaids/7029.cfm.

57. Bill and Melinda Gates Foundation, "HIV/AIDS," 2011, http://www.gates foundation.org/hivaids/Pages/default.aspx; Erika Baehr, *U.S. Philanthropic Support to Address HIV/AIDS in 2009* (Arlington, VA: Funders Concerned about AIDS, 2009); Erika Baehr, *European Philanthropic Support to Address HIV/AIDS in 2009* (Brussels: European HIV/AIDS Funders Group [EFG], 2009).

58. UNAIDS, "New Reports Show That Despite Commitment, Total Philanthropic Funding for AIDS in Slight Decline," press release, November 16, 2010, http://www.unaids.org/en/resources/presscentre/pressreleaseandstatement archive/2010/november/20101116prphilanthropicfunding/.

59. The full text of the press conference is reproduced in Kontaratos, *Dissecting a Discovery*, 395–401.

60. Jon Cohen, *Shots in the Dark: The Wayward Search for an AIDS Vaccine* (New York: W. W. Norton, 2001), 43–77.

61. Ibid., 68–68.

62. Ibid., 68–69.

63. D. Zagury et al., "Immunization against AIDS in Humans," *Nature* 326, no. 6110 (March 19, 1987): 249–50; D. Zagury et al., "A Group Specific Anamnestic Immune Reaction against HIV-1 Induced by a Candidate Vaccine against AIDS," *Nature* 332, no. 6166 (April 21, 1988): 728–31; J. A. Berzofsky et al., "Antigenic Peptides Recognized by T Lymphocytes from AIDS Viral Envelope-Immune Humans," *Nature* 334, no. 6184 (August 25, 1988): 706–8.

64. AIDS Epidemic: Hearing before the Committee on Labor and Human Resources on Reviewing Federal Efforts Being Conducted toward Combating the AIDS Epidemic, 100th Cong. (1987).

65. Ibid.; Cohen, *Shots in the Dark*, 70–73.

66. Cohen, *Shots in the Dark*, 139.

67. National Institutes of Health, "The NIH Almanac, 2010," U.S. Department of Health and Human Services, 2010, http://www.nih.gov/about/almanac/nobel/ index.htm#content; Buhm Soon Park, "The Development of the Intramural Research Program at the National Institutes of Health after World War II," *Perspectives in Biology and Medicine* 46, no. 3 (2003): 383–402.

68. There is a large literature on this topic. With respect to the AIDS epidemic, see Victoria A. Harden and Dennis Rodrigues, "Context for a New Disease: Aspects of Biomedical Research Policy in the United States before AIDS," in *AIDS and Contemporary History*, 182–202.

69. Cohen, *Shots in the Dark*, 186.

70. A Pulitzer Prize–winning history of polio is David M. Oshinsky, *Polio: An American Story* (New York: Oxford University Press, 2005).

71. National Institutes of Health Revitalization Act of 1993, Pub. L. No. 103-43, Title 18 (1993), http://www.history.nih.gov/research/downloads/PL103-43.pdf.

72. Cohen, *Shots in the Dark*, 139–41.

73. Ibid., 165–74.

74. Katherine Harmon, "Renewed Hope for an AIDS Vaccine," *Sci. Am.*, November 16, 2009; Supachai Rerks-Ngarm et al., "Vaccination with ALVAC and AIDSVAX to Prevent HIV-1 Infection in Thailand," *N. Engl. J. Med.* 361 (2009): 2209–20; Adel Benlahrech et al., "Adenovirus Vector Vaccination Induces Expansion of Memory CD4 T Cells with a Mucosal Homing Phenotype That Are Readily Susceptible to HIV-1," *Proc. Natl. Acad. Sci.* 106 (2009): 19940–45. See also the British journalist Brian Deer's critique of the AIDSVAX trial: "The VaxGen Experiment: Brian Deer Investigates An 'AIDS Vaccine,'" October 3, 1999, http://briandeer.com/aidsvax.htm.

75. NIAID, "NIAID Announces Revised Priorities for HIV Vaccine Research," news release, July 24, 2008, http://www.niaid.nih.gov/news/newsreleases/2008/Pages/hiv_vax_priorities.aspx; Ruslan Medzhitov and Dan Littman, "HIV Immunology Needs a New Direction," *Nature* 455, no. 7213 (October 2, 2008): 591; A. S. Fauci et al., "HIV Vaccine Research: The Way Forward," *Science* 321, no. 5888 (July 2008): 530–32.

76. Kevin Sack, "Economy Wreaks Havoc on Federal AIDS Drug Program," *New York Times*, June 30, 2010, *New York Times* Online AIDS Colection.

77. "A Living History of AIDS Vaccine Research" International AIDS Vaccine Initiative Report, March–April 2009, http://www.iavireport.org/archives/2009/Documents/IR_Fauci_SpecialFeature.pdf.

78. "Dale and Betty Bumpers Vaccine Research Center," NIAID, July 1, 2011, http://www3.niaid.nih.gov/about/organization/vrc/default.htm; Rockfeller Foundation, *HIV Vaccines—Accelerating Development of Preventive HIV Vaccines for the World, Summary Report and Recommendations of an International Meeting, March 7–11, 1994, Belagio, Italy*, http://www.iavi.org/Lists/IAVIPublications/attachments/d8dd04c6-b24f-46de-9d28-0468beed9c0e/IAVI_Bellagio_Report_1994_ENG.pdf; International AIDS Vaccine Initiative, "About the International AIDS Vaccine Initiative," Info Sheet, 2010, http://www.iavi.org/Lists/IAVIPublications/attachments/ce2ccdcb-3a3a-4543-be2d-334f2fc3db45/IAVI_About_IAVI_2010_ENG.pdf; International AIDS Vaccine Initiative, 2009 Annual Report, 2009, http://www.iavi.org/about-IAVI/Documents/IAVI_APR_2009.pdf; Rutgers University, "AIDS Vaccine Gets Closer: Targeting Virus' Achilles Heel," ScienceDaily, March 13, 2009, http://www.sciencedaily.com/releases/2009/03/090312114801.htm; George Makedonas and Michael R. Betts, "Living in a House of Cards: Re-evaluating CD8+ T-Cell Immune Correlates against HIV," *Immunological Reviews* (*Immunol.*

Rev. hereafter) 239, no. 1 (January 2011): 109–24; Marcela F. Pasetti et al., "Immunology of Gut Mucosal Vaccines," *Immunol. Rev.* 239, no. 1 (2011): 125–48.

79. Carina Storrs, "Clean-Cut: Study Finds Circumcision Helps Prevent HIV and Other Infections: Scientific American," *Sci. Am.*, January 13, 2010; Jorge Sánchez et al., "Male Circumcision and Risk of HIV Acquisition among MSM," *AIDS (London)* 25, no. 4 (February 20, 2011): 519–23; Maria J. Wawer et al., "Male Circumcision as a Component of Human Immunodeficiency Virus Prevention," *American Journal of Preventive Medicine* 40, no. 3 (March 2011): e7–8; Lance B. Price et al., "The Effects of Circumcision on the Penis Microbiome," *Public Library of Science One* 5, no. 1 (2010): e8422.

80. "Statement of Anthony S. Fauci, M.D. Director, National Institute of Allergy and Infectious Diseases National Institutes of Health on Results from the CA-PRISA 004 Microbicide HIV Prevention Study," NIH News, July 20, 2010, http://www.nih.gov/news/health/jul2010/niaid-20.htm. David Brown, "Gel Found to Reduce AIDS Risk in Women," *Washington Post*, July 20, 2010; Jon Cohen, "HIV/AIDS: At Last, Vaginal Gel Scores Victory against HIV," *Science* 329, no. 5990 (July 23, 2010): 374–75; Quarraisha Abdool Karim et al., "Effectiveness and Safety of Tenofovir Gel, an Antiretroviral Microbicide, for the Prevention of HIV Infection in Women," *Science* 329, no. 5996 (September 3, 2010): 1168–74; Sten H. Vermund and Lut Van Damme, "HIV Prevention in Women: Next Steps," *Science* 331, no. 6015 (January 21, 2011): 284. On rate of infection of women in sub-Saharan Africa, see *UNAIDS Report on the Global AIDS Epidemic 2010*, 131, figs. 5.6 and 5.7.

81. NIAID, "Treating HIV-Infected People with Antiretrovirals Protects Partners from Infection," press release, May 12, 2011, http://www.niaid.nih.gov/news/newsreleases/2011/Pages/HPTN052.aspx; David Brown, "HIV Drugs Sharply Cut Risk of Transmission, Study Finds," *Washington Post*, May 12, 2011.

82. Fauci quotation from NIAID, "Treating HIV-Infected People"; Chan and Sidebe quotations from Julie Steenhuysen, "UPDATE 2-Early Drug Treatment Greatly Cuts Spread of HIV," Reuters, May 12, 2011, http://www.reuters.com/article/2011/05/12/aids-drugs-idUSN1227849820110512.

83. Ian McNicholl, "Adverse Effects of Antiretroviral Drugs," HIV InSite, July 2010, http://hivinsite.ucsf.edu/InSite?page=ar-05-01.

84. NIAID, "NIH Study Examines Best Time for Healthy HIV-Infected People to Begin Antiretrovirals," press release, March 7, 2011, http://www.niaid.nih.gov/news/newsreleases/2011/Pages/START.aspx.

85. WHO/UNAIDS, "The 3 by 5 Initiative. Access to HIV Treatment Continues to Accelerate in Developing Countries, but Bottlenecks Persist, Says WHO/UNAIDS Report," press release, June 29, 2005, http://www.who.int/3by5/progressreportJune2005/en/.

86. Gregory K. Folkers and Anthony S. Fauci, "Controlling and Ultimately Ending the HIV/AIDS Pandemic: A Feasible Goal," *JAMA* 304 (2010): 350–51.

Epilogue: AIDS at 30

1. *UNAIDS, Report on the Global AIDS Epidemic*, 12.

2. See U.S. Food and Drug Administration, "HIV/AIDS Related Therapies: Approved Therapies, Treatment Guidelines," August 19, 2009, http://www.fda

.gov/ForConsumers/ByAudience/ForPatientAdvocates/HIVandAIDS
Activities/ucm117891.htm.

3. Sam Whiting, "Life Before the Lifeboat," *San Francisco Chronicle*, November 27, 2009, http://articles.sfgate.com/2009-11-27/movies/17181524_1_world-aids
    -day-aids-clinic-aids-virus.

4. Robert M. Wachter, "AIDS, Activism, and the Politics of Health," *N. Engl. J. Med.* 326 (1992): 128–33; Steven Epstein, "The Construction of Lay Expertise: AIDS Activism and the Forging of Credibility in the Reform of Clinical Trials," *Science, Technology and Human Values* 20 (1995): 408–37; Bettyann Kevles, *Naked to the Bone: Medical Imaging in the Twentieth Century* (New Brunswick: Rutgers University Press, 1997), 258. On the AIDS red ribbon, see Nigel Wrench, "Why a Red Ribbon Means AIDS," *BBC News*, November 7, 2003, http://news.bbc.co.uk/2/hi/health/3250251.stm.

5. Sharma Howard, "Standing at the Nexus of a History," *Norwich Bulletin*, June 28, 2008, http://www.norwichbulletin.com/lifeevents/x1743983550/Standing-at-the-nexus-of-a-history#axzz1FjyygYhN; John-Manuel Andriote, *Victory Deferred: How AIDS Changed Gay Life in America* (Chicago: University of Chicago Press, 1999).

6. "Uganda Considers Death Penalty for Gays," *The Root*, December 9, 2009, http://www.theroot.com/buzz/uganda-considers-making-homosexuality
    -capital-offense; "Obituary: David Kato," *Economist*, February 10, 2011, 96; Marc Epprecht, *Heterosexual Africa? The History of an Idea from the Age of Exploration to the Age of AIDS* (Athens: Ohio University Press, 2008).

7. Jose Antonio Vargas and Darryl Fears, "At Least 3 Percent of D.C. Residents Have HIV or AIDS, City Study Finds; Rate Up 22% From 2006," *Washington Post*, March 15, 2009; Lena H. Sun, "D.C.'s Leading Provider of Clean Needles to Drug Addicts to Close Feb. 25," *Washington Post*, February 10, 2011; Petula Dvorak, "End of Needle Exchange Marks Loss of a Bulwark in D.C.'s AIDS Fight," *Washington Post*, February 24, 2011.

8. Piot interviews, NIH AIDS Oral Histories.

9. Bruce R. Schackman, "Implementation Science for the Prevention and Treatment of HIV/AIDS," *J. Acquir. Immune Defic. Syndr.* 55, Suppl. 1 (2010): S27–S31.

Index

3TC, 150
4-H groups, 31, 267n54
6000 a Day: An Account of a Catastrophe Foretold, 176

Aaron Diamond AIDS Research Center of the New York University School of Medicine, 151, 154, 238
Abbott Laboratories, 89, 90, **91**, 150, 151
ABC television network, 167
Abdur-Rahman, Zahra, 152
Absolutely Positive, 176
Accelerating Access Initiative, 227, 228
Acer, David, 82, 83
Achmat, Zackie, 177, 224
    acquired immune deficiency syndrome (AIDS)
    alternative theories about, 181–84
    annual AIDS-related deaths by region, 1990–2009, **246**
    defined, 1, 253, 267n42
    drugs access as economic issue, 227–29
    as international economic issue, 221
    as international security issue, 217, 300n3
    global prevalence in 2010, **201**
    named in July 1982, 34
    and quackery, 182
ACT UP. *See* AIDS Coalition to Unleash Power (ACT UP)
activists, 247
    1988 demonstration at the FDA, 143
    demonstrations over foscarnet approval process, 144–45
    overview, 112–15

adolescent AIDS, 138–39
Advocate (San Francisco), 21
Afghanistan, AIDS in, 200–203
Africa, AIDS in, 198
Africa's solution, 182
African AIDS Epidemic: A History, The (Iliffe), 192
African Americans and AIDS, 119–20
African National Congress (ANC), support for Virodene, 222–27
African swine fever virus (ASFV), 168, 253
Against the Odds: The Story of AIDS Drug Development, Politics, and Profits (Arno and Feiden), 142
AID Atlanta, 179
AIDES (France), 115, 122
AIDS. *See* acquired immune deficiency syndrome
AIDS Action Committee (Boston), 112
AIDS: An Expanding Tragedy (National Commission on AIDS), 111, **113**
AIDS and Its Metaphors (Sontag), 123
AIDS awareness trading cards, **179**
AIDS Coalition to Unleash Power (ACT UP), 114, 168, 176, 237
    1988 demonstration at the FDA, 143
    1990 demonstration at NIH, **116**
    and demonstrations about foscarnet approval process, 144–45
    protests over price of AZT, 136–37
AIDS denialists, 145–49, 181–84
    and South African government, 222–27
AIDS from the Beginning (JAMA), 164
AIDS History Group, 291n1

AIDS in the Industrialized Democracies: Passions, Politics, and Policies (Kirp and Bayer), 109
AIDS in the World (Mann), 199
AIDS Jaago (film), 177
AIDS Law Project (South Africa), 224
AIDS Medical Foundation (U.S.), 122
AIDS Memorandum (NIAID), 44
AIDS orphans, 250
AIDS Pandemic in Latin America, The (Smallman), 208
AIDS Project Los Angeles, 112
AIDS Quilt, 120–21, **121**, 176
AIDS red ribbon, 211, **220**, 306n4
AIDS Society of the Philippines, 206
AIDS test kit, **91**
AIDS Treatment News (James), 141
AIDS: Papers from Science, 1982–1985 (AAAS), 164
AIDS-associated retrovirus (ARV), 60, 67, 127, 253. *See also* Levy, Jay
AIDSVAX, 240
AL-721, 141
Alda, Alan, 170
"Alive and Well: AIDS Alternatives" website, 182
Altman, Lawrence K., 63, 166, 215
ALVAC-HIV, 240
American Association for the Advancement of Science (AAAS), 164, 247
American Association for the History of Medicine, 291n1
American Association of Blood Banks, 163
American Foundation for AIDS Research (amfAR), 118, 122, 176
American Public Health Association (APHA), 24, 36
American Society of Newspaper Editors, 164
Amin, Idi, 194
amyl nitrite drugs ("poppers") as possible cause of AIDS, 41
An Early Frost (film), 175
And the Band Played On: Politics, People, and the AIDS Epidemic (Shilts), 15, 168, 176
Anderson, Warwick, 117
Andriote, John-Manuel, 247
Angels in America (Kushner), 174, 175
animal models for AIDS, 274n49
Annan, Kofi, 178, 216, 217, 229
Antara news agency, 203
antibiotics, 2
antibody, 253

antigen, 253
antiretroviral therapy (ART), 156, 168, 177, 182–84, 215, 222, 243, 253
Argentina, AIDS in, 207–9
Arno, Peter S., 136, 142
Aronson, David, 87
ART. *See* antiretroviral therapy (ART)
Arthur Ashe Institute for Urban Health, 82
Ashe, Arthur, 82
Asociación Civil Impacta Salud y Educación (Impacta, Peru), 208
assay, 253
Astra Pharmaceutical Products, 144–45
Aventis-Pasteur, 240
Avon, Lord, 107
azidothymidine (AZT), 65, 107, 129, 144, 149–50, 171, 223, 253
    development of, 130–35
    dispute over price of, 136–38
    litigation over patent for, 137–38
    trade name Retrovir, 135
AZT. *See* azidothymidine

B cells, 253. *See also* immune system, humoral
Bahamas, AIDS in, 207
Baird, Barbara Fabian, 77, 78, 80
Baltimore, David, 51
Bangladesh, AIDS in, 200–203
Bardhan, Niilanjana, 165
Barnard, Christiaan, 223
Barr Laboratories, 137
Barré-Sinoussi, Françoise, 45, 51, **52**, 58, 69, 270n12
Barrows, Walter L., 214
Bassin, Robert, 51
bathhouse closure, 109–10
    and formation of GLAAD, 113
Bay Area Reporter (San Francisco), **156**, 157
Bayer, Ronald, 83, 106, 109
Bayh-Dole Act, 65
Behring, Emil von, 13, 149
Belgian Institute of Tropical Medicine (ITM), 188–91
Belgium, early AIDS case identified in, 8
Belize, AIDS in, 207
Bell, Frederic, **27**
Bergalis, Kimberly, 82, 83
Berger, Edward A., 152–54
Berridge, Virginia, 106, 107, 108
Bhengu, Nozipho, 182
Bianculli, David, 175

Bill and Melinda Gates Foundation, 177–78,
    230–32
bioethical issues and AIDS. *See* eithical issues
    and AIDS
Blattner, William, 41, 147
*Blood Feuds: AIDS, Blood, and the Politics of
    Medical Disaster* (Feldman and Bayer), 83
blood infected with HIV
    early response of blood bankers to pos-
        sibility, 34
    scandal in France, 91–92
    scandal in Japan, 92
    scandals in other industrialized coun-
        tries, 92–93
blood test for HIV, as developed in U.S. and
    France, 64
blood-banking policy, 71
    before AIDS, 85–86
    donation restrictions in 2011, 93
    donor voluntary disqualification form, **88**
Bollinger, Robert, 205
Bolognesi, Dani, 132
Botswana, AIDS in, 195–97
branched-DNA test (b-DNA), 150
Brandt, Alan, 105
Brandt, Edward, 99, 100
Brazil, AIDS in, 207–9, 219
Bressan, Arthur J., Jr., 175
Brink, Anthony, 225
Bristol-Myers-Squibb, 139
British Broadcasting Corporation (BBC), 178
British Medical Journal, 173
Broder, Samuel, **49**, 129–39, **131**, 171, 238
Brooks, Philip, 176–77
Brown, Timothy, 155
Brundtland, Gro Harlem, 227
Brun-Vézinet, Françoise, 54
Buddies, 175
Burkina Faso, AIDS in, 197–98
Burma. *See* Myanmar
Burroughs Wellcome Company, 132–36,
    142, 171
    and litigation over patent for AZT, 137–38
Burton, Lawrence, 141
Burundi, AIDS in, 193–95
Bush, George H. W., 103, 137, 200
Bush, George W., 231

Cabradilla, Cirilo (Cy), 57
Cáceres, Carlos, 208–9
California HealthCare Foundation, 120
Cambodia, 207

Cameron, Edwin, 227
Cameroon, AIDS in, 192–93
Campbell, Bobbi, 38
candidiasis, 3, 20, 41, 77, 253
capsid, viral, 253
Caribbean, AIDS in, 207–9
Catholic Church and AIDS in Latin
    America, 208
Catsoulis, Jeannette, 184
CCR-5, 152, 253
CD4, 254
CDC. *See* U.S. Centers for Disease Control
    and Prevention
Cedars-Sinai Hospital, Los Angeles, 1
celebrities and AIDS, 81–83
cellular immune system, **19**, 254
Center for Attitudinal Healing (California),
    179
Central African Republic, AIDS in, 192–93
Central Asia, AIDS in, 209–10
*Challenge of HIV/AIDS in Communities
    of Color, The* (Watkins Commission re-
    port), 111
Chamberland, Mary, **27**
Chan, Margaret, 242
chemokines, 154, 254
Chermann, John-Claude, 45, 51–52, **52**, 54,
    58, 69, 270n12
Chicago Tribune, 172
Chile, 221
chimpanzee (*Pan troglodytes troglodytes*), 5
China, AIDS in, 206–7
    state television network (CCTV), 177
Chirac, Jacques, 66
Chiron Corporation, 60, 150
Cholera Years, The (Rosenberg), 123
Cipla pharmaceutical company, 228
circumcision of males to prevent AIDS,
    231, 241
Claude Bernard Hospital (Paris), 54, 58
clinical associate program at NIH, 32, 46,
    49, 73
clinical research on AIDS, 72–77
clinical trials, 140
Clinton, Bill, 176, 237
clone, 254
CNN television network, 167
codon, genetic, 254
cofactor theories as cause of AIDS, 41–42
Cohen, Jon, 172, 188, 207, 209, 233–36
Cohen, Myron, 242
Colebunders, Robert, **189**, 191

Colombia, AIDS in, 207–9
Columbia Journalism Review, 183
Columbia University, 90
Common Threads: Stories from the Quilt
   (film), 176
Conant, Marcus, 21, 23
condoms, funding for under PEPFAR, 231
Confronting AIDS (Institute of Medicine
   report), 110
Congo Brazzaville. *See* Republic of Congo
Congo Kinshasa. *See* Democratic Republic
   of Congo (DRC)
Cooper, Ted, 238
Copeland, Terry D., 149
Corey, Lawrence, 266n33
Cornell University Medical College, 73, 187
Côte d'Ivoire, AIDS in, 197–98, 221
*Covering the Plague: AIDS and the
   American Media* (Kinsella), 165
Cowal, Sally Grooms, 221
Cravero, Kathleen, 218, 220
Crewdson, John, 172–74
Crixivan, 150
cryptosporidiosis, 22, 41, 254
Curie Institute (Paris), 51
Curran, James, 27–29, 36–37, 53–54, 87, 99,
   119, 188, **189**, 190–91
CXCR-4, 152, 254
cytokines, 254
cytomegalovirus (CMV), 21–22, 40, 72, 76,
   80, 141, 254

d4T, 145
Dana-Farber Cancer Institute (Boston), 154
data and safety monitoring board (DSMB),
   133–35, 242, 254
Davis, Karen, 98
Davison, Irwin, **27**
Defert, Daniel, 98
Delaney, Martin, 145, 170
Delhi University (India), 59
Demme, Jonathan, 176
Democratic Republic of Congo, 6–8, 188,
   191, 192–93. *See also* Zaire
denialists, AIDS, 146–49
Denmark, 22, 32, 198
Denver Principles, 38
*Denying AIDS: Conspiracy Theories,
   Pseudoscience, and Human Tragedy*
   (Kalichman), 148
Department of Health and Social Security
   AIDS Unit (U.K.), 107

dermatology, 21, 22
Destiny of Me, The (Kramer), 174
DeVita, Vincent T., 33, 63, 130
Devork, Petula, 249
diagnostic test for HIV, **91**, 246. *See also*
   ELISA test, Western blot
   and travel ban on HIV-infected people,
     106
   developed, 64, 89
   patent dispute over, 65-66
Diana, Princess of Wales, Memorial
   Lecture, 216
dideoxycytidine (ddC), 139
dideoxyinosine (ddI),139
Dingell, John, 173
"discovery" in science, 55–57
diseases
   names of, 2
   theories of, 12
*Dissecting a Discovery: The Real Story of
   How the Race to Uncover the Cause of
   AIDS Turned Scientists against Disease,
   Politics against Science, Nation against
   Nation* (Kontaratos), 174
Djibouti, AIDS in, 193–95
DNA, 254
Does Anyone Die of AIDS Anymore? (film), 177
Dominant 7 film company, 176
Dominican Republic, 7
Doms, Robert, 154
Donahue, Phil, 115
Douglas-Brown, Laura, 157
Dowdle, Walter, 199
Drake, Donald C., 86
Dritz, Selma, 11, 30, 31
Drug Access Initiative, 227
drug research, antiviral drugs before AIDS, 128
drug trials
   placebo-controlled, double-blind, 133
   process of bringing a drug to market, **134**
   phases of, 257–58
Duesberg, Peter, 108, 145–49, 168, 183
Dugas, Gaetan, 169
Duke University, 23, 132–33, 136
Dulbecco, Renato, 50
Dunlop, David, 151
Duvalier, François (Papa Doc), 6

Eastern Europe, AIDS in, 209–10
Eberstadt, Nicholas, 202
Ebola fever, 25
efficacy, 254

Eigo, Jim, 145
electron microscope, 59
ELISA test, 89, 204, 254
Elizabeth Taylor HIV/AIDS Foundation, 122
Elton John AIDS Foundation, 122
enfuvirtide, 155
ephemera about AIDS, 178–81, **179**, **180**
epidemic, 254
Epidemic Intelligence Service (EIS), 26,
    28–29
epidemic of fear, 77–81, 183
Equatorial Guinea, AIDS in, 192–93
Eritrea, AIDS in, 25, 193
Erman, John, 175
Ermarth, Fritz, 214
Essex, Myron (Max), **49**, 57, 63, 197, 227
ethical issues and AIDS, 9, 14, 57, 66, 135,
    138–43, 163–64, 244
Ethiopia, AIDS in, 25, 193–95
etiology, 255
European HIV/AIDS Funders Group, 231

Fabius, Laurent, 90, 92
FACS machine, 255
factor IX (blood clotting factor), 85, 90
factor VIII (blood clotting factor), 30, 64,
    85, 90
"Facts About AIDS" poster, **180**
Fahey, John, 24
Falwell, Jerry, 123
Fan, Peng Thim, 20
Farber, Celia, 183
Fauci, Anthony S., 71, 73–76, **74**, 79, 104,
    116, 141–45, 154, 167, 235, 238, 240–43
Feachem, Richard, 230
fear, epidemic of, 77–81
Feiden, Karyn, 142
Feldman, Eric A., 83, 92
Feldman, Marvin, 120
feline leukemia virus, 57
Ferencic, Nina, 211
Figueroa, Elisabeth Manipoud, 211
film treatments of AIDS, 175–78
Fischinger, Peter, 270n12
fluorescence-activated cell sorter (FACS), 53
Foege, William, 31, 33
Fortovase, 150
foscarnet, 76, 144-45
Francis, Donald, 57, 63, 87, 170–72, 239–40
Francis, Henry (Skip), **189**, 191
Franco-Prussian War, 55
Fréchette, Louise, 217

French Polynesia, AIDS in, 205–6
French Working Group (FWG), 54, 58
Friedman, Milton and Rose, 97
Friedman-Kien, Alvin, 21, 29, 32
Fumento, Michael, 108
Funders Concerned about AIDS, 231
funding for AIDS in the third decade,
    229–32
fund-raising activities for AIDS charities, 122
fungal toxin as possible cause of AIDS, 41
fusion, 152
Fuzeon, 155
Futures Group International (Washington,
    D.C.), 229

G8 economic summit, 228
Gabon, AIDS in, 192–93
Gajdusek, D. Carleton, 77
Gallo laboratory, **49**, 59–60, 64–68
Gallo, Robert C., 45–46, **48**, **49**, 51–54,
    57–70, 89, 125, 131–32, 147–48, 153,
    170–74, 255
    and memoir, *Virus Hunting*, 54, 270n12
ganciclovir, 76, 141–44
Gates Foundation. *See* Bill and Melinda
    Gates Foundation
Gates, Bill, 213
Gay and Lesbian Alliance against
    Defamation (GLAAD, U.S.), 113
gay bowel syndrome, 264n12
gay compromise syndrome, 23
Gay Men's Health Crisis(GMHC), 16, 38,
    112, 114, 175, 178
Gazprom-Media, Russia, 178
Gebbie, Kristine, 110
Geffen, Nathan, 182
Gellman, Barton, 214
gene, 255
Genentech, 235, 239, 240
George, Greg, 152
germ theory of infectious disease, 12 13, 55
Gevisser, Mark, 226
Ghana, AIDS in, 197–98
GHESKIO. *See* Haitian Group for the Study
    of Kaposi's Sarcoma and Opportunistic
    Infections (GHESKIO)
Gift, The (film), 177
Gillespie, Duff, 215
Gilmartin, Ray, 227
Glaser, Elizabeth Meyer, 82, 122
    pediatric AIDS foundation, 82
Glaser, Paul Michael, 82

Glaxo-Wellcome company, 223
GlaxoSmithKline, 138
Gliad, Sherry, 90
global business council and AIDS, 221
Global Fund, 230, 229–30, 231
Global Health Initiative (United States), 231
Global Media AIDS Initiative, 178
Global Programme on AIDS (WHO). *See*
   World Health Organization (WHO)
Goedert, James, 41
Goines, David Lance, 180
Golden Triangle, 206
Good Intentions: How Big Business and the
   Medical Establishment Are Corrupting the
   Fight against AIDS (Nussbaum), 171
Gordon, Robert, 85, 99
Gore, Albert (Al), 217
Gottlieb, Michael, 20, 23–24, 26, 163
Gould, Stephen J., 95, 160
gp, 255
Grady, Christine, 80
Gray, Peter B., 200
"Great AIDS Quest," 172
Green Cross company (Japan), 92
Greenberg, Daniel S., 174
GRID (Gay Related Immune Deficiency), 23
Groopman, Jerome, 60
Guyana, AIDS in, 207

H. F. Verwoerd Hospital (Pretoria), 223
HAART. *See* highly active anti-retroviral
   therapy.
Haiti, 6–7, 185–87, 207
Haitian Group for the Study of Kaposi's
   Sarcoma and Opportunistic Infections
   (GHESKIO), 187
Haitians, 31
   as member of the 4-H group, 37, 40,
     267n55
   right to give blood reinstated, 89
Hall, Katherine J., 214
Hanks, Tom, 176
Hansen, Gerhard, 123
Hansen's disease, 123
harm reduction, 96
Harper's, 183
Hartford Hospital (Connecticut), 72
Hartl, John, 175
Hartley, Janet, 50
Harvard University, 60, 200
   School of Public Health, **49**, 57, 163,
     197, 227

Hastings Center, 163
Haverkos, Harry, 186
HBO television network, 177
health care policy issues raised by AIDS
   epidemic, 109
Health Education Resource Organization
   (Baltimore), 112
Healy, Bernadine, 62, 238
Heckler, Margaret, 62–64, 99, 232
Hein, Karen, 138
Helfand, William, 178, 181
Hellman, Hal, 55
helper T cells, 255
hemophilia, 2–3
Hemophilia Foundation, 34, 86, 92
hemophiliacs, 30–31, 37–39, 60, 64, 71, 81,
   84–85
   as part of 4-H group, 31
   compensation for infection via contami-
     nated blood, 90–93
Henderson, David, 78
Henry J. Kaiser Family Foundation, 178
hepatitis A, 2
hepatitis B, 2, 5, 45, 54, 78, 81, 86
herpes viruses, 3, 255
Heywood, Mark, 224
highly active antiretroviral therapy (HAART),
   168, 255
     development of, 149–52
     shortened to ART, 156
Hill, James C., 104
Hilliman, Maurice, 237
Hitchcock, Heath, 84
Hitchcock, Priscilla, 84, 85
HIV. *See* human immunodeficiency virus
   (HIV)
HIV Drug Access Initiative, 221–22
Ho, David, 151, 154, 238
Hoffmann–La Roche, 149, 155
Hogarth, Louise, 177
Holbrooke, Richard, 217
Holmes, King K., 25
homophobia, 78, 79
homosexual men
   4-H group, as part of, 31
   AIDS first recognized in, 15–16
   early community support efforts, 37–38
Hong Kong flu, 52
Hoover Institution, 97
Hopital de l'Université d'Etat d'Haiti, 186,
   295n3
Horowitz, Jerome, 129

House of Numbers, 183Howard Hughes
  Medical Institute, 154
HPA-23, 140
HTLV-III. *See* human lymphatropic virus III
Hudson, Rock, 81, 82, 107, 140, 167, 175, 176
  impact of death on Reagan administra-
    tion, 104–5
Huebner, Robert, 44, 49, 50
Hughes, Sally Smith, 30, 50
Human Genome Project, 236
human immunodeficiency virus (HIV)
  becomes name of AIDS virus, 67–68
  diagram of, **128**
  HIV-1, 5, 6, 255
  HIV-2, 5, 197, 255
  life cycle as known in 1987, **129**
  life cycle as known in 2009, **153**
  second receptor needed for infection
    identified, 152–53
  transmission, 5–6
  visualized in three dimensions, **248**
human lymphotropic virus III (HTLV-III),
  59–60, 67–68, 127, 255
  HTLV-IIIB, 68
human T-cell leukemia virus (HTLV-I), 48,
  54, 58–59
human T-cell lymphoma virus II (HTLV-
  II), 48, 58–59
humoral immune system, **18**, 255
Hussein, Warls, 176
Hütter, Gero, 155
Hvidovre Hospital, 22

iceberg image for AIDS epidemic, 36, 203
influenza, 5
Iliffe, John, 192–96
immune system, 16–19
  cellular immunity, **19**, 76
  helper T cell, 76, 255
  humoral immunity, **18**,76
  memory B cells, 17–18, 257
  plasma B cells, 75, 258
  suppressor T cell, 259
in vitro, 255
in vivo, 255
IND, 256
IND, treatment, 256
India, AIDS in, 203–5
Indian Council of Medical Research
  (ICMR), 204
Indian National AIDS Control
  Organization, 205

indinavir, 150, 151
indirect immune fluorescence test, 59
Indonesia, AIDS in, 200–203, 205–6
Indonesia Mujahiddin Council, 203
Ingelfinger rule, 163
Ingelfinger, Franz J., 163
injecting drug users and AIDS, 30–31, 37,
  106. *See also* needle exchange, Vienna
  declaration
  4-H group, part of, 31
  in China, 206, 249–50
  in Central Asia, Eastern Europe, and
    Russia, 209, 246
  in Indonesia, 203
  in India, 204–5
  and needle-exchange programs, 115–19
  in Southeast Asia, 206, 240
  in Spain, 108
Institute for Global Health, California, 230
Institute for Human Virology (Baltimore), 173
Institute of Medicine. *See* U.S. National
  Academy of Sciences
Institute of Virology (Glasgow), 50
institutional review board, 256
integrase, 127, 256
interferon, 44, 51, 76, 256
interleukin-2, 46, 54, 76, 256
international AIDS conferences
  1990, boycott of San Francisco confer-
    ence, 106
  1996, announcement of HAART thera-
    py, 211–15
  1996, developing world on agenda,
    215–16
  2010, Vienna Declaration, 209–10
International AIDS Vaccine Initiative
  (IAVI), 241
International Committee on the Taxonomy
  of Viruses, 68
International Olympic Committee, 230
International Partnership against AIDS in
  Africa, 216
Intimate Contact (film), 176
Inventing the AIDS Virus (Duesberg), 146
Invirase, 150
Isentress, 155
Islam and AIDS, 200–203
isoprinosine, 140
It's My Life (film), 177

Jacob, François, 65
Jacobson, Frank, 23

JAMA: The Journal of the American Medical Association, 161, 164
James, John S., 141
Japan, 32, 92
Jefferson Medical College, 46
Jinnah Postgraduate Medical Center (Karachi), 202
John, Elton, 122
John, T. Jacob, 204
Johns Hopkins University School of Medicine, 151, 205
Johnson, Earvin (Magic), 82
Johnson, Lyndon B., 35
Joint United Nations Programme on AIDS (UNAIDS), 8, 178, 185, 213, 215, 245, 249–50
   and Accelerating Access Initiative, 227–28
   created, 210–11
   and Drug Access Initiative, 221–22
   and Global Media AIDS Initiative, 178
   Global Report, 2010, 245
   making AIDS an economic issue, 216–17, 221, 228–29
   presentation at UN Security Council, 216–17
   presentation at UNGASS, 219–20
   three ones principles, 229
   three-by-five initiative, 243
Jonathan, Ronald, 203
Jones, Cleve, 120
Jordon, Frank, 117
   journalism and AIDS, 164–68

Kaiser Foundation. *See* Henry J. Kaiser Family Foundation
Kaleeba, Noerine, 176
Kalichman, Seth, 148
Kalyanaraman, V. S. (Kaly), 63
Kan, Naoto, 92
Kapita, Bila, 188, **189**, 190
Kaposi's sarcoma (KS), 256
Kaposi's Sarcoma Research and Education Foundation, 23
Kaposi's Sarcoma Clinic, UCSF, 38
Kawata, Paul A., 112
Kelley, Laura M., 202
Kellner, Aaron, 87
Kelsey, Frances, 143
Kennedy, Rory, 177
Kenya, AIDS in, 193–95
Kessler, David, 93, 150, 238

Kinsella, James, 165, 166, 167
Kinshasa General Hospital, 188
Kirp, David L., 106, 109
Kitasato, Shibasaburo, 13
Klein, Harvey, 34
Koch, Edward, **27**, 117
Koch, Robert, 12, 27, 55, 56, 57, 70
Koch's postulates, 12, **56**, 56–57, 146–47, 256
Kontaratos, Nikolas, 174
Koop, C. Everett, 35–36, 99–102, **100**, 119
   Surgeon General's Report on AIDS, 101–2, **103**
Koplan, Jeffrey, 34, 99
Kouchner, Bernard, 176
Kramer, Larry, 16, 38, 114, 125, 145, 168, **169**, 174
Krause, Richard, 73, 186, 188
Kreiss, Joan, 266n33
Krim, Mathilde, 122, 176
Kulstad, Ruth M., 161–63
Kushner, Tony, 174

laboratory instrumentation available in 1981, 52–53
Laboratory of Tumor Cell Biology, U.S. National Cancer Institute, **49**
lamivudine, 228
LaMontagne, John, **189**
Lancet, 23, 60, 161, 168
Landau, Nathaniel R., 154
Lane, H. Clifford, 73–76, **74**, 141, 186
Laos, 207
Lasker, Albert Prize, 53, 69
Lassa fever, 25
Latin America, AIDS in, 207–9
Laubenstein, Linda, 21
LAV, 256. *See also* Montagnier laboratory
Lavender Hill Mob, 113–14
Legionella pneumophila, 25
Legionnaires' disease, 20, 25–27, 39, 114
Leibovitch, Jacques, 22, **49**, 54
Lekatsas, Anastasia, **27**
lentivirus, 68, 256
Leonard, John, 175
Levi Strauss and Co., 221
Levy, Jay, 45, 49–50, 60–61, 67–68, 152, 172, 253, 270n12
   names AIDS virus ARV, 67
Lewin, Roger, 171
Liberace, 82
Life Before the Lifeboat (film), 247
Lister, Joseph, 13

Literary Gazette (Moscow), 183
Littman, Dan R., 154
London School of Hygiene and Tropical
   Medicine, 229, 230
Long, Russell, 238
long-term nonprogressors, 154–56, 256
Longtime Companion (film), 176
Lord, Katherine, **27**
Louganis, Greg, 82, 176
   Breaking the Surface: The Greg Louganis
      Story, 82
Lwegaba, Anthony, 191
lymphadenopathy associated virus (LAV),
   58, 67–68, 127
   LAV-BRU, 68
   LAV-LAI, 68
lymphocyte, 256
lymphokine, 16–17, 256
Lyons, Maryinez, 194

MacPherson, Ian, 50
macrophage, 17, 77, 256–57
Madlala-Routledge, Nozizwe, 227
Maggiore, Christine, 182
Magic Johnson Foundation (U.S.), 122
Mahler, Halfdan, 108, 198, 199
Maison Martin Margiela AIDS T-shirts, 122
Malasia, AIDS in, 205–6
Malawi, AIDS in, 195–97
Mali, AIDS in, 197–98
Mama Yemo Hospital, 188
Mandela, Makgatho, 226
Mandela, Nelson, 221–22, 225–26
Mane, Purnima, 211
Manhattan Project for AIDS, 237
Mann, Jonathan, 108, **189**, 191, 210–11, 235
   death of, 199
   and WHO Global Programme on AIDS,
      198–200
maraviroc, 155
Marburg fever, 25
Martin, David, 235
Martyn, Christopher, 173
Mason, James O., 63, 100, 102, 282n19
Mass, Larry, 167
Masur, Henry, 79
Mbeki, Thabo, 177, 222–25, 239
McCormick, Joseph, 188, **189**, 199
McNeill, William H., 1
measles, 5
Medical Research Council laboratories
   (Carshalton, England), 50

medical writing about AIDS, 160–64
Medicines Control Council (MCC),South
   Africa, 223
Medicins Sans Frontières, 211
memory B cells, 257
men who have sex with men (MSM), 93,
   208, 257
Mendez, Enrique, Jr., 238
Merck Research Laboratories, 149–51, 155, 227
Merson, Michael, 199, 200, 210
Messinger, Delfi, 191
Mexico, AIDS in, 207–9
miasma, 2, 12
microbicide to prevent AIDS, 231, 241
MicroGeneSys, 239, 239
military attitude toward AIDS prevention, 217
Milk, Harvey, 120, 168
Miller, David, 199
Milwaukee AIDS Project, 179
MIP-1α, 153, 257
MIP-1β, 153, 257
Mitisi, John, 72
Mitsuya, Hiroaki (Mitch), 130–32, **131**,
   138–39
Mlambo-Ngcuka, Phumzile, 226
MMWR. See Morbidity and Mortality
   Weekly Reports
Mobuto Sese Seko, 188, 191
molecular biology, 257
molecular immunology, 16–17, **18**, **19**
molecular virology, 126–27
Mongolia, 207
monkey, sooty mangaby (*Cercocebus atys*), 5
monocyte, 77, 257
Montagnier laboratory, 67
   names AIDS virus LAV, 67
Montagnier, Luc, 50–54, **52**, 58, 61–70, 152,
   172, 225, 256, 270n12
   Virus, 51, 270n12
Monzon, Ofelia T., 206
Moodie, Rob, 211
Morbidity and Mortality Weekly Reports
   (MMWR), 20–22, 84, 87, 99, 161, **162**,
   163–64
Morgan, Doris, 46
Moscone, George, 120
MSM. *See* men who have sex with men
   (MSM)
MTV, 221
Muhammadiyah University (East Java), 203
Mullis, Kary, 148
Murdoch, Rupert, 178

murine animals, 257
Murphy, Philip, 154
Myanmar, 204–7
Myburgh, James, 222, 225
Myth of Heterosexual AIDS, The (Fumento), 108

Nakajima, Hiroshi, 199, 214
NAMES Project Foundation, 120–21, 176. *See also* AIDS quilt
Nation, The (magazine), 183
National AIDS Control Organization (India), 204
National AIDS Control Programme (Pakistan), 203
National AIDS Network (U.S.), 112
National AIDS Research Foundation (U.S.), 122
National AIDS Research Institute (Pune, India), 205
National AIDS Trust (U.K.), 108
National Bureau of Asian Research, 202
National Condom Week (Indonesia), 203
National Foundation for Infantile Paralysis (U.S.), 237
National Gay Task Force (U.S.), 34
National Institute for Health and Medical Research, France (INSERM), 51
National Institute of Biomedical Research (INRB), Kinshasa, 191
National Institute of Public Health (Mexico), 229
National Minority AIDS Council (U.S.), 112
National Public Radio (NPR), 175
Nature, 66, 68, 161, 235
NBC television network, 175
NDA, 257
needle exchange, 106, 115–19, **118**, 249
Nelson, Ann Marie, **189**
Netherlands, 32, 117
nevirapine, 226, 228
New England Deaconess Hospital, 60
New England Journal of Medicine, 20–21, 30, 161, 163
New Scientist, 62, 174
New York Blood Center, 87
New York City Department of Health, 24, **27**, 31
New York magazine, 175
New York Native, 15, 16, 167
   and theory that African swine fever virus was cause of AIDS, 168

New York Stock Exchange, 137
New York Times, 63, 83, 114–15, 151, 166, 174, 183, 215
Ngali, Bosenga, **189**
Nichols, Mike, 175
Nicholson, William, 176
Niger, AIDS in, 197–98
Nigeria, 8, 25
   AIDS in, 197, 200–203
NIH intramural, 257
NIH, extramural, 257
Nipomo Community Medical Center (California), 179
Nixon, Richard, 35, 45, 172, 236
"No Obits" headline, **156**, 157
Nobel prize, 13, 51, 69, 70
   awarded for discovery of AIDS virus, 69–70
Noble, Gary, 100
Normal Heart, The (Kramer), 114, 125, 174
Norvir, 150
Novopharm Ltd, 137
Nowinski, Robert, 240
Nussbaum, Bruce, 171–72
Nussenblatt, Robert B., 76, 142
Nyswane, Ron, 176
Nzila, Eugène Nzilamabi, **189**

O'Connor, Basil, 237
O'Connor, Cardinal John, 118
Obama, Barack, 231
Office of AIDS Research, NIH. *See* U.S. National Institutes of Health
Oleske, James, 164
oncovirus, 68, 257
Oppenheimer, Gerald, 25
Oregon State University, 208
Organization for African Unity, 229
Oroszlan, Stephen, 149
Ortleb, Chuck, 167, 168
Osborn, June, 111

p (e.g., p24, p25), 257
Pakistan, AIDS in, 200–203
Palestine, Alan, 76, 142
Pan American Health Organization (PAHO), 186
pandemic, 257
Pandemic: Facing AIDS (film), 177
Pape, Jean, 187, 295n3
parallel track, 145–46
Parent Teacher Association, 102

Parker, Jon, 117
Parmentier, Marc, 154
Parting Glances (film), 175
Pasteur Diagnostics, 89–90
Pasteur Institute, 50–59, 62–67, 89, 140,
    170, 172–73, 225, 233, 256
    laboratory at Marne-la-Coquette, 51,
    271n22
Pasteur, Louis, 12, 50, 55
pathophysiology, 14, 257
patient zero, 169
Patriot, The (newspaper), 183
Paul, William, 154
PBS television network, 208
PCP, 257
PCR, 257
pediatric AIDS, 138–39
peer review, 20, 42, 161, 257
pentamidine isethionate, 28
People of Color Against AIDS, 180
People with AIDS (PWA), 38
Peru, AIDS prevention research, 208–9
Pfizer, 155
Philadelphia (film), 176
Philadelphia Inquirer, 87
Philippines, AIDS in, 203, 205–6
Pierre and Marie Curie University (Paris), 234
Piot, Peter, 8, 176, **189**, 199, 210, 211, **218**,
    242, 249, 266n33, 296n11
    and founding of UNAIDS, 210–11
    and Projet SIDA, 188–91
    and work of UNAIDS, 213–29
Pizzo, Phillip, 138
placebo, 133, 258
placebo-controlled, double-blind drug
    trial, 258
plasma, 258
plasma B cells, 258
PLUS, the Coalition Internationale SIDA, 122
Pneumocystis carinii, 2, 17, 40, 257, 258
pneumonia (PCP), 20, 21, 22, 23, 28–29,
    72–73
Point Defiance AIDS Project (Tacoma,
    Washington), 117
Politicsweb.co.za, 222
polymerase chain reaction (PCR), 53, 68, 126
    quantitative test (Q-PCR), 150
Pool, Judith Graham, 85
Pope Benedict XVI, 208
Popovic, Mikulas (Mika), **49**, 59, 66, 132, 173
Popper, Karl R., 39
poppers. *See* amyl nitrite drugs

Porter, Roy, 119
Power to the People, 182
Pozalski, Irving, 20
Presidential Commission on the Human
    Immunodeficiency Virus Epidemic
    (Watkins Comission), 110
    suggested name change, 111
Pretoria High Court (South Africa), 226
Prevention Point (San Francisco), 117
PreventionWorks (Washington, D.C.), 249
Project Inform, 145, 170
Projet SIDA, 187–91, **189**, 199, 210, 235
protease, 258
protease inhibitors in combination therapy
    for AIDS, 149–52
protocol, medical research, 258
Public Health Laboratory Service (U.K.), 107
Purchase, Dave, 117
PWA, 258

Qaddafi, Muammar al-, 101
quackery and AIDS, 140, 181–84
Quilt, AIDS, 120–21, **121**, 176
Quinn, Thomas, 186–88, **189**, 191, 203–5,
    266n33

raltegravir, 155
Ramalingaswami, Vulimiri, 204
RANTES, 153, 258
Ray brothers (Ricky, Robert, and Randy),
    81, 83, 105
Raymond Poincare Hospital (France), 49
Reagan administration
    budget policies related to AIDS, 104
    Domestic Policy Council's views on
    AIDS, 101
    domestic policy priorities, 98–99
    first public mention of AIDS, 105
    Rock Hudson's death, impact on, 104–5
    ignores Watkins commission report, 111
Reagan, Ronald, 32–36, 62, 66, 97, 101, 105,
    106, 110, 114
reagent, biological, 258
recombinant DNA technology, 258
red ribbon, 247
Redfearn, Martin, 62
Reitz, Marvin, **49**
religious views about AIDS, 98
Relman, Arnold S., 20, 163
Republic of Congo, AIDS in, 192–93
Resio, Don, 25, 75, 76
Resio, Ron, 75, 76, 77, 79, 141

Retrovir. *See* AZT
retrovirus, 5, **47**, 258
Reuters news agency, 205
reverse transcriptase, 47, 51, 54, 57, 58,
    127, 258
reverse transcription inhibitor drugs,
    139–40
ribavirin, 140
ribonucleic acid, 5
Richards, Greg, 107
Rickettsia rickettsii, 4
Ricky Ray Hemophilia Relief Fund Act, 93
Rio group, 219
ritonavir, 150
Ritter, Don, 84
RNA, 259
Robbins, Fred, 238
Rockefeller Foundation, 241
Rocky Mountain spotted fever, 4, 274n65
Roe v. Wade, 97, 100
Root-Bernstein, Robert, 148
Rosenberg, Charles, 96, 123
Rosenthal, Abe, 166
Rossi, Giovanni Battista, 60
Rous sarcoma virus, 51, 67
Rowe, Wallace, 50
Rowland, Roy, 111
Royal National Hospital (Bournemouth,
    U.K.) 22
Rozenbaum, Willy, 22, 58
Ruschetti, Frank, 46
Russia, AIDS in, 209–10
Rwanda, AIDS in, 193–95
Ryan White Care Act, 103
Ryder, Robin, **189**

safari research, 190
Sagabiel, Stephanie, **189**
Salk, Jonas, 234
Salzman, Lois, 80–81
San Francisco AIDS Foundation, 112,
    117, 120
San Francisco Chronicle, 168
San Francisco General Hospital, 23, 50,
    120, 144
San Francisco Health Department, 30
Sánchez, Jorge, 208–9
Sanders, Kingsley, 50
saquinavir, 150
Sarang, Anya, 209
Sarngadharan, M. G. (Sarang), **49**, 59, 66
SARS. *See* severe acute respiratory syndrome

Save the Children Fund, 211
Sawye, Eric, 176
Saxon, Andrew, 20
Schanker, Howard M., 20
Schlafly, Phyllis, 102
Schultz, George, 101
Schüpbach, Jörg, **49**, 59
Schwartz, Maxime, 173
Science, 57–60, 62, 68, 126, 146–48, 161,
    163, 172, 188, 207, 209, 229, 247
*Science Fictions: A Scientific Mystery, A
    Massive Coverup, and the Dark Legacy of
    Robert Gallo* (Crewdson), 173
Sell, Kenneth, 41
selzentry, 155
Sencer, David J., 26, **27**, 87, 109, 117
Senegal, AIDS in, 197–98
sequence, 259
serum, 259
Serwadda, David, 192
severe acute respiratory syndrome (SARS), 207
Shandera, Wayne, 20, 26
Shaw, George, 151
Shearer, Gene, 131
Sherry, James, 214
Sherwood, Bill, 175
Shilts, Randy, 15, 168–70
Shots in the Dark, 233, 236
SIDA, 259
Sidibe, Michel, 242
Silverman, Mervyn, 118
simian immunodeficiency virus (SIV), 5, 259
Singapore, AIDS in, 205–6
SIV. *See* simian immunodeficiency virus
Skirball Institute of Biomolecular Medi-
    cine, New York University School of
    Medicine, 154
slim disease, 191–92
Sloan-Kettering Institute (New York), 50
Smallman, Shawn, 208
Smart, Rose, 223
Smith, Phillip, 77
Smith., Mark D., 120
Snopes.com, 183
Society of Professional Journalists, 164
Sodroski, Joseph, 154
Somalia, AIDS in, 193–95
Sonnabend, Joseph, 148
Sontag, Susan, 123–24
South Africa, AIDS in, 195–97
South African Broadcasting Corporation
    (SABC), 178

South African Health Department, 225
South African National AIDS Council, 226
South African Treatment Action Group, 182
South America, AIDS in, 207–9
Southern Illinois University at Carbondale, 165
Spain, AIDS in, 32, 60
Special Programme on AIDS (WHO). *See* World Health Organization (WHO)
Special Virus Cancer Program. *See* U.S. National Cancer Institute
Sri Lanka, AIDS in, 205–6
St. Martin's Press, 168
Staphylococcus aureus, 25
Star Group Ltd. (India) 178
stavudine, 145, 228
Steffen, Monika, 89
Stoker, Michael, 50
Stoneburner, Rand, **27**
Stonewall Inn, 15
"Storm the NIH" demonstration, **116**
Strait, George, 167
Sturchio, Jeffrey, 215
Suarez, Ray, 208
Sudan, AIDS in, 25, 195
suppressor T cells, 259
Surgeon General's Report on AIDS, 102, **103**
Sutton, Terry, 144
Sweet As You Are (TV production), 176
syndrome, 259
Syntex Company, 142, 143

T cells, 259. *See also* immune system, cellular
Takehiko Kawano, 92
Tanzania, AIDS in, 193–95
Tanzanian National Institute for Medical Research, 225
Taylor, Elizabeth, 122
T-cell growth factor. *See* interleukin-2
television and AIDS, 166–67, 177–78
Temin, Howard, 51, 68, 147, 148
Terrence Higgins Trust (U.K.), 115
Thai Ministry of Public Health, 223
Thailand, AIDS in, 205–7, 210
"That's What Friends Are For" song, 122
Thatcher government policies on AIDS, 107
Thatcher, Margaret, 97
The AIDS Support Organization (TASO), Uganda, 176
theatrical treatment of AIDS, 174–78
Thomas, Polly, **27**
Thurman, Sandra, 176
Tilley, Brian, 177

Time magazine, 205
Titmuss, Richard, 85
Tonga, AIDS in, 205–6
toxic-shock syndrome, 25–27, 114
toxoplasmosis, 41, 259
Trans-African highways, **195**
travel ban on HIV-infected people. *See* diagnostic test for HIV
Treatment Action Campaign (TAC), South Africa, 177, 224, 226, 228
Treatment Action Group (TAG), U.S., 237
treatment IND, 135, 136, 143, 145
Trimeris Inc., 155
Trinidad and Tobago, AIDS in, 207
Tshabalala-Msimang, Manto, 225
Tuskegee experiment, 119, 120

Understanding AIDS (report), 102, **103**
U.S. Agency for International Development (USAID), 215
U.S. Centers for Disease Control and Prevention (CDC), 3, 15, 20–37, 63, 161, 163, 223
    and AZT dosage study in Thailand, 223
    budget reduced in 1980s, 99
    and contamination of U.S. blood supply, 34, 83–89
    definitions of AIDS, 3–4
    epidemiological definition of AIDS, 27–34
    first guidelines for prevention of AIDS issued, 37
    in Haiti, surveillance of AIDS, 185–87, 295n3
    and needle exchange projects support, 119
    and Projet SIDA, 187–91
    publication of *MMWR*, 161, 163,
    task force on AIDS, 27, 33, 53, 99
    and travel ban on HIV-infected people, 106
    and *Understanding AIDS* mailing, 102–3
U.S. Central Intelligence Agency (CIA), 214
U.S. Department of Defense, 238
U.S. Department of Health and Human Services (DHHS), 32, **43**, 62–65, 99, 101, 104
    1980s AIDS policies, 103
    Federal Coordinating Committee on AIDS Information, Education, and Risk Reduction, 100–101
    Intragovernmental Task Force on AIDS Health Care Delivery, 101
U.S. Food and Drug Administration (FDA), 151, 157, 171, 246, 255, 256

ACT UP demonstration against drug approval policies of, 114–15, 143
and AZT approval, 131–35, 137–38
budget and regulatory responsibilities reduced in 1980s, 35, 99
and contamination of U.S. blood supply, 86–89, 93
and ddI and ddC approval, 139–40
and foscarnet approval, 144–45
and gancyclovir approval, 141–44
and parallel track concept, 145–46
and protease inhibitors approval, 151–51
and VaxSyn candidate vaccine , 238
U.S. Freedom of Information Act (FOIA), 171–73
U.S. House of Representatives, 173
U.S. National Academy of Sciences, 146, 148
Institute of Medicine of, 93, 110
U.S. National Cancer Act (1971), 45, 236
U.S. National Cancer Institute (NCI), 28, 32, 41, 236, 241
background on NCI research in viruses and cancer, 44–46
and chemokines, 154
and development of AZT, 130–38
and diagnostic tests for AIDS virus, 89
and dispute over patent for AIDS diagnostic test, 64–65
establishes task force on AIDS, 99
first NCI intramural AIDS patient, 72–73
and first liaison with CDC AIDS task force, 33
and Heckler press conference, 62–64
National Cancer Advisory Board, 53
National Cancer Program, 236
and pediatric AIDS, 139
as target of criticism about AIDS research, 171–74
Special Virus Cancer Program, 44–45, 236, 270n12
U.S. National Commission on AIDS, 111
final report, **113**
position on travel ban for HIV-infected people, 106
reports and recommendations, 111–12
U.S. National Eye Institute (NEI), 42, 76
U.S. National Institute of Allergy and Infectious Diseases (NIAID), 42, 151, 238, 241
and AIDS in Haiti, 186–87

and AIDS research in India, 205
and AIDS research in Peru, 209
background on, 44
establishes task force on AIDS, 99
first NIAID intramural AIDS patient, 73
National Cooperative Vaccine Development Groups, 235
and parallel track, 145–46
and Projet SIDA, 187–91
returns to basic research on AIDS vaccine, 240
and second receptor for HIV, 153–54
seeks increased funding for AIDS research, 104
and trial of ART as preventive, 242–43
and VaxSyn proposal, 238–39
U.S. National Institute of Dental Research (NIDR), 77, 80
U.S. National Institute of Neurological and Communicative Disorders and Stroke (NINCDS), 77
U.S. National Institutes of Health (NIH)
and AZT litigation, 137–38
and balance between basic and applied research, 236
budget stagnant in 1980s, 35, 99
clinical associate program, 46
Clinical Center and research on AIDS, 72–79, 130, 136
and contamination of U.S. blood supply, 85–87
and epidemic of fear, 77–81
establishes working group on AIDS, 31, 99
extramural (grants) program, 42
and Heckler press conference, 63
and increased funding for AIDS research, 104
intramural research program, 43–44, 52
Office of AIDS Research (OAR), 104, 155, 237–38, 241
organization of, 42–44
and patent dispute over AIDS diagnostic test, 65–66
and phase I trial of AZT, 133
reauthorization act of 1993, 106
and Robert C. Gallo investigation, 172–73
as target of criticism about AIDS research, 171
Vaccine Research Center (VRC), 241
and VaxSyn proposal, 238–39

U.S. National Library of Medicine, 22, 178
U.S. National Science Foundation, 247
U.S. Patent Office, 65
U.S. President's Emergency Plan for AIDS
    Relief (PEPFAR), 231
U.S. Presidential Commission on the
    Human Immunodeficiency Virus
    Epidemic (Watkins Commission),
    110–11
U.S. Public Health Service (PHS), 32, 35, 42,
    73, 99, 135, 186
    AIDS Executive Committee, 99
    AIDS Operational Plan, 104
    Commissioned Corps revitalization
        effort, 99
    Executive Task Force on AIDS, 100
    hospitals closed, 99
    and Tuskegee experiment, 119, 120
U.S. Technology Transfer Act, 65, 66, 137
U.S. Walter Reed Army Institute of
    Research, 238
Uganda, AIDS in, 193–95, 210, 221
UN. See United Nations (UN)
UN Population Fund, 227
UNAIDS. See Joint United Nations
    Programme on AIDS (UNAIDS)
UNICEF. See United Nations International
    Children's Emergency Fund (UNICEF)
United Kingdom (U.K.) AIDS policies, 106–8
United Nations (UN), 178
    2001 Declaration of Commitment on
        HIV/AIDS, 219–20
    building with AIDS red ribbon, **220**
    General Assembly Special Session
        (UNGASS), 108, 213, 218–20
    Millennium Declaration, 219
    position on travel ban for HIV-infected
        people, 106
    Secretary General Kofi Annan decides
        to make AIDS a priority, 216–17
    Security Council session on AIDS,
        2000, 216–17
United Nations Development Program
    (UNDP), 210
United Nations International Children's
    Emergency Fund (UNICEF), 210, 211,
    214, 227
Universidad Peruana Cayetano Heredia
    (Lima), 208–9
Université Libre de Bruxelles, 154
University Methodist Temple (Seattle), **118**
University of Alabama–Birmingham, 151

University of California–Berkeley, 180, 230
University of California–Los Angeles
    (UCLA), 1, 20, 23–24
University of California–San Francisco
    (UCSF), 23–24, 31, 38, 49–50, 154, 230
University of Capetown, 182
University of Chicago, 46
University of Copenhagen, 22
University of Grenoble, 89–90
University of Maryland School of Med-
    icine, 173
University of North Carolina–Chapel Hill, 242
University of Pennsylvania, 154
University of Southern California, 202
University of Washington, 25
University of Wisconsin–Madison, 147
Upjohn Company, 238
urban legends about AIDS, 181–84

vaccine against AIDS, search for, 232–41
Vaccine Research Center (VRC). See U.S.
    National Institutes of Health (NIH)
vaccines, 2, 232–33
vaginal microbicide gel to prevent AIDS, 241
Van der Mass, Tine, 182
Varmus, Harold, 68
vasculitis, 259
Vatican position on condoms to prevent
    AIDS, 208
VaxGen, 240
VaxSyn, 238, 239
Vennström, Björn, 69
Verhof, Hans Paul, 106
Vézinet-Brun, Françoise, 58
Viacom Media Networks, 178
*Victory Deferred: How AIDS Changed Gay
    Life in America* (Andriote), 247
Vienna Declaration, 209–10
Vietnam, AIDS in, 207, 221
Vietnam War, 35
VIH, 259
Village Voice, 166
viral load, 150–51, 259
Virchow, Rudolf, 34
Virodene PO58, 222–27, 239
virus, 259
    naming systems, 67–68, 272n26
    replication of retrovirus, **47**
    replication of RNA virus, **46**
*Virus: The Codiscoverer of HIV Tracks Its
    Rampage and Charts the Future* (Mon-
    tagnier), 51, 270n12

Virus Hunting: AIDS, Cancer and the Human Retrovirus: A Story of Scientific Discovery (Gallo), 54, 271n14
Visser, Jacques Siegfried (Zigi), 222–27
Visser, Olga, 222–27
Visual AIDS, 247
Visual Science Company, 247
Volberding, Paul, 50, 247
Volvovitz, Frank, 238

Wahl, Sharon, 77
Waldmann, Thomas, 72–73, 130
Wall Street Journal, 207
"War on Cancer," 45
war on drugs, 115
Warwick, Dionne, 122
Washington Post, 214
Washington, Denzel, 176
Watkins, James D., 110
Waxman, Henry, 36
Webster, William H., 214
Weekly Epidemiological Record, 206
Wegener's granulomatosis, 73, 74
Weisman, Joel D., 20
Weiss, Robin, 60, 152
Western blot, 59, 89, 204, 260, 279n54
Western, Karl, 186
What If Everything You Thought You Knew about AIDS Was Wrong? (Maggiore), 182
White House Conference on HIV/AIDS, 4
White, Ryan, 81, 83, 176
WHO. *See* World Health Organization
Wikipedia, 183
Williams, Judith, 8
Winterthur Insurance/Credit Suisse Group, 230
Wolff, Sheldon M., 73

Women's Health Initiative, 237
women and AIDS, 3, 21, 23, 30, 39, 119, 152, 179, 186–89, 193–97, 204–5, 223–26, 230, 234–36, 240–41
Wong-Staal, Flossie, **49**
World AIDS Day, 199
World AIDS Foundation, 66
World Bank, 203, 210, 227
Multicountry AIDS Program (MAP), 230
World Economic Forum, 221
World Health Organization (WHO), 3, 108, 172, 186, 198, 206, 208, 211, 223, 227, 242
Global Programme on AIDS, 108, 110, 198–200, 210, 235
International Classification of Diseases, 3
and reluctance to make AIDS a top priority, 214
Special Programme on AIDS, 108
Wu, Yi, 207
Wyeth-Ayerst, 239
Wyngaarden, James, 63

xenotropic viruses, 50

Yarchoan, Robert, 130–33, **131**, 138–39
yellow fever, 5
Young, Frank, 114, 143
Young, James Harvey, 141

Zagury, Daniel, 234, 235
Zaire, 25
AIDS in, 187–91
Zambia, AIDS in, 195–97
"zap" action, 113
Zimbabwe, AIDS in, 195–97
zoonosis, 4, 260
Zulu, 196
Zuma, Nkosazane, 222, 223, 224

About the Author

Victoria A. Harden retired in January 2006 as director of the Office of NIH History and the Stetten Museum at the National Institutes of Health, an office she created during the 1986–1987 observance of the NIH centennial. She continues to serve the office as a special volunteer.

Harden received her BA and PhD degrees in American history at Emory University (1966, 1983) and conducted much of her dissertation research as a fellow at the National Museum of American History of the Smithsonian Institution. During a post-doctoral year at the Institute for the History of Medicine at the Johns Hopkins University School of Medicine, she was supported by a grant from the National Library of Medicine and completed work on *Inventing the NIH: Federal Biomedical Research Policy, 1887–1937* (Johns Hopkins University Press, 1986).

From 1984 to 1986, Harden was on the staff of the National Institute of Allergy and Infectious Diseases, researching and writing *Rocky Mountain Spotted Fever: History of a Twentieth-Century Disease* (Johns Hopkins University Press, 1990). It won the 1991 Henry Adams Prize of the Society for History in the Federal Government.

In 1989 and 1993 she organized conferences on the history of AIDS. The proceedings were published as *AIDS and the Historian* (Government Printing Office, 1991) and *AIDS and the Public Debate: Historical and Contemporary Perspectives* (IOS Press, 1995). In June 2001, she launched the website "In Their Own Words: NIH Researchers Recall the Early Years of AIDS" (http://www

.history.nih.gov/NIHInOwnWords/), commemorating the twentieth anniversary of the first publication about AIDS.

Harden also oversaw the creation and development of the Stetten Museum at NIH, which collects and exhibits biomedical research instruments and memorabilia related to the National Institutes of Health. *Windows into NIH History,* a series of exhibits prepared for the NIH centennial, won the 1989 John Wesley Powell Prize of the Society for History in the Federal Government. The Office of NIH History website, http://history.nih.gov, now makes many of the exhibits available in a virtual format.

Harden is an active member of many professional societies. She has served on the executive councils of the American Historical Association and the American Association for the History of Medicine. From 1993 to 1994 she served as president of the Washington Society for the History of Medicine and in 1998–1999 as president of the Society for History in the Federal Government. In 2006 she was awarded the Herbert Feis Prize by the American Historical Association, and in 2007 the Lifetime Achievement Award of the American Association for the History of Medicine.